Government Procedures and Operations

snova
New York

Government Procedures and Operations

COVID-19 in Nursing Homes: Impact, Transmission and Prevention
Fred C. Wallace (Editor)
2023. ISBN: 979-8-88697-673-1 (Hardcover)
2023. ISBN: 979-8-88697-683-0 (eBook)

The Significance of the COVID Pandemic in Nursing Homes
John S. Gill (Editor)
2023. ISBN: 979-8-88697-660-1 (Hardcover)
2023. ISBN: 979-8-88697-682-3 (eBook)

Putting an End to Surprise Medical Billing
Danial E. Tackett (Editor)
2022. ISBN: 979-8-88697-296-2 (Hardcover)
2022. ISBN: 979-8-88697-327-3 (eBook)

Abortion Rights, Access, and Legislative Response
Jorge P. Sandford (Editor)
2022. ISBN: 979-8-88697-258-0 (Softcover)
2022. ISBN: 979-8-88697-294-8 (eBook)

Review of Capitol Police Procedures During the Capitol Attack
Rafael B. Phillips (Editor)
2022. ISBN: 979-8-88697-260-3 (Hardcover)
2022. ISBN: 978-1-53617-478-6 (eBook)

More information about this series can be found at
https://novapublishers.com/product-category/series/government-procedures-and-operations/

Jack M. Lee
Editor

New Policies on Marijuana's Status

snova
New York

Library of Congress Cataloging-in-Publication Data

ISBN: 979-8-88697-870-4

Published by Nova Science Publishers, Inc. † New York

Contents

Preface

A half century ago, Congress listed cannabis as a highly controlled schedule I substance. Other schedule I drugs include heroin, LSD and ecstasy. Schedule I drugs have no medical value and high potential for abuse. The schedule I designation restricts legitimate medical research about cannabis. Over the years, several entities have submitted petitions to the DEA to reschedule marijuana. This book looks at key issues related to the Schedule I status of marijuana and the gap between federal and state marijuana policies.

Chapter 1

Cannabis Policies for the New Decade*

Committee on Energy and Commerce

Wednesday, January 15, 2020
House of Representatives, Subcommittee on Health,
Committee on Energy and Commerce,
Washington, DC.

The subcommittee met, pursuant to call, at 10:01 a.m., in the John D. Dingell Room 2123, Rayburn House Office Building, Hon. Anna G. Eshoo (chairman of the subcommittee) presiding.

Present: Representatives Eshoo, Engel, Butterfield, Matsui, Castor, Sarbanes, Luján, Schrader, Kennedy, Cárdenas, Ruiz, Dingell, Kuster, Kelly, Barraga´n, Blunt Rochester, Rush, Pallone (ex officio), Burgess (subcommittee ranking member), Upton, Shimkus, Guthrie, Griffith, Bilirakis, Long, Bucshon, Brooks, Hudson, Carter, Gianforte, and Walden (ex officio).

Also Present: Representatives Schakowsky and Rodgers.

Staff Present: Joe Banez, Professional Staff Member; Jeffrey C. Carroll, Staff Director; Waverly Gordon, Deputy Chief Counsel; Tod Guidry, Health Fellow; Meghan Mullon, Policy Analyst; Tim Robinson, Chief Counsel; Rebecca Tomilchik, Staff Assistant; Kimberlee Trzeciak, Chief Health Advisor; C. J. Young, Press Secretary; Madison Wendell, Intern; S. K. Bowen, Minority Press Assistant; Jordan Davis, Minority Senior Advisor; Theresa Gambo, Minority Human Resources/Office Administrator; Tyler Greenberg,

* This is an edited, reformatted and augmented version of Hearing before the Subcommittee on Health, of the Committee on Energy and Commerce, House of Representatives, One Hundred Sixteenth Congress, Second Session, Serial No. 116–89, dated January 15, 2020.

In: New Policies on Marijuana's Status
Editor: Jack M. Lee
ISBN: 979-8-88697-870-4

Minority Staff Assistant; Peter Kielty, Minority General Counsel; Ryan Long, Minority Deputy Staff Director; Brannon Rains, Minority Legislative Clerk; Kristin Seum, Minority Counsel, Health; and Kristen Shatynski, Minority Professional Staff Member, Health.

Ms. ESHOO. Good morning, everyone. The Subcommittee on Health will now come to order. Welcome to everyone who is here in the hearing room.

The Chair now recognizes herself for 5 minutes for an opening statement.

Opening Statement of Hon. Anna G. Eshoo, a Representative in Congress from the State of California

According to the Department of Health and Human Services' National Survey on Drug Use, 44 million Americans reported using cannabis in the last year. Thirty-three States now allow the medicinal use of cannabis and 11 States in the District of Columbia have legalized cannabis for adult use.

But State laws and Federal policy are a 1,000 miles apart. As more States allow cannabis, the Federal Government still strictly controls and prohibits it, even restricting legitimate medical research.

Given the widespread availability of cannabis, the purpose of today's hearing is to examine the pressing need for medical research about cannabis and its chemical compounds with CBD being one of them.

A half century ago, Congress listed cannabis as a highly controlled schedule I substance. Other schedule I drugs include heroin, LSD and ecstasy. Schedule I drugs have no medical value and high potential for abuse. Schedule II drugs, such as cocaine and Vicodin through schedule V drugs, such as Robitussin, all have some medical value but differ in ranking depending on their potential for abuse.

The schedule I designation restricts legitimate medical research about cannabis. Today scientists who wish to study cannabis must seek approval from three Federal agencies: the NIH, the FDA and the DEA. Once scientists are federally approved, which can take more than a year, they are allowed to only research cannabis grown by a government-authorized farm at the University of Mississippi.

This cannabis lacks the properties and potency of commercially available cannabis and leads to inadequate research. So researchers are in a catch-22, they can't conduct cannabis research until they show cannabis has a medical use, but they can't demonstrate cannabis as a medical use until they can conduct research. It doesn't make sense, at least to me.

So why is it concerning that research about cannabis is blocked by Federal law? First, cannabis has therapeutic potential for chronic pain, nausea, and the treatment of neurological disorders such as seizures. In 2018, the FDA approved the first cannabis-derived medication, Epidiolex, which treats seizures in patients two years of age or older. Second, the restrictions on cannabis research has led to unanswered questions about the safety and quality of products containing CBD.

In December 2018, the farm bill removed hemp, including CBD derived from hemp, from the Controlled Substances Act. The farm bill explicitly preserved the FDA's authority over CBD products, but the FDA has yet to issue regulations due to its unanswered questions about the intrinsic safety of the CBD. The FDA says it will take three to five years to finalize CBD regulations. And in the meantime, the CBD market is predicted to reach $20 billion in sales by 2024. Meanwhile, CBD is now available in everything from fast food hamburgers, to scented lotions, to over-the-counter pills.

Today, we are considering six bills that offer a range of solutions to update Federal policy to advance research on cannabis and its compounds. I want to thank the leaders of the bills. Representatives Barbara Lee and Congressman Earl Blumenauer who have joined us. They are sitting in the front row. Thank you for being here and for your work. Congressman Jerry Nadler, Hakeem Jeffries, Matt Gaetz, and our fellow subcommittee member Congressman Morgan Griffith: Thank you to each one of you for your good work.

Now I would like to yield to Mr. Kennedy for the remainder of my time.

[The prepared statement of Ms. Eshoo follows:]

Prepared Statement of Hon. Anna G. Eshoo

According to the Department of Health and Human Services National Survey on Drug Use, 44 million Americans reported using cannabis in the past year. Thirty-three states now allow the medicinal use of cannabis and 11 states and the District of Columbia have legalized cannabis for adult use.

But states' laws and federal policy are a thousand miles apart. As more states allow cannabis, the Federal Government still strictly controls and prohibits it, even restricting legitimate medical research.

Given the widespread availability of cannabis, the purpose of today's hearing is to examine the pressing need for medical research about cannabis and its chemical compounds with CBD being one of them.

Fifty years ago, Congress listed cannabis as a highly-controlled Schedule I substance. Other schedule I drugs include heroin, LSD, and ecstasy.

Schedule 1 drugs have no medical value and high potential for abuse. Schedule 2 drugs (for example, cocaine and Vicodin) through Schedule 5 drugs (for example, Robitussin) all have some medical value but differ in ranking depending on their potential for abuse.

The Schedule I designation restricts legitimate medical research about cannabis. For example, scientists who wish to study cannabis must seek approval from three federal agencies—the NIH, the FDA, and the DEA.

Once scientists are federally approved, which can take more than a year, they're allowed to only research cannabis grown by a government-authorized farm at the University of Mississippi. This cannabis lacks the properties and potency of commercially available cannabis and leads to inadequate research.

Researchers are in a catch-22. They can't conduct cannabis research until they show cannabis has a medical use, but they can't show cannabis has a medical use until they can conduct research.

Why is it concerning that research about cannabis is blocked by federal law?

First, cannabis has therapeutic potential for chronic pain or nausea and the treatment of neurological disorders such as seizures. For example, in 2018, the FDA approved the first cannabis-derived medication, Epidolex, which treats seizures in patients two years of age or older.

Second, the restrictions on cannabis research has led to unanswered questions about the safety and quality of products containing CBD.

In December 2018, the Farm Bill removed hemp, including CBD derived from hemp, from the Controlled Substances Act. The Farm Bill explicitly preserved the FDA's authority over CBD products, but the FDA has yet to issue regulations due to its unanswered questions about the intrinsic safety of CBD.

The FDA says it will take three to five years to finalize CBD regulations, and in the meantime, the CBD market is predicted to reach $20 billion in sales by 2024. CBD is now available in everything from fast food hamburgers, to scented lotions, to over-the-counter pills.

Today we'll consider six bills that offer a range of solutions to update federal policy to advance research on cannabis and its compounds.

I thank the leaders of the bills for their work: Representatives Barbara Lee and Earl Blumenauer, who have joined us in the audience today, as well as Representatives Jerry Nadler, Hakeem Jeffries, Matt Gaetz, and our fellow Subcommittee Member Representative Morgan Griffith.

Working together, I hope our Subcommittee can move forward on a commonsense proposal that stops the Federal Government from impeding medical research and allows Americans to have access to the information they need about the harmful and therapeutic effects of cannabis.

I yield the remainder of my time to Representative Kennedy.

* * *

Mr. KENNEDY. Thank you, Madam Chair. I want to thank you for the time for yielding.

This is a critical debate, and it is long overdue. Federal prohibition has failed, from our criminal justice system, to our healthcare system, to our State and local governments that are forced to navigate an impossible landscape. To that end, government officials and elected representatives are important witnesses and bring an important perspective to this conversation.

But there are also critical stakeholders who are missing, those who lives have been directly touched by our broken marijuana policies. The people unjustly incarcerated, patients who rely on medical cannabis, and researchers with expertise yearning to learn more, small businesses owners trying to find fair footing in a new industry.

I am grateful for woman who is committed to continue working with us on a second hearing that will center those voices in this debate.

Thank you, Madam Chair. I yield back.

Ms. ESHOO. The gentleman yields back. It is a pleasure to recognize Dr. Burgess, the ranking member of our subcommittee for his opening statement.

Opening Statement of Hon. Michael C. Burgess, a Representative in Congress from the State of Texas

Mr. BURGESS. And I thank the Chair. I appreciate—and thanks to our witnesses who are here with us today to help advise us in this important matter. I appreciate that we are holding the hearing today to discuss this policy. It is a topic that is of interest to many members of this subcommittee. In fact, that was evidenced when we had our discussion on the smokeless tobacco products. At the end of last year, some of the Republican members of the full Energy and Commerce Committee and myself sent a letter to request a hearing on three of the bills before us today that focus on easing pathways to marijuana research. So I am glad that we followed through with that. It included H.R. 171, the Legitimate Use of Medical Marijuana Act; H.R. 601, The Medical Cannabis Research Act of 2019; and H.R. 3797, the Medical Marijuana Research Act of 2019 in this hearing.

States and localities across the country have moved forward, they have different policies to address marijuana, including both recreational and medicinal. I am concerned that there is a lack of available research on the benefits and the risks of the medical and recreational use of this product and that we really don't justify the actions that some of the States have taken. Thus far the Food and Drug Administration, the National Academies have found that there is a lack of evidence to demonstrate effective medical use for marijuana. So certainly we need more research.

It is concerning that there are arguments over what may or may not be a great medicinal use for marijuana, but we don't have any data. So it is time to get the data and let the decision be driven by the data. Additionally, some of the data that we do have includes some concerning results. For example, a study conducted by researchers at Kaiser Permanente in northern California found that cannabis use among pregnant mothers nearly doubled between 2009 and 2016. Research has also found that prenatal marijuana may impair fetal growth and neural development but added that more studies are necessary as the THC potency continues to vary, but appears to be continuing to rise. So, as someone who has practiced obstetrics for a number of years, I worry about the health of the mothers and their babies that could be at risk.

So one of the key hurdles to research is that researchers require DEA approval. And for decades they have only been allowed to obtain marijuana from one source, the University of Mississippi, which is the only contract that the National Institute on Drug Abuse has for research-grade cannabis.

In the past, it may have made some sense to have this single source for research purposes. Certainly if there are variations in quality or gradation, that could be minimized by having that single source. But because of the diversity now of the quality potency and other aspects of the marijuana that is available for individuals to obtain from medical and recreational purposes, and it does vary across the United States, research using the single-source marijuana may not adequately assess what the current landscape represents. Not to mention, it is difficult to obtain the quantity necessary to conduct research in the existing structure.

To that point, the Drug Enforcement Agency—we are grateful that you are with us this morning—announced in 2016 that it would establish a new policy to increase the number of approved sources of research grade marijuana, but I don't think that has quite gotten across the finish line. Maybe we can hear about that today. I hope that we will get an update on the administrative efforts to streamline the research process today. I hope that we can identify ways to work together to achieve that goal.

While three of the bills before us today aim to enhance research efforts, there are two that may go a step too far. H.R. 2843 and H.R. 3884 completely remove marijuana from the controlled substances list. It is worth noting and I believe the Food and Drug Administration will explain this in more detail, that in order for the Drug Enforcement Agency to reschedule a drug, doing it administratively without congressional direction, the Food & Drug Administration must conduct a medical evaluation of the drug and provide a recommendation to the Drug Enforcement Agency as to what the scheduling should be. This recommendation is binding; therefore, the DEA must do what the FDA recommends. My opinion, completing descheduling marijuana using or congressional authority, which can override this scenario, could possibly be a dangerous move, especially given the lack of research to back up the decision.

So it is critical that the American public, the medical community understands what marijuana does to our bodies and our brains at different potencies throughout our lifecycle. We have a way to go before we have a full understanding of all of these factors. Some of the bills before us are a step in the right direction. Some go a step too far, but I look forward to learning more about the issues of our Federal agencies and the efforts they are taking to work on this problem.

Thank you all for being here, and I yield back my time.

[The prepared statement of Mr. Burgess follows:]

Prepared Statement of Hon. Michael C. Burgess

Thank you, Madame Chair. I appreciate that we are holding this hearing today to discuss marijuana policy, a topic that is of interest to many Members on this subcommittee. At the end of last year, a few Republican Members of the full Energy & Commerce Committee and I sent a letter to request a hearing on three of the bills before us today that focus on easing pathways to marijuana research. I am glad that you have followed through and included H.R. 171, the Legitimate Use of Medicinal Marijuana Act, H.R. 601, Medical Cannabis Research Act of 2019, and H.R. 3797, Medical Marijuana Research Act of 2019, in this hearing.

States and localities across the country have moved forward with different policies to address marijuana, including both recreational and medical use.

As a physician, I am concerned that the available research on the benefits and risks of marijuana, both medical and recreational, do not adequately justify the actions states have taken. Thus far, the Food and Drug Administration and the National Academies have found that there is a lack of evidence to demonstrate effective medical use for marijuana. That being said, we need more research.

It is concerning that there are arguments over what may or may not be a great medicinal use for marijuana, but we don't even have the data. It's time to get the data and let the decision be driven by the data. Additionally, some of the data that we do have includes some concerning results. For example, a study conducted by researchers at Kaiser Permanente in Northern California found that cannabis use among pregnant mothers nearly double between 2009 and 2016.

Researchers also found that "prenatal marijuana may impair fetal growth and neurodevelopment," but added that more studies are necessary as THC potency continues to rise. As an OB/GYN, I worry that the health of mothers and their babies could be at risk.

One of the key hurdles to research is that researchers require DEA-approval, and for decades they have only been allowed to obtain their marijuana from one source— the University of Mississippi—which is the only contract that the National Institute on Drug Abuse has for research-grade cannabis.

In the past it may have made sense to have a single source for research purposes. However, because the diversity of the quality, potency, and other aspects of marijuana that individuals obtain for medical and recreational purposes varies across the United States, research using this sole source of marijuana may not adequately assess the current landscape. Not to mention that it is difficult to obtain the quantity necessary to conduct research under the existing structure.

To that point, the Drug Enforcement Agency announced in 2016 that it would establish a new policy to increase the number of approved sources of research-grade marijuana but has failed to do so. I hope that the DEA will update us on its administrative efforts to streamline the research process today, and that we can identify ways to work together to achieve that goal.

While three of the bills before us today aim to enhance research efforts, there are two that take a step too far. H.R. 2843 and H.R. 3884 completely remove marijuana from the list of Controlled Substances.

It is worth noting, and I believe that the Food and Drug Administration will explain this in more detail, that in order for the Drug Enforcement Agency to reschedule a drug administratively without Congressional direction, the Food and Drug Administration must conduct a medical evaluation of the drug and provide a recommendation to the DEA as to what the rescheduling should be. That recommendation is binding; therefore, the DEA must do what the FDA recommends. I think that completely descheduling marijuana using our Congressional authority is a dangerous move, especially given the lack of research to back up that decision.

It is critical that the American public, and the medical community, understand what marijuana does to our bodies and to our brains, at different potencies, and throughout our life cycle. We have a way to go before we will have a full understanding all of those factors, but some of the bills before us are a step in the right direction.

I look forward to learning more about the issues our federal agencies are facing and the current efforts they are working on. Thank you to all of our agency witnesses for being here today to discuss this important topic. I yield back.

Ms. ESHOO. The gentleman yields back.

It is a pleasure to yield 5 minutes to the chairman of the full committee, Mr. Pallone, for his opening statement.

Opening Statement of Hon. Frank Pallone, Jr., a Representative in Congress from the State of New Jersey

Mr. PALLONE. Thank you, Chairwoman Eshoo.

Today the subcommittee will have an important hearing about Federal cannabis policies. While State laws and public perception around cannabis and its derivatives have evolved over the years, much of the Federal framework that regulates cannabis has stayed the same. In my home State of New Jersey, for example, State law allows for the use of medical cannabis, and at the end of last year, State lawmakers passed a referendum that will put the question of legalizing adult cannabis use to New Jersey voters on the 2020 ballot this coming November.

New Jersey is not alone in its State-level changes, in fact the National Conference of State Legislatures reports that 33 States, as well as Puerto Rico, Guam, the U.S. Virgin Islands, and the District of Columbia approved medical cannabis programs while 11 States, DC, Guam, the Northern Mariana Islands approved adultuse cannabis. And although some States have changed their own policies, national laws, such as the Controlled Substances Act, have yet to change in the same way. And that is why we are looking forward to this hearing from a panel of agency witnesses who agreed to appear before the subcommittee today. The Drug Enforcement Agency, the FDA, the National Institute on Drug Abuse all play crucial roles on the Federal cannabis policy. From researching its benefits and harms to protecting the American public from bad actors. And I hope that we can learn about what the agencies believe works and what needs to be changed.

We will discuss six bills offered by both Democrats and Republicans, some bipartisan. These bills propose various policy changes, such as rescheduling or descheduling marijuana, providing a safe harbor for patients and veterans who use medical marijuana, and streamlining cannabis research processes.

Given the evolving landscape in the States, these bills are worthy of further discussion. And I am particularly interested in hearing about how Federal agencies are reducing barriers to research and enabling research on cannabis to thrive. I am also interested in how the agencies are working together to regulate a cannabis derivative recently removed from the Controlled Substances Act, and that is CBD or cannabidiol, I guess is how it is pronounced.

Before I conclude, I did want to recognize, as Ms. Eshoo did, Representatives—first—Blumenauer and Representative Barbara Lee. I know they have talked to many us on a regular basis, and we are pleased to see that you are here in the audience today. And they are the co-chairs of the bipartisan Cannabis Caucus with Representatives Young and Joyce. Together they foster a continued dialogue on cannabis issues and both have offered bills before us today. And I thank them for joining us and commend them for their ongoing leadership in this area.

Thank you again, Madam Chair. I don't know if anybody are— I have two minutes left if anybody wants it. If not, I yield back.

[The prepared statement of Mr. Pallone follows:]

Prepared Statement of Hon. Frank Pallone, Jr.

Today the Subcommittee will have an important hearing about federal cannabis policies. While state laws and public perception around cannabis and its derivatives have evolved over the years, much of the federal framework that regulates cannabis has stayed the same.

In my home state of New Jersey, for example, state law allows for the use of medical cannabis and, at the end of last year, state lawmakers passed a referendum that will put the question of legalizing adult cannabis use to New Jersey voters on the 2020 ballot.

New Jersey is not alone in its state-level changes. In fact, the National Conference of State Legislatures reports that 33 states as well as Puerto Rico, Guam, the U.S. Virgin Islands, and the District of Columbia approved medical cannabis programs while 11 states, the District of Columbia, Guam, and the Northern Mariana Islands approved adult-use cannabis. Although some states have changed their own policies, national laws, such as the Controlled Substances Act, have yet to change in the same way.

That is why I am looking forward to hearing from the panel of agency witnesses who agreed to appear before the Subcommittee today. The Drug Enforcement Agency, the Food and Drug Administration, and the National Institute on Drug Abuse all play crucial roles on federal cannabis policy—from researching its benefits and harms to protecting the American public from bad actors. I hope that we can learn about what the agencies believe works, and what needs to be changed.

We will discuss six bills offered by both Democrats and Republicans, and some bipartisan in nature. These bills propose various policy changes such as rescheduling or descheduling marijuana, providing a safe harbor for patients and veterans who use medical marijuana, and streamlining cannabis research processes.

Given the evolving landscape in the states, these bills are worthy of further discussion. I am particularly interested in hearing about how federal agencies are reducing barriers to research and enabling research on cannabis to thrive. I am also interested in how the agencies are working together to regulate a cannabis derivative recently removed from the Controlled Substances Act—cannabidiol, or CBD.

Before I conclude, I would like to recognize Representatives Lee and Blumenauer, who are joining us in the audience today. They serve as the cochairs of the bipartisan Cannabis Caucus with Representatives Young and Joyce. Together they foster a continued dialogue on cannabis issues, and both helped author bills before us today. I thank them for joining us and commend them for their ongoing leadership in this area.

Thank you again to the witnesses for testifying before us. I am looking forward to this discussion. Thank you, and I yield back.

* * *

Mr. GRIFFITH. Mr. Chairman, will take it.

I appreciate that. As one of the sponsors of the bills, a lot of times people think, why does a conservative Republican get into this and champion it?

Well, let me tell you a story. When I was a young man in the 1980s, some of my friends were smuggling marijuana into the hospital in our community there in the Roanoke Valley because there was an individual whom I did not know who was dying of cancer, but he wanted to spend every day he could with his son who was about two at the time. And that formed my policy that we need to have a rational medical marijuana policy; thus the LUMMA bill.

But I decided when I got to Congress that, you know, well, it is kind of controversial, and maybe I shouldn't do that. But I would talk about it. And when I was at a high school townhall as I call them—I go to the high schools and talk to students—they ask about marijuana policy.

I told them my position on medical marijuana, which I went public with in 1998 on the floor of the Virginia House of Delegates. And I was standing there, and I thought—all the hands went up, and I thought one of the kids was going to say to me, "Well, what about for just for recreational use or for fun?" And I will never forgot it: I was in Wise, Virginia, and a young man on this side of the room raised his hand, and I went to him expecting to get the recreational question. And he said, "They did that for my daddy, too." Now my district is a big district. These two communities, 20 years apart—30 years apart, and hours apart from one another. And yet doctors were turning a blind eye to allow marijuana to be brought into the hospital because they recognized for those patients who were dying, this was the only way they could have a little bit of relief and get the nutrients that they needed to stay alive a little bit longer to spend a little bit more time with their children. I came back to DC, and I said: You know what? I am in Congress now. I can do something about the DEA and the FDA not making marijuana available for patients who need it. And today is that day.

I yield back.

Mr. PALLONE. And I yield back, Madam Chair.

Ms. ESHOO. The gentleman yields back. There is nothing like a real-life story.

It is a pleasure to recognize the ranking member of the full committee, my friend Mr. Walden, for 5 minutes for his opening statement.

Opening Statement of Hon. Greg Walden, a Representative in Congress from the State of Oregon

Mr. WALDEN. Thank you, Madam Chair.

We appreciate the hearing today because we will finally have an opportunity to review initiates aimed at improving federally sanctioned research on cannabis. Representatives Burgess, Griffith, Rodgers, and others, we sent a letter asking for this hearing. We appreciate your willingness to have it, Madam Chair.

Federally sanctioned reached on cannabis is challenging. It is a schedule I controlled substance under the Controlled Substances Act. This means that researchers seeking to investigate cannabis must work with the Food & Drug Administration, the National Institute of Drug Abuse and the drug enforcement administration just to meet the Federal guidelines, requirements specified in the CSA to conduct research. In addition, international obligations set forth in the United Nations drug control treaties impose additional requirements on the substance impacting the supply of research-grade cannabis.

So researchers now can only use cannabis for products sourced through the NIDA's drug supply program single DEA licensee, the University of Mississippi.

Now, unfortunately, that cannabis is distinct from what is commercially available from State legal dispensaries, such as in my home State of Oregon, meaning that we have little to no data on the health impacts of products in States that have legalized cannabis for medical or recreational use.

Now, in Oregon, you can purchase a range of THC-infused products, like these cookies we have a photo of right there. If you look up on the screen behind you, I guess, it is sort of stereo on this other side, but right there. And each of you, by the way, has a cookie in front of you. I have a pizza stand opening in an hour out in a hallway. Don't worry; I didn't get that carried away. You can actually eat these, as far as I know. Unless Safeway inserted something beyond the normal ingredients, it is just a cookie.

The question is, how do you know if your child stumbled upon it? So serious side. Oregon, these cookies in this photo are limited to five milligrams of THC per serving, 50 milligrams per package. Now, if you go across the Columbia River to Washington State, you find they have a different limit, ten milligrams and 100 milligrams per package. The difference is arbitrary. You see we lack data. We do not know—what we do know is there have been an elevated number of cannabis-related poison center calls, emergency room visits, and impaired driving incidents. But we need the research that reflects the reality of what is on today's market.

Additionally, products containing CBD derived from the hemp plant have become commonplace across the country in pharmacies, food health stores, even fast food chains since hemp was removed from the CSA in 2018 farm bill. Now these products often contain claims they can effectively treat depression, inflammation, and even cancer or Alzheimer's. However, none of these claims have been evaluated or approved by the Food and Drug Administration, which means patients may be relying on the unsubstantiated claims of CBD products and foregoing other proven medical treatments.

And while there is potential for CBD to provide real patient benefit, the research and science lags far behind the market, and the agencies are struggling to catch up.

So nationwide exposure in youth is increasing. From 2006 to 2013, children's exposure to marijuana products rose 147.5 percent nationwide. And in States that have legalized medical marijuana, exposure has risen 610 percent. And while alcohol use is going down in teens, last month, NIDA reported record numbers of eighth through twelfth grade students regularly vaping marijuana, a subject we have talked about before this committee.

So we need more research, and we need more data. Americans are consuming more cannabis, and policy decisions on this substance has been made in a virtual information vacuum. States that have legalized marijuana, such as my State, have done so with far less information than they have on legal substances that are easily abused, such as alcohol or tobacco. Rescheduling cannabis may help improve the research landscape and allow for more medical treatments. However, administrative rescheduling necessitates robust data on potential medical uses, and the current research restrictions on fully studying cannabis have effectively created a catch-22 in this rescheduling debate. Evaluations by the FDA and the National Academies have both concluded that lack of research was a significant factor in denying previous rescheduling petitions.

So I would like to note that two of the six bills we are reviewing today completely descheduled cannabis, removing it from the Controlled Substances Act, even though we do not have the necessary data to justify doing so, in my opinion. Descheduling cannabis is a step too far and a step I cannot support because descheduling removes it from the Controlled Substances Act and cuts the DEA completely out of the picture. So any discussion of descheduling must be preceded by a fuller understanding of the potential risks associated with cannabis use, which we currently do not have.

Research is the first step in making it easier to get our research on cannabis. It is common ground we should pursue as we improve the Federal-State relationship and the marijuana policy gap.

And, with that, Madam Chair, I yield back.

And you can eat your cookies now.

[The prepared statement of Mr. Walden follows:]

Prepared Statement of Hon. Greg Walden

At today's hearing, we will have the opportunity to review initiatives aimed at improving federally-sanctioned research on cannabis. Republican Leader, Burgess, Reps. Griffith, Rodgers and I sent a letter requesting this hearing last month, and I'd like to thank the Majority for responding and getting a hearing on the books in such a timely fashion.

Federally sanctioned research on cannabis is challenging. It is a Schedule I controlled substance under the Controlled Substances Act (CSA). This means that researchers seeking to investigate cannabis must work with the Food and Drug Administration (FDA), the National Institute on Drug Abuse (NIDA), and the Drug Enforcement Administration (DEA) to meet the federal requirements specified in the CSA to conduct research. In addition, international obligations set forth in three United Nations (U.N.) drug control treaties impose requirements on the substance, impacting the supply of research-grade cannabis.

Currently, researchers can only use cannabis products sourced through the NIDA's Drug Supply Program single DEA licensee: the University of Mississippi. Unfortunately, that cannabis is distinct from what is commercially available from state-legal dispensaries, such as in my home state of Oregon, meaning that we have little to no data on the health impacts of products in states that have legalized cannabis for medical or recreational use.

In Oregon, you can purchase a range of THC infused products, like these cookies we have a photo of here.

Now everyone on the dais has a cookie in front of them that looks a lot like this photo. Don't worry, yours are just from Safeway. But how would you know if you, or a child, stumbled upon it.

That serious concern aside, in Oregon, the cookies in this photo are limited to 5mg of THC per serving. 50mg per package. Washington state has limits of 10mg and 100mg.

The difference is largely arbitrary. We lack data. We do know there have elevated numbers of cannabis-related poison center calls, emergency room visits, and impaired driving incidents.[1] We need research that reflects the reality of what's on the market.

Additionally, products containing CBD derived from the hemp plant, have become commonplace across the country in pharmacies, health food stores, and even fast food chains since hemp was removed from the CSA in the 2018 Farm Bill. These products often contain claims that they can effectively treat depression, inflammation, and even cancer or Alzheimer's. However, none of these claims have been evaluated or approved by the FDA, meaning patients may be relying on the unsubstantiated claims of CBD products and forgoing other, proven, medical treatments. While there is potential for CBD to provide real patient benefit, the research and science lags far behind the market and the agencies are struggling to catch up.

Nationwide, exposure in youth is increasing. From 2006 to 2013, children's exposure to marijuana products rose 147.5 percent nationwide. In states that have legalized medical marijuana, exposure has risen 610 percent.[2] And while alcohol use is going down in teens, last month NIDA reported record numbers of eighth through 12th grade students regularly vaping marijuana.[3]

We need more research and better data. Americans are consuming more cannabis and policy decisions on this substance have been made in a virtual information vacuum. States that have legalized marijuana have done so with far less information than they have on legal substances that are easily abused, such as alcohol or tobacco. Rescheduling cannabis may help improve the research landscape and allow for more medical treatments. However, administrative rescheduling necessitates robust data on potential medical uses;

---

[1] https://www.oregon.gov/oha/PH/PREVENTIONWELLNESS/MARIJUANA/Documents/fact-sheet-marijuana-consequences.pdf.

[2] https://journals.sagepub.com/doi/abs/10.1177/0009922815589912.

[3] https://www.nih.gov/news-events/news-releases/vaping-marijuana-rise-among-teens.

and the current research restrictions on fully studying cannabis have effectively created a Catch-22 in the rescheduling debate. Evaluations by the FDA and the National Academies have both concluded that lack of research was a significant factor in denying previous rescheduling petitions.[4]

I would like to note that two of the six bills we are reviewing today completely de-schedule cannabis, removing it from the Controlled Substances Act, even though we do not have the necessary data to justify doing so. De-scheduling cannabis is a step too far and is something I cannot support, as de-scheduling removes it from the Controlled Substances Act and cuts the DEA completely out of the picture.

Any discussion of de-scheduling MUST be preceded by a fuller understanding of the potential risks associated with cannabis use—which we currently do not have. Research is the critical first step. Making it easier to conduct research on cannabis is common ground that we can pursue together in improving the state-federal marijuana policy gap, and I'm looking forward to hearing from our distinguished federal witnesses on potential solutions to help improve the research landscape.

* * *

Ms. ESHOO. The gentleman yields back. The Chair would like to remind Members that, pursuant to committee rules, all members' written opening statements shall be made part of the record.

Now I would like to introduce our witnesses for today's hearing and to thank each one of you for being with us today. Dr. Nora Volkow is the director of the National Institute of Drug Abuse at the National Institutes of Health.

Thank you to you.

Dr. Douglas Throckmorton is the deputy director for regulatory programs at the Center for Drug Evaluation and Research at the FDA, at the Food & Drug Administration.

And Mr. Matthew Strait is senior policy adviser for the Diversion Control Division of the Drug Enforcement Administration.

So welcome to each one of you. Thank you for essentially your life's work that brings you to the table to testify today. We look forward to the testimony that each one of you are going to offer.

---

[4]https://www.nap.edu/catalog/24625/the-health-effects-of-cannabis-and-cannabinoids-the-current-state.

I think you are familiar with the lights. It is like a traffic system. Green is go. Yellow is caution, and when red turns up, it is time to stop.

So we will start with Dr. Volkow.

You are recognized for your 5 minutes of testimony. And, again, thank you not only for your work, but for being here with us today. Turn your microphone on.

Statement of Nora D. Volkow, M.D. Director, National Institute on Drug Abuse, National Institutes of Health

Dr. VOLKOW. I want to say good morning to everybody, and I want to than Chairwoman Eshoo, Ranking Member Burgess, and all of the members of the subcommittee for inviting us to discuss cannabis research.

Cannabis is the most widely used illicit drug in the world and in the United States. THC is responsible for cannabis rewarding and addictive effects. And it is content has tripled in the past two decades. On the other hand, the content of cannabidiol, or CBD, which is not rewarding but of interest because of its potential therapeutic effects, has decreased in cannabis plants while food, drinks, and other products containing it have proliferated it.

THC exerts its effects by interacting with cannabinoid receptors, which are part of our own endogenous cannabinoid system. The system is involved in brain development and multiple brain functions, memory, emotions, reward, among others. Cannabinoid receptors also modulate immune, inflammatory, hormonal, metabolic processes in our body. Thus, it is not surprising that cannabis, which basically hijacks that systems can negatively affect health. Of particular concern are its effects on the developing fetal and adolescent brain. Cannabis exposure, as was mentioned before, during pregnancy has increased and is associated with fetal growth restriction, lower birth rate, and preterm delivery. In adolescents, cannabis use has been consistently associated with lower academic achievement, higher risk of dropping out of school, lower IQ, disruptions in brain connectivity and structure as the brain transitions into adulthood. Cannabis use at a young age increases the risk of addiction to cannabis and to other drugs.

Another area of major concern is the association of cannabis use with psychosis, the risk of which increases with consumption of high-content THC. While most episodes of psychosis are short lasting, they can become chronic.

Concerns have also emerged regarding higher risk for depression and suicide, though these associations have been less studied.

The availability of high-THC products has markedly increased emergency department visits and hospital admissions associated with cannabis exposures. Vehicle-related injuries while driving under the influence of THC are one of the main causes. Another frequent cause is severe cycles of nausea, vomiting, and abdominal pain referred to as cannabis hyperemesis syndrome.

However, our understanding of the adverse effects of cannabis is incomplete. This was made clearly evident by the outbreak of e-cigarette or vaping product use associated lung injury or EVALI, a condition reported in June 2019 predominantly associated with THC vaping that has, over six months, resulted in 2,500 more hospitalizations and 55 deaths.

Consumption of cannabis edibles packaged in food and drinks disproportionately accounts for cannabis-related emergency department visits. The slow absorption can prompt the user to take further doses, resulting in very high THC levels. Toxicity was frequently manifest as acute psychosis, severe anxiety, and cardiovascular complaints, and they also contribute increasingly to intoxication in children. Cannabis plants have been legalized for medical use for multiple indications in many States, even though FDA has not approved any of them for any indication.

Though not meeting FDA requirements, there is evidence though that cannabis may be effective for treating spasticity multiple sclerosis and for pain, but otherwise there is little evidence for other indications for which patients are using it.

NIH is helping to close this knowledge gap, including supporting stories to examine CBD for treating pain, inflammation, PTSD, and addiction. Understanding the effects of cannabis on brain development is a NIDA priority. And the adolescent brain cognitive development study will follow more than 11,000 children into early adulthood to investigate how cannabis affects their brains.

Despite the urgency for advancing research, the fact that cannabis is a schedule I substance proposes major challenges. NIDA's contract with the University of Mississippi is currently the only DEA source of research cannabis, and researchers are unable to access cannabis for research from dispensaries and other sources resulting in a gap in our understanding of their impact on health.

Cannabis research is urgently needed both to guide policy and to develop therapeutics; thus the importance of facilitating their ability to do so.

Thank you very much.

[The prepared statement of Dr. Volkow follows:]

Prepared Statement of Nora Volkow, M.D.

Chairwoman Eshoo, Ranking Member Burgess, and members of the Subcommittee, thank you for inviting the National Institute on Drug Abuse (NIDA), a component of the National Institutes of Health (NIH), to participate in this hearing. I am pleased to address the state of the science on cannabis and its constituent compounds and the process for conducting research with cannabis and other Schedule I drugs.

Background

In 2018, 43.5 million people reported using cannabis in the past year, making it the most commonly-used illicit drug in the United States. Cannabis contains hundreds of constituent compounds, including the cannabinoids delta-9-tetrahydrocannabinol (THC) and cannabidiol (CBD). Cannabinoids exert their effects on the body mainly by interacting with two types of receptors: CB1 and CB2 receptors. CB1 receptors are located mainly on neurons and glial cells in the brain and in several other organs in the body. CB2 receptors are found mainly on immune cells and are less common in the brain than CB1 receptors.[5] Whereas the euphoric effects of cannabis are caused by THC's activation of CB1 receptors, CBD has a very low affinity for these receptors (100-fold less than THC), and when it binds to them it produces little to no effect. Consequently, CBD, unlike THC, does not appear to produce euphoria, intoxication, or addiction. CBD acts on other brain signaling systems and on the immune system, and it is these actions that are thought to be important to its potential therapeutic effects.[6]

Cannabis products with varying concentrations of THC, CBD, and other chemicals have proliferated. The cannabis available today is much more potent than what was available in the past. The THC concentration in commonly cultivated cannabis plants increased three-fold between 1995 and

---

[5] Drysdale AJ, Platt B. Cannabinoids: mechanisms and therapeutic applications in the CNS. *Curr Med Chem.* 2003;10(24):2719-2732.

[6] Borgelt LM, Franson KL, Nussbaum AM, Wang GS. The Pharmacologic and Clinical Effects of Medical Cannabis. *Pharmacother J Hum Pharmacol Drug Ther.* 2013;33(2):195-209. doi:10.1002/phar.1187.

2014 (an increase from 4 to 12 percent in that period),[7] and cannabis available in dispensaries in some states has average concentrations of THC between 17.7 percent and 23.2 percent.[8] Concentrated products, commonly known as dabs or waxes, are widely available in some states and may contain between 23.7 percent and 75.9 percent THC.[9] CBD is ubiquitous, and it is possible to purchase CBD extracts as well as food, drinks, cosmetics, and other CBD-containing products, which are sometimes marketed with health and wellness claims that are not backed by science. Given the widespread availability of cannabis, its increasing potency, and the fact that many Americans are using cannabis products for medical and/or other purposes, there is a pressing need for research on the health consequences of cannabis and its constituent compounds, including CBD.

Adverse Health Effect of Cannabis

Prenatal and Adolescent Development

Cannabis is not a benign substance, and cannabis exposure carries particular risk early in life. The body's endocannabinoid system—on which cannabis acts—appears relatively early during fetal development. As the fetal brain grows, this system influences how brain cells develop and connect with one another, and it plays a major role in the formation of brain circuits including those important for decision making, mood, and responding to stress.[10] THC freely crosses the placenta resulting in fetal exposure.[11] Animal studies have shown that *in utero* exposure to cannabis can interfere with the proper development and regulation of brain circuitry.[12] In humans, fetal exposure is

[7] Elsohly, M. A., Mehmedic, Z., Foster, S. (2016). Changes in Cannabis Potency Over the Last 2 Decades (1995-2014): Analysis of Current Data in the United States. Biological Psychiatry, 79(7), 613-619. doi:10.1016/j.biopsych.2016.01.004.

[8] Jikomes, N., & Zoorob, M. (2018). The Cannabinoid Content of Legal Cannabis in Washington State Varies Systematically Across Testing Facilities and Popular Consumer Products. Scientific reports, 8(1), 4519. doi:10.1038/s41598-018-22755-2.

[9] Alzghari, S. K., Fung, V., Rickner, S. S., Chacko, L., & Fleming, S. W. (2017). To Dab or Not to Dab: Rising Concerns Regarding the Toxicity of Cannabis Concentrates. Cureus, 9(9), e1676. doi:10.7759/cureus.1676.

[10] Brents L. K. (2016). Marijuana, the Endocannabinoid System and the Female Reproductive System. The Yale journal of biology and medicine, 89(2), 175–191.

[11] Bailey JR, Cunny HC, Paule MG, Slikker W Jr. Fetal disposition of delta 9-tetrahydrocannabinol (THC) during late pregnancy in the rhesus monkey. Toxicol Appl Pharmacol. 1987 Sep 15;90(2):315-21.

[12] de Salas-Quiroga A, Díaz-Alonso J, García-Rincón D, Remmers F, Vega D, Gómez-Cañas M, Lutz B, Guzmán M, Galve-Roperh I. Prenatal exposure to cannabinoids evokes long-lasting

associated with significant negative outcomes including fetal growth restriction,[13,14] lower birth weight,[15] and preterm delivery.[10]

Adolescents, whose brains are also undergoing major developmental changes, are also particularly vulnerable to the negative effects of cannabis. Preclinical studies have found that THC exposure during adolescence increases subsequent sensitivity to the rewarding effects of other drugs,[16] which could be one reason why those who use cannabis at a young age are more vulnerable to cannabis and other drug addiction later in life. Epidemiological studies have found that youth who regularly use cannabis have lower academic achievements and a higher risk of dropping out of school.[17] Frequent cannabis use during adolescence is associated with changes in areas of the brain involved in attention, memory, emotions, and motivation.[18] These changes may account for the adverse cognitive and behavioral effects associated with youth cannabis use, although there is likely also a role for peer and family influences, among others.

Cannabis Use Disorder

Cannabis use can lead to cannabis use disorder and, in severe cases, addiction. Data suggest that nearly 10 percent of people who use cannabis will become dependent on it.[19] People who begin using cannabis before the age of 18 are

---

functional alterations by targeting CB1 receptors on developing cortical neurons. Proc Natl Acad Sci U S A. 2015 Nov 3;112(44):13693-8.

[13] Petrangelo A, Czuzoj-Shulman N, Balayla J, Abenhaim HA. Cannabis Abuse or Dependence During Pregnancy: A Population-Based Cohort Study on 12 Million Births. J Obstet Gynaecol Can. 2019 May;41(5):623-630.

[14] Corsi DJ, Walsh L, Weiss D, Hsu H, El-Chaar D, Hawken S, Fell DB, Walker M. Association Between Self-reported Prenatal Cannabis Use and Maternal, Perinatal, and Neonatal Outcomes. JAMA. 2019 Jul 9;322(2):145-152.

[15] National Academies of Sciences, Engineering, and Medicine 2017. The Health Effects of Cannabis and Cannabinoids: The Current State of Evidence and Recommendations for Research. Washington, DC: The National Academies Press.

[16] Ellgren M, Spano SM, Hurd YL. Adolescent cannabis exposure alters opiate intake and opioid limbic neuronal populations in adult rats. Neuropsychopharmacology. 2007 Mar;32(3):607-15.

[17] McCaffrey DF, Pacula RL, Han B, Ellickson P. Marijuana use and high school dropout: the influence of unobservables. Health Econ. 2010;19(11):1281–1299.

[18] Jacobus J, Tapert SF. Effects of cannabis on the adolescent brain. Curr Pharm Des. 2014;20(13):2186–2193.

[19] Hasin DS, Saha TD, Kerridge BT, et al. Prevalence of Marijuana Use Disorders in the United States Between 2001-2002 and 2012-2013. JAMA Psychiatry. 2015;72(12):1235-1242. doi:10.1001/jamapsychiatry.2015.1858.

four to seven times more likely to develop cannabis use disorder than adults.[20] The risks of physical dependence, addiction, and other negative consequences increase with frequent use and exposure to high concentrations of THC.[21]

Mental Illness

The association between cannabis use and mental illness is another major concern, particularly in light of the higher content of THC in today's cannabis. Serious mental illnesses and suicides are on the rise in our country,[22] and while multiple factors very likely contribute to this rise, it is imperative to understand if exposure to cannabis in adolescence is one of them. High doses of THC can trigger acute psychotic episodes, which is one of the main causes for emergency department visits associated with cannabis use.[23] Most of these episodes are short lasting, but some can last from days to weeks after use.[24] While overall risk of developing a lasting psychotic disorder is low, multiple studies have associated adolescent cannabis use (especially use of high potency products) with an increased overall risk for, and early onset of, chronic psychosis such as schizophrenia,[25,26] particularly in those with other

---

[20] Winters KC, Lee C-YS. Likelihood of developing an alcohol and cannabis use disorder during youth: Association with recent use and age. Drug Alcohol Depend. 2008;92(1-3):239-247. doi:10.1016/j.drugalcdep.2007.08.005.

[21] Freeman, T. P., & Winstock, A. R. (2015). Examining the profile of high-potency cannabis and its association with severity of cannabis dependence. Psychological medicine, 45(15), 3181– 3189. doi:10.1017/S0033291715001178.

[22] Substance Abuse and Mental Health Services Administration. (2019). Key substance use and mental health indicators in the United States: Results from the 2018 National Survey on Drug Use and Health (HHS Publication No. PEP19-5068, NSDUH Series H-54). Rockville, MD: Center for Behavioral Health Statistics and Quality, Substance Abuse and Mental Health Services Administration.

[23] De Aquino JP, Sherif M, Radhakrishnan R, Cahill JD, Ranganathan M, D'Souza DC. The Psychiatric Consequences of Cannabinoids. Clin Ther. 2018 Sep;40(9):1448-1456.

[24] Pearson NT, Berry JH. Cannabis and Psychosis Through the Lens of DSM-5. *Int J Environ Res Public Health*. 2019;16(21):4149.

[25] Arseneault L, Cannon M, Witton J, Murray RM. Causal association between cannabis and psychosis: examination of the evidence. Br J Psychiatry. 2004 Feb;184:110-7. Review.

[26] Di Forti M, Sallis H, Allegri F, Trotta A, Ferraro L, Stilo SA, Marconi A, La Cascia C, Reis Marques T, Pariante C, Dazzan P, Mondelli V, Paparelli A, Kolliakou A, Prata D, Gaughran F, David AS, Morgan C, Stahl D, Khondoker M, MacCabe JH, Murray RM. Daily use, especially of high-potency cannabis, drives the earlier onset of psychosis in cannabis users. Schizophr Bull. 2014 Nov;40(6):1509-17.

risk factors.[27] Adolescent cannabis use is also associated with increased risk of suicidal behavior.[28]

Lung Injuries

Inhalation of vaporized THC has been implicated in the outbreak of e-cigarette, or vaping, product use-associated lung injury (EVALI) that was first reported in June of 2019. EVALI results in an acute respiratory illness characterized by respiratory, gastrointestinal, and constitutional (e.g., chills, fever) symptoms, which has resulted in more than 2,500 hospitalizations and 55 deaths across the country over a 6 month period.[29] Most EVALI patients report vaping THC-containing products.[30] Vitamin E acetate, frequently found as an additive to vaped THC, is closely associated with EVALI. This substance, while safe to ingest or apply topically, may damage the lungs when heated and inhaled. Vitamin E acetate has a similar viscosity to THC, and the timing of its appearance as an additive to illicit THC-containing vaping products corresponds to the EVALI outbreak.[31]

Other Medical Complications

Different cannabis products (e.g., plant, THC concentrates) and routes of administration (e.g., inhalation, ingestion) pose unique risks. For example, eating cannabis can increase the risk of taking unintentionally high amounts

---

[27] Caspi A, Moffitt TE, Cannon M, McClay J, Murray R, Harrington H, Taylor A, Arseneault L, Williams B, Braithwaite A, Poulton R, Craig IW. Moderation of the effect of adolescent-onset cannabis use on adult psychosis by a functional polymorphism in the catechol-O-methyltransferase gene: longitudinal evidence of a gene X environment interaction. Biol Psychiatry. 2005 May 15;57(10):1117-27.

[28] Silins E, Horwood LJ, Patton GC, Fergusson DM, Olsson CA, Hutchinson DM, Spry E, Toumbourou JW, Degenhardt L, Swift W, Coffey C, Tait RJ, Letcher P, Copeland J, Mattick RP; Cannabis Cohorts Research Consortium. Young adult sequelae of adolescent cannabis use: an integrative analysis. Lancet Psychiatry. 2014 Sep;1(4):286-93.

[29] https://www.cdc.gov/tobacco/basic_information/e-cigarettes/severe-lung-disease/need-to-know/index.html.

[30] Lozier MJ, Wallace B, Anderson K, et al. Update: Demographic, Product, and Substance-Use Characteristics of Hospitalized Patients in a Nationwide Outbreak of E-cigarette, or Vaping, Product Use–Associated Lung Injuries — United States, December 2019. MMWR Morb Mortal Wkly Rep 2019;68:1142–1148.

[31] Blount BC, Karwowski MP, Shields PG, Morel-Espinosa M, Valentin-Blasini L, Gardner M, Braselton M, Brosius CR, Caron KT, Chambers D, Corstvet J, Cowan E, De Jesús VR, Espinosa P, Fernandez C, Holder C, Kuklenyik Z, Kusovschi JD, Newman C, Reis GB, Rees J, Reese C, Silva L, Seyler T, Song MA, Sosnoff C, Spitzer CR, Tevis D, Wang L, Watson C, Wewers MD, Xia B, Heitkemper DT, Ghinai I, Layden J, Briss P, King BA, Delaney LJ, Jones CM, Baldwin GT, Patel A, Meaney-Delman D, Rose D, Krishnasamy V, Barr JR, Thomas J, Pirkle JL; Lung Injury Response Laboratory Working Group. Vitamin E Acetate in Bronchoalveolar-Lavage Fluid Associated with EVALI. N Engl J Med. 2019 Dec 20.

due to its lengthy absorption time and delayed effect, which may prompt users to take more. This can result in aversive psychiatric and cardiac symptoms; edibles are, therefore, responsible for a disproportionate number of cannabis-related emergency department visits.[32] Edibles are often in the form of desserts or snacks and have increasingly been a cause of accidental ingestion by children[33] and adolescents.[34]

An additional medical complication that can result from chronic use of cannabis is known as cannabinoid hyperemesis syndrome, which is marked by severe cycles of nausea and vomiting.[35] The increase in the THC content of cannabis has led to a worrisome upward trend in the rate of calls to poison control centers and emergency department visits, especially in States that have legalized the drug.[36,37]

Impaired Driving

Cannabis significantly impairs judgment, motor coordination, and reaction time, and studies have found a direct relationship between blood THC concentration and impaired driving ability.[38,39,40] Several meta-analyses found that the risk of being involved in a crash significantly increased after cannabis use.[41] However, in a large case-control study, the significance of cannabis use

---

[32] Monte AA, Shelton SK, Mills E, et al. Acute Illness Associated With Cannabis Use, by Route of Exposure: An Observational Study. Ann Intern Med. 2019;170:531–537.

[33] Richards, J.R., Smith N.E., Moulin, A.K. Unintentional Cannabis Ingestion in Children: A Systematic Review. *J Pediatr* 2017; 190:142-52.

[34] Cao, D., Sahaphume, S., Bronstein, A.C., Hoyte, C.O., Characterization of edible marijuana product exposures reported to the United States poison centers. *Clinical Toxicology*, 54:9, 840-846, DOI: 10.1080/15563650.2016.1209761.

[35] Galli, J.A., Sawaya, R.A., Friedenberg, F.K. Cannabinoid Hyperemesis Syndrome. Curr Drug Abuse Rev. 2011 Dec; 4(4): 241–249.

[36] Wang GS, Hall K, Vigil D, Banerji S, Monte A, VanDyke M. Marijuana and acute health care contacts in Colorado. Prev Med. 2017 Nov;104:24-30.

[37] Whitehill JM, Harrington C, Lang CJ, Chary M, Bhutta WA, Burns MM. Incidence of Pediatric Cannabis Exposure Among Children and Teenagers Aged 0 to 19 Years Before and After Medical Marijuana Legalization in Massachusetts. JAMA Netw Open. 2019 Aug 2;2(8):e199456.

[38] Lenné MG et al. The effects of cannabis and alcohol on simulated arterial driving: Influences of driving experience and task demand. Accid Anal Prev. 2010;42(3):859-866. doi:10.1016/j.aap.2009.04.021.

[39] Hartman RL, Huestis MA. Cannabis effects on driving skills. Clin Chem. 2013;59(3):478-492. doi:10.1373/clinchem.2012.194381.

[40] Hartman RL, Brown TL, Milavetz G, et al. Cannabis effects on driving lateral control with and without alcohol. Drug Alcohol Depend. 2015;154:25-37. doi:10.1016/j.drugalcdep.2015.06.015.

[41] Elvik R. Risk of road accident associated with the use of drugs: a systematic review and meta-analysis of evidence from epidemiological studies. Accid Anal Prev. 2013;60:254-267.

disappeared after controlling for drivers' age, gender, race, and the presence of alcohol.[42] A complicating factor in determining crash risk is the difficulty of assessing cannabis impairment in the field, particularly compared to assessing impairment due to alcohol. Blood alcohol concentration is easily determined in a breath sample and reliably reflects impairment level.[43] Cannabis, however, is rapidly absorbed by fat cells; this means that blood levels drop rapidly after smoking and that cannabis may be detected in frequent users long after its impairing effects have subsided.[44]

Therapeutic Potential of Cannabis and Its Constituent Cannabinoids

While cannabis has been legalized for medical use in many states, it remains a Schedule I substance under the Federal Controlled Substances Act (CSA), and it does not have FDA approval for any indication. Some synthetic forms of THC are FDA approved (i.e., Marinol and Syndros) for the treatment of anorexia and weight loss in AIDS patients and for nausea and vomiting associated with cancer treatment. The FDA also approved Cesamet, which contains the active ingredient nabilone, a synthetic chemical similar to THC, for treating nausea and vomiting related to cancer chemotherapy.

Epidiolex is the first cannabis-derived medication and contains a highly purified form of CBD. It has been approved by the FDA for the treatment of seizures associated with Lennox-Gastaut and Dravet syndromes in patients two years of age and older. Research is underway to assess the therapeutic potential of CBD to treat multiple health conditions including, pain, inflammation, posttraumatic stress disorder, HIV, digestive disorders, and substance use disorders.[45] Outside of standard drug development there has been a proliferation of purported dietary supplements and food products that contain CBD.

A recent report published by the National Academies of Sciences, Engineering, and Medicine, which was sponsored by the Centers for Disease

---

[42] Compton RP, Berning A. Drug and Alcohol Crash Risk. Washington, DC: National Highway Traffic Safety Administration; 2015. DOT HA 812 117.

[43] Van Dyke NA, Fillmore MT. Laboratory analysis of risky driving at 0.05% and 0.08% blood alcohol concentration. Drug Alcohol Depend. 2017;175:127–132.

[44] Hartman RL, Brown TL, Milavetz G, et al. Effect of blood collection time on measured Δ9-tetrahydrocannabinol concentrations: implications for driving interpretation and drug policy. Clin Chem2016;62:367–77.

[45] https://projectreporter.nih.gov/Reporter_Viewsh.cfm?sl=15E1C90E468AC7D17598B8961CAA4A01A2FFCEB861BF.

Control and Prevention, NIDA, the National Cancer Institute (NCI), FDA, and other stakeholders, concluded that there is substantial evidence that cannabis or cannabinoids are effective for treating chronic pain and improving patient-reported spasticity symptoms in multiple sclerosis. However, in general, adequate and well-controlled studies are lacking, which means that individuals across the country are using cannabis strains and extracts that have not undergone the rigorous clinical trials required to show they are safe and effective for medical use, and are not regulated for consistency or quality.

Research Supported by the National Institutes of Health's (NIH) National Institute on Drug Abuse (NIDA)

Research supported by NIH is helping to close the gaps in our understanding of the risks and potential benefits associated with cannabis product use. In fiscal year 2018, NIH Institutes and Centers supported $147 million in cannabinoid research, broadly, including $38 million on therapeutic cannabinoid research and $19 million on studies involving CBD.[46] Although most of this research is supported by NIDA, several other NIH Institutes and Centers fund cannabinoid research relevant to their respective missions. NIDA's portfolio includes research on the pharmacology of THC and other cannabinoids; the changes in the brain at the molecular, cellular, and systems levels associated with cannabis addiction and other adverse effects; the potentially beneficial effects of cannabis and its constituent compounds; preventing and treating cannabis misuse and addiction; and research to elucidate the prevalence and patterns of cannabis use and how cannabis policies affect public health.

Several important areas of interest across NIH include evaluating the endocannabinoid system as a new target for pain and addiction therapies,[47] disentangling the distinct therapeutic benefits and potential health risks of different component compounds within cannabis as they relate to pain,[48,49] and evaluating the effects of cannabis and exposures to other substances during vulnerable periods of development. The Adolescent Brain Cognitive Development (ABCD) study has great potential to advance knowledge on the developmental effects of cannabis exposure during adolescence. The largest

---

[46] https://report.nih.gov/categorical_spending.aspx.
[47] https://grants.nih.gov/grants/guide/pa-files/pa-18-465.html.
[48] https://grants.nih.gov/grants/guide/rfa-files/rfa-at-19-008.html.
[49] https://nccih.nih.gov/news/press/09192019.

long-term study of brain development and child health, the ABCD study will follow more than 11,000 children ages 9-10 into young adulthood. Researchers will assess their development, including how it may be affected by cannabis and other drug use, through brain imaging, genetic and other biological markers, and psychological, behavioral, and other health assessments. Complementing ABCD is the HEALthy Brain and Child Development (HBCD) Study. Currently in its planning phase, the HBCD study will advance knowledge on prenatal exposure to cannabis and other substances.

Conducting Research with Schedule I Substances

The increasing availability and potency of cannabis along with the proliferation of new cannabis products and methods for consuming them raise serious public health concerns. We know from other drug research that potency and route of administration are important factors in understanding the consequences of drug use, yet there is a relative dearth of research on these newer products. Rigorous research is essential for understanding how the changing cannabis landscape will affect public health and, ultimately, for guiding evidence-based policy. Despite the public health urgency, legal and regulatory barriers continue to present challenges to advancing cannabis research.

Obtaining and Modifying a Registration to Conduct Research with Cannabis and Other Schedule I Drugs is Challenging

Under the CSA, cannabis and its constituent compounds, excluding hemp, are classified as Schedule I controlled substances – defined as having no currently accepted medical use in the United States, a lack of accepted safety for use under medical supervision, and a high potential for abuse.[50] Obtaining or modifying a Schedule I registration involves significant administrative challenges, and researchers report that obtaining a new registration can take more than a year. Adding new substances to an existing registration can also be time consuming.

It would be useful to clarify aspects of the CSA that have been sources of confusion and administrative burden for the research community, including that it is permissible for one individual to hold a Schedule I registration under which colleagues from the same institution may work even if those colleagues do not work directly for the registrant (e.g., as members of their laboratory);

---

[50] https://www.deadiversion.usdoj.gov/schedules/.

that registered researchers may store, administer, and work with any substances for which they hold a researcher registration at multiple practice sites on a single contiguous campus; and that if a person is registered to conduct research with a controlled substance and applies to conduct research with a second controlled substance that is in the same schedule or in a schedule with a higher numerical designation, an inspection that was performed for purposes of the existing registration shall be sufficient to support the application.

Lastly, and specifically relevant to cannabis research, it would be helpful to clarify that individuals registered to conduct research with a controlled substance who need to perform limited manufacturing activities on small quantities of that substance consistent with their research protocol (for example, creating a particular dosage formulation for research purposes) are not required to obtain a separate manufacturing registration. This would be especially helpful in cases in which researchers are required to create dosage formulations in their own laboratories from cannabis products supplied through the NIDA Drug Supply Program.

NIDA Is the Only Source of Cannabis in the United States Permitted for Research

Although the CSA permits importation of cannabis and cannabis related substances for research, the University of Mississippi is the only entity in the United States currently registered with the DEA to cultivate cannabis for research purposes, which it does under a contract with NIDA. Having only a single domestic source of research cannabis limits the diversity of products and formulations available to researchers and slows the development of cannabis-based medications. Although the University of Mississippi supplies cannabis for clinical trials, it does not have the capacity to manufacture a broad array of cannabis-derived formulations for research or to supply these cannabis products for commercial development. Moreover, it is not clear how entities seeking to develop these products for commercial purposes would demonstrate equivalency between the University of Mississippi cannabis used in clinical trials and the drug product that would ultimately be approved by the FDA for marketing and sale. NIDA was pleased that on August 26, 2019, the DEA signaled that it is moving forward with its review of additional grower applications[51] and that it would promulgate new regulations governing

[51]https://www.dea.gov/press-releases/2019/08/26/dea-announces-steps-necessary-improve-access-marijuana-research.

cannabis cultivation. NIDA looks forward to opportunities to provide input to the DEA as it develops a new regulatory framework that ensures an adequate and diverse supply of cannabis for research.

Researchers Are Unable to Access Marketed Cannabis Products

Under Federal law, researchers supported by NIDA and other federal agencies are unable to access marketed cannabis products through state marijuana dispensaries. There is a significant gap in our understanding of their impact on health. The recent outbreaks of e-cigarette or vaping product use associated lung injury (EVALI), which has been linked to informally-sourced THC-containing vape products, underscores the critical importance of facilitating researcher access to different product sources.

NIDA appreciates this opportunity to discuss our work to advance research on cannabis and its constituent compounds. Rigorous research is essential for understanding how the changing cannabis landscape will affect public health, for guiding evidence-based policy and to help advance therapeutics. I look forward to answering any questions the Subcommittee may have on this important issue.

* * *

Ms. ESHOO. Thank you, Doctor.

We will now recognize Dr. Throckmorton for his 5 minutes of testimony.

And thank you again for being here today. Do you have your microphone on?

Dr. THROCKMORTON. I do. Thanks.

Ms. ESHOO. You are recognized.

Statement of Douglas C. Throckmorton, M.D. Deputy Director for Regulatory Programs, Center for Drug Evaluation and Research, Food and Drug Administration

Dr. THROCKMORTON. Chairman Eshoo, Ranking Member Burgess, and members of the subcommittee, I am Dr. Douglas Throckmorton Morton from the Center for Drug Evaluation and Research at the Food & Drug Administration. Thank for the opportunity to be here today to discuss the important role that FDA plays in research involving cannabis and cannabis-derived compounds for potential medical uses in the United States.

I would also like to discuss the recent work the FDA is doing to respond to the recent legislation affecting the availability of compounds derived from cannabis, such as cannabidiol.

First, with regards to drug development, FDA continues to believe that the drug approval process represents the best way to ensure that safe and effective new medicines, including medicines derived from cannabis, are available for patients. FDA stands ready today provide information to investigators on the progress and process and specific requirements needed to develop a human drug that is derived from plants such as cannabis. For example, FDA has ways to speed drug development programs, including programs such as fast track, breakthrough therapy, accelerated approval, and priority review, all designed to facilitate the development of and to expedite the approval of novel and effective drug products.

We have also established a botanical review team to assist the development of plant-based drugs, including those derived from cannabis. Using these resources, the FDA has successfully approved one cannabis-derived drug product, Epidiolex, containing cannabidiol or CBD, and three synthetic cannabis-derived drug products: Marinol, Syndros and Cesamet.

While FDA is aware of the activities of States in this area, to date FDA has not approved any other cannabis, cannabis-derived, or CBD products currently available on the market. Turning our activities through recent work under legislation, in December of 2018, the farm bill removed hemp defined as cannabis and its derivatives with extremely low concentrations of THC from the definition of marijuana in the Controlled Substances Act. The farm bill explicitly preserved FDA's authorities over products derived from hemp, such as CBD, which means the products must still meet any applicable FDA requirements and standards just like any other FDA-regulated product. Because we understand the broad interest in making compounds found in cannabis more widely available to the public, FDA is working hard to respond to these changes quickly and appropriately.

For example, we have reached several conclusions about the use of CBD in nondrug products. First, it is prohibited under our statute to introduce into interstate commerce any human or animal food to which certain drug ingredients have been added. In addition, drug ingredients are excluded from the definition of dietary supplement. Because CBD is an active ingredient of an approved drug, these restrictions apply to products made with CBD.

These provisions make sense. It is easy it to understand why we generally don't want blood pressure medicines or pain medicines in our food are in our dietary supplements. Additionally, FDA is concerned that the marketing of CBD in nondrug products could put consumers at risk, such as by making unsubstantiated claims to prevent or cure serious diseases such as cancer or Alzheimer's disease. The proliferation of such products may deter consumers from seeking proven, safe medical therapies for serious illnesses.

We also know that CBD can cause adverse effects, including drug interactions, sleepiness that could impair driving, and potential liver injury. There are many unanswered questions about the safety and quality of products containing CBD, and the agency has made it a priority to address these questions, including questions about the safety of long-term use of CBD by different populations. For example, we have very little information about the use of CBD by pregnant women, by children, and by the elderly. To address these gaps, FDA is in the process of systematically collecting all of the data that are available to us to make the best science based and public-health-focused decisions about the availability of the compounds in hemp.

To close, FDA understands the broad interest in making that compounds more available to the public and is considering the possibilities and new legal pathways for CBD products. However, it is important to maintain adequate incentives for drug development as we do so. Drugs have important therapeutic value and are approved after rigorous scientific studies that provide important, new information about their safety and effectiveness. It is critical that we continue to do what we can to support quality science needed to develop new products in cannabis.

With that, I thank you and look forward to answering any questions I can.

[The prepared statement of Dr. Throckmorton follows:]

Prepared Statement of Douglas C. Throckmorton

Introduction

Chairwoman Eshoo, Ranking Member Burgess, and Members of the Subcommittee, I am Dr. Douglas Throckmorton, Deputy Director of the Center for Drug Evaluation and Research (CDER) at the Food and Drug Administration (FDA or the Agency), which is part of the Department of Health and Human Services (HHS). Thank you for the opportunity to be here today to discuss the important role that FDA plays in research involving cannabis and cannabis-derived compounds for potential medical uses in the United States, as part of FDA's mission to protect and promote the public health by ensuring the safety, efficacy, and quality of medical products, including drugs.

FDA has an important role to play in supporting scientific research into the medical uses of cannabis and its constituents in scientifically valid investigations as part of the Agency's drug review and approval process. As a part of this role, FDA supports those in the medical research community who intend to study cannabis by:

1) Providing information on the process needed to conduct clinical research using cannabis.
2) Providing information on the specific requirements needed to develop a human drug that is derived from a plant such as cannabis. In December 2016, FDA updated its Guidance for Industry: Botanical Drug Development,[52] which provides sponsors with guidance on submitting investigational new drug (IND) applications for botanical drug products.
3) Providing specific support for investigators interested in conducting clinical research using cannabis and its constituents as a part of the IND process through meetings and regular interactions throughout the drug development process.
4) Providing general support to investigators to help them understand and follow the procedures to conduct clinical research through the FDA Center for Drug Evaluation and Research (CDER) Small Business and Industry Assistance group.

To conduct clinical research that can lead to an approved new drug, including research using materials from plants such as cannabis, researchers need to work with FDA and submit an IND application to CDER. The IND application process gives researchers a path to follow that includes regular interactions with FDA to support efficient drug development while protecting the patients who are enrolled in the trials. An IND includes protocols describing proposed studies, the qualifications of the investigators who will conduct the clinical studies, and assurances of informed consent and

---

[52] https://www.fda.gov/regulatory-information/search-fda-guidance-documents/botanical-drug-development-guidance-industry.

protection of the rights, safety, and welfare of the human subjects. FDA reviews the IND to ensure that the proposed studies, generally referred to as "clinical trials," do not place human subjects at an unreasonable risk of harm. FDA also requires obtaining the informed consent of trial subjects and human subject protection in the conduct of the clinical trials.

To date, FDA has not approved a marketing application for cannabis for the treatment of any disease or condition. The Agency has, however, approved one cannabis-derived drug product: Epidiolex (cannabidiol), and three synthetic cannabis-related drug products: Marinol (dronabinol), Syndros (dronabinol), and Cesamet (nabilone). These approved drug products are only available with a prescription from a licensed healthcare provider. Importantly, FDA has not approved any other cannabis, cannabis-derived, or cannabidiol (CBD) products currently available on the market.

FDA has programs such as Fast Track, Breakthrough Therapy, Accelerated Approval and Priority Review that are designed to facilitate the development of and expedite the approval of drug products. In addition, FDA's expanded access (sometimes called "compassionate use") statutory and regulatory provisions are designed to facilitate the availability of investigational products to patients with serious diseases or conditions when there is no comparable or satisfactory alternative therapy available, either because the patients have exhausted treatment with or are intolerant of approved therapies, or when the patients are not eligible for an ongoing clinical trial. Finally, recognizing the unique challenges presented by products derived from plants such as cannabis, FDA has established a Botanical Review Team that is available to assist with the development of plant-based drugs.

FDA continues to believe the drug approval process represents the best way to ensure that safe and effective new medicines, including any drugs derived from cannabis, are available to patients in need of appropriate medical therapy. The Agency is committed to supporting the development of new drugs, including cannabis and cannabis-derived drugs, through the investigational new drug and drug approval process.

Under section 202 of the Controlled Substances Act (CSA), certain types and parts of the *Cannabis sativa L.* plant are controlled under the drug class "marijuana." Schedule I includes those substances that have a high potential for abuse, have no currently accepted medical use in treatment in the United States, and lack accepted safety for use under medical supervision. Nevertheless, Schedule I substances, including drugs that are derived from botanical sources such as cannabis, can be and are the subject of clinical trials under the Federal Food, Drug, and Cosmetic Act, provided, among other things, that the sponsor successfully submits an IND to FDA and successfully registers with the Drug Enforcement Administration (DEA).

In December 2018, the Agriculture Improvement Act of 2018 (also known as the Farm Bill) removed hemp, defined as cannabis (*Cannabis sativa L.*) and derivatives of cannabis with extremely low concentrations of the psychoactive compound delta-9-tetrahydrocannabinol (THC) (no more than 0.3 percent THC on a dry weight basis), from the definition of marijuana in the CSA. Because the Farm Bill explicitly preserved FDA's authorities over hemp and other low-THC cannabis products, including cannabidiol (CBD), these products must meet any applicable FDA requirements and standards, just like any other FDA-regulated product. For example, FDA's existing authorities over foods, dietary supplements, human and veterinary drugs, and cosmetics apply to hemp and CBD products to the extent such products fall within those categories. These safeguards help ensure that Americans have access to safe and accurately labeled hemp products, and, in the case of drugs, that patients can depend on the effectiveness of these products.

Nonetheless, the misperception persists that all products made from or containing hemp, including those made with CBD, are now legal to sell in interstate commerce. The result has been that storefronts and online retailers have flooded the market with these products, many with unsubstantiated therapeutic claims. FDA has seen CBD appear in a wide variety of products including those purporting to be foods, dietary supplements, veterinary products, and cosmetics. As this new market emerges, we have seen substantial interest from industry, consumers, and Congress. However, FDA's role remains the same: to protect and promote the public health.

At present, any food containing CBD or purported CBD dietary supplement product in interstate commerce is in violation of the FD&C Act under the statutory provisions discussed above. FDA's biggest concern is the marketing of CBD products that put consumers at risk, such as by making unsubstantiated therapeutic claims to prevent, diagnose, mitigate, treat, or cure serious diseases, but that have not obtained new drug approvals. For example, FDA has seen various CBD products with claims of curing cancer or treating Alzheimer's disease. The proliferation of such products may deter consumers from seeking proven, safe medical therapies for serious illnesses – potentially endangering their health or life. FDA's commitment to protect consumers from these unsubstantiated therapeutic claims does not just apply to CBD products – it is a longstanding commitment of the Agency across all the products we regulate.

There are also many unanswered questions about the science, safety, and quality of products containing CBD. The Agency is working on answering these questions through ongoing efforts including feedback from a recent FDA hearing and information and data gathering through a public docket. Although FDA has approved one drug, Epidiolex, that contains CBD, it is only approved for use in a limited population at a specific dose, was studied for safety and efficacy in rigorous randomized clinical trials, and is available only by a prescription from a licensed medical professional. When considering the use of CBD in non-drug products, such as conventional foods and dietary supplements, FDA must evaluate different factors than for a prescription drug product. CBD food and dietary supplement products would be directly available to a wide range of consumers, which could potentially include pregnant or nursing mothers, children, the elderly, those with chronic illnesses, and those taking medications that might interact with CBD. These would also be available without discussions with a doctor or other medical professional. Given this, FDA must consider the potential safety implications of long-term use of CBD by different populations.

Consumers should be aware of the potential risks associated with using CBD products. Some of these can occur without awareness, such as:

- *Liver Injury:* During its review of the marketing application for Epidiolex, FDA identified certain safety risks, including the potential for liver injury. This serious risk can be managed when an FDA-approved CBD drug product is taken under medical supervision, but it is less clear how it might be managed when CBD is used far more widely, without medical supervision, and not in accordance with FDA-approved labeling. Although this risk was increased when taken with other drugs that impact the liver, signs of liver injury were seen also in patients not on those drugs. The occurrence of this liver injury was identified through blood tests, as is often the case with early problems with the liver. Liver injury was also seen in other studies of CBD in published literature. We are concerned about potential liver injury associated with CBD use that could go undetected if not monitored by a healthcare provider.
- *Drug Interactions:* Information from studies of Epidiolex show that there is a risk of CBD impacting other medicines a consumer takes – or that other medicines could impact the dose of CBD that can safely be used. Taking CBD with other medications may increase or decrease the effects of the other medications. This may lead to an

increased chance of adverse effects from, or decreased effectiveness of, the other medications. Drug interactions were also seen in other studies of CBD in published literature. We are concerned about the potential safety of taking other medicines with CBD when the consumer is not being monitored by a healthcare provider. In addition, there is limited research on the interactions between CBD products and herbs or botanicals in dietary supplements. Consumers should use caution when combining CBD products with herbs or dietary supplements.

- *Male Reproductive Toxicity:* Studies in laboratory animals showed male reproductive toxicity, including in the male offspring of CBD-treated pregnant females. The changes seen include decrease in testicular size, inhibition of sperm growth and development, and decreased circulating testosterone, among others. Because these findings were only seen in animals, it is not yet clear what these findings mean for humans and the impact it could have on men (or the male children of pregnant women) who take CBD. For instance, these findings raise the concern that CBD could negatively affect a man's fertility. Further testing and evaluation are needed to better understand this potential risk.

In addition, CBD can cause side effects. These side effects should diminish when CBD is stopped or when the amount ingested is reduced. Side effects may include changes in alertness, most commonly experienced as somnolence (sleepiness), but this could also include insomnia; gastrointestinal distress, most commonly experienced as diarrhea and/or decreased appetite, but could also include abdominal pain or upset stomach; and changes in mood, most commonly experienced as irritability and agitation.

FDA is actively working to learn more about the safety of CBD and CBD products, including the risks identified above and other topics, such as:

- *Cumulative Exposure:* The cumulative exposure to CBD if people access it across a broad range of consumer products. For example, what happens if you eat food with CBD in it, use CBD-infused skin cream and take other CBD-based products on the same day? How much CBD is absorbed from your skin cream? What if you use these products daily for a week or a month?

- *Special Populations:* The effects of CBD on other special populations (e.g., the elderly, children, adolescents, pregnant and lactating women).
- *CBD and Animals:* The safety of CBD use in pets and other animals, including considerations of species, breed, or class and the safety of the resulting human food products (e.g., meat milk, or eggs) from food-producing species.

FDA is considering questions not only about the intrinsic safety of CBD, but also about potentially unsafe manufacturing processes for products containing CBD. FDA knows from CBD products we have tested that they may not contain the amount of CBD indicated on a label, or they may contain other potentially dangerous compounds that are not listed on the label. Therefore, FDA must consider questions related to good manufacturing practices for CBD products and potential labeling that might be appropriate for these products to address any potential risks to consumers.

FDA has made it a priority to address these questions, and we are working diligently to do so. We are also working diligently to consider whether and how legal pathways might be established to allow the safe marketing of certain dietary supplements and/or food products containing CBD.

While FDA is considering the possibility of new legal pathways for CBD products, we know that it is important to maintain adequate incentives for drug research and development. Drugs have important therapeutic value and are approved after rigorous scientific studies that provide important new information about therapeutic uses. It is critical that we continue to do what we can to support the science needed to develop new drugs from cannabis.

FDA appreciates this opportunity to discuss our work in the regulation of cannabis for potential medical uses in the United States, which is a part of FDA's core mission to protect and promote the public health by ensuring the safety, efficacy, and quality of medical products, including drugs. FDA will continue to use its available authorities to ensure that any such new therapies are safe, effective, and manufactured to a high quality, applying the drug development paradigm that continues to provide new medicines that meet these standards for patients. This paradigm, grounded in rigorous scientific research, is essential to determining any appropriate uses of cannabis and its constituents in the treatment of human disease. The drug approval process remains the best way to identify new treatments that are safe and effective for patients and to protect patients from products that are not what they purport to be.

Thank you for your interest in this important topic, and I am happy to answer any questions.

* * *

Ms. ESHOO. Thank you, Doctor.

Now it is a pleasure to recognize Mr. Matthew Strait for his 5 minutes of testimony.

And thank you again for joining us today.

Statement of Matthew J. Strait, Senior Policy Advisor, Diversion Control Division, Drug Enforcement Administration

Mr. STRAIT. Thank you. Chairwoman Eshoo, Ranking Member Burgess, and distinguished members of committee, on behalf of the Administrator Dillon and 9,000 men and women of the Drug Enforcement Administration. I appreciate the invitation to be here today to discuss DEA's regulatory requirements for those who perform research with schedule I controlled substances, including marijuana.

Much like our partners at HHS, the Department of Justice and DEA fully support research into the effects of marijuana and the potential medical utility of its component. The procedures for evaluating an application for registration by statute is an interagency process. At HHS, the Food and Drug Administration conducts a review of the qualifications and competency of the researcher as well the merits of the scientific protocol. The DEA is charged with ensuring that adequate steps are in place to safeguard against diversion. These procedures have been in place for several decades, and in my 20 years, there has not been a single incident in which a researcher who has put forth a valid research protocol and has implemented safeguards to prevent diversion has been denied.

Given the public interest in marijuana research, DEA has taken a number of proactive steps to do its part in improving research with marijuana. First, in December 2015, DEA executed a change intended to ease the requirements to modify existing registrations in order to conduct research with cannabidiol or CBD, which at the time was being investigated for use in children with certain epilepsy disorders. I believe this action ultimately contributed to the 2018 approval of Epidiolex.

Second, in August 2016, the Department of Justice and DEA took steps to increase the number of entities registered under the Controlled Substances Act to grow marijuana to supply researchers. To ensure that this program is consistent with applicable laws and treaties, the Department, in consultation with other Federal agencies, continues to be engaged in a policy review process. In August 2019, DEA published a list of the 33 entities who have applied for registration and whose applications remain pending to grow marijuana pursuant to that policy. A forthcoming proposed rule, which has been drafted and submitted to the Office of Management and Budget, remains under development at this time.

Third, in February 2018, DEA announced its development of and implementation of an online portal for researchers to safely and securely submit their research protocol, curriculum vitae, and institutional approval, materials required by DEA regulations to be submitted for FDA and DEA review. This online portal has streamlined the process and improved the amount of time for obtaining a schedule I research registration. Presently the average time it takes to approve a new application is 52 days, while the time required to modify an existing registration is far less.

Finally, two months ago, DEA increased the aggregate production quota for marijuana to 3,200 kilograms. The increase was based on a close collaboration with NIDA, who provides high-quality marijuana to NIH and non-NIH-funded researchers. The 2020 quota represents a 575-percent increase for marijuana since 2017.

I believe these efforts are working. Today DEA has 829 active researchers; 70 percent of those researchers, 605 in total, are performing research with marijuana or its constituent parts, making it far and away the most researched schedule I controlled substance in the United States.

Despite these efforts and our successes the multistep process for approving research with schedule I controlled substances is perceived as onerous by some of the research community. Unfortunately, this perception has translated into a false narrative that DEA does not support research. I am here today to tell you that this is simply not true. This belief has hampered efforts to pass practical commonsense legislation aimed at addressing the more than 30,000 overdose deaths in the United States from fentanyl and fentanyl-related substances. In just 23 days, DEA's temporary scheduling action which placed schedule I controls on substances chemically similar to fentanyl will expire unless Congress acts. DEA and the Department of Justice have worked with HHS and ONDCP to put forth a proposal that addresses this public health emergency while improving access for research. On behalf of the Department of Justice, I urge the committee to take up this important legislation.

In conclusion, DEA is fully committed to supporting research for schedule I controlled substance. We will continue to work with our partners within the administration to find commonsense approaches to improve and enhance research of marijuana.

Thank you and I look forward to your questions.

[The prepared statement of Mr. Strait follows:]

Prepared Statement of the U.S. Department of Justice, Matthew J. Strait

Chairman Eshoo, Ranking Member Burgess, and distinguished members of the Subcommittee, as the Senior Policy Advisor of the Diversion Control Division, Drug Enforcement Administration (DEA), within the Department of Justice (Department), I am integrally involved in the Department's efforts to expand access to research with controlled substances. The Diversion Control Division is charged with the responsibility to prevent, detect, and investigate the diversion of controlled pharmaceuticals and listed chemicals from legitimate sources while ensuring an adequate and uninterrupted supply for legitimate medical, commercial, and scientific needs. I appreciate the opportunity to share with you an update on the actions that DEA has taken as well as those that are intended to be undertaken in the near future with the goal of improving access to marijuana to meet the research needs of the United States.

Much like our partners at the Department of Health and Human Services (HHS), the Department and DEA fully support research into the effects of marijuana and the potential medical utility of its chemical constituents. In the last few years, the Department and DEA, in close collaboration with HHS and the Office of National Drug Control Policy (ONDCP), have made great strides in improving research with marijuana and its constituent parts. For example:

- In December 2015, DEA announced to all existing schedule I researchers that it was easing the requirements for obtaining a modification of their existing registration for those who wished to conduct research with cannabidiol (CBD), an effort directly aimed at improving research on the substance which ultimately contributed to the subsequent approval by Food and Drug Administration (FDA) of Epidiolex for use in the treatment of certain childhood epilepsy syndromes.[53]

- In early 2018, DEA announced that it had developed and implemented an online portal for researchers to safely and securely submit their qualifications, research protocol and institutional approvals for a proposed schedule I research registration thereby streamlining the acquisition of information necessary to process each application. Presently, the average time it takes for DEA and the FDA to review/approve an application is 52 days.
- Between 2017 and 2020, DEA increased the aggregate production quota[54] for marijuana by 575 percent from 472 kg in 2017 to 3,200 kg in 2020. The increase has directly supported the National Institute on Drug Abuse's (NIDA) provision of various strains of marijuana to researchers in the United States.
- Over the last 5 years, there has been a 155 percent increase in the number of active researchers registered with DEA to conduct research with marijuana, marijuana extracts and marijuana derivatives (from 237 in November 2014 to 605 in October 2019).
- At present, more research is conducted on marijuana, marijuana extracts, and marijuana derivatives than any other Schedule I substance in the United States. More than 70 percent of DEA's total Schedule I research registrant population (605 of 829 as of December 2019) conducts research on these substances.

As detailed below, to further expand medical and scientific research, the Department and DEA are taking a number of actions to increase the number of registered marijuana manufacturers (or growers), consistent with applicable law, to meet a demonstrated need for different varieties.

The Controlled Substances Act and Marijuana

Under the Controlled Substances Act (CSA), every controlled substance is classified into one of five schedules based upon its potential for abuse, its

---

[53] See https://www.fda.gov/news-events/press-announcements/fda-approves-first-drug-comprised-active-ingredient-derived-marijuanamarihuana-treat-rare-severe-forms.

[54] The "aggregate production quota" for schedule I and II controlled substances.

currently accepted medical use in treatment in the United States, and the degree of dependence the drug or other substance may cause. 21 U.S.C. § 812. The initial schedules of controlled substances established by Congress are found at 21 U.S.C. § 812(c), and the current list of all scheduled substances is published at 21 CFR part 1308. Substances in Schedule I are those that have a high potential for abuse, no currently accepted medical use in treatment in the United States, and a lack of accepted safety for use under medical supervision. 21 U.S.C. § 812(b)(1).

Congress specifically placed "marijuana" in Schedule I of the CSA in 1970[55] and defined "marijuana" as all parts of the plant Cannabis sativa L., with certain exceptions for the parts of the plant that are not the source of cannabinoids. Among the parts of the cannabis plant included in the definition of marijuana are: the flowering tops, the leaves, viable seeds, and the resin extracted from any part of the plant, and every compound, manufacture, salt, derivative, mixture, or preparation of the plant, its seeds or resin. 21 U.S.C. § 812(c) Schedule I; 21 U.S.C. § 802(16); 21 C.F.R. § 1308.11(d).

The Agriculture Improvement Act of 2018 (Pub.L. 115-334, referred to as the AIA) was signed into law on December 20, 2018. It provided a new statutory definition of "hemp" and amended the definition of "marijuana" under the CSA. The AIA modified the definition by adding that the "term 'marijuana' does not include hemp, as defined in section 1639*o* of Title 7." 21 U.S.C. § 802(16)(B). Furthermore, the AIA added a definition of "hemp" to 7 U.S.C. 1639o, which reads as follows:

> The term "hemp" means the plant Cannabis sativa L. and any part of the plant including the seeds thereof and all derivatives, extracts, cannabinoids, isomers, acids, salts, and salts of isomers, whether growing or not, with a deltat-9-tetrahydrocannabinol concentration of not more than 0.3% on a dry weight basis.

The CSA and the Federal Food, Drug, and Cosmetic Act (FDCA) contain provisions that are specifically designed to allow for both clinical research with, and treatment uses of, investigational drugs containing controlled substances, provided certain steps are taken to protect the rights, safety, and welfare of human subjects. The FDA drug approval process, as established and modified by Congress, ensures that safe and effective new medicines are

---

[55] Controlled Substances Act, Section 100 of the Comprehensive Drug Abuse Prevention and Control Act of 1970, Pub.L. 91-513 Oct. 27, 1970.

available as soon as possible for the largest numbers of patients; DEA and the Department stand committed to assist our federal partners in this process.

Current Statutory Framework Governing the Registration of Certain Individuals Handling Marijuana under the CSA

Under the CSA, DEA is responsible for registering growers who can produce an adequate and uninterrupted supply of marijuana under adequately competitive conditions for such research.[56] The University of Mississippi (UMiss) has, for several decades, applied for and received a registration from DEA to grow marijuana. This work is performed pursuant to a contractual agreement with NIDA for the production of research-grade marijuana for federally-approved research.[57] Presently, there are no other DEA-registered bulk manufacturers of marijuana authorized to cultivate marijuana for research purposes. The DEA is actively taking steps to expand the program, which should result in additional registered growers and a larger, more diverse variety of marijuana for research.

The CSA requires all individuals who wish to perform research with marijuana to register with DEA. In those instances, DEA's role is to ensure that proper safeguards are in place to prevent diversion (e.g., security and recordkeeping), while HHS (delegated to FDA) is charged with determining the qualifications and competency of the researcher as well as reviewing the merits of the protocol.[58] Those who wish to perform research with marijuana (or any schedule I controlled substance) must submit certain information to assist DEA and HHS with their respective roles:

1) Information about the Investigator – name, address, curriculum vitae and institutional affiliation
2) Information about the Research Project – Purpose, description of the research (i.e., protocol), the location for the research and security
3) Authority – Document approval by the research institution

Importantly, the applicant also provides information about the name of the substance under investigation, the amount required and the proposed source of supply.[59] With regard to this provision, DEA and HHS work in concert to

---

[56] 21 U.S.C. 823(a)(1). https://www.deadiversion.usdoj.gov/21cfr/21usc/823.htm.

[57] NIDA has established procedures governing the process for providing marijuana to non-federally approved researchers as well.

[58] 21 U.S.C. 823(f). https://www.deadiversion.usdoj.gov/21cfr/21usc/823.htm.

[59] 21 CFR 1301.18.

ensure that the source of the schedule I controlled substance is from a DEA registrant to ensure that the substance was produced in accordance with state, federal, and international law. Furthermore, as coincident activity a DEA registered schedule I researcher, may import marijuana for research purposes so long as the activity is consistent with their protocol and from a legitimate source as authorized through the regulated importation process.

DEA has never denied an application to conduct bona fide research with marijuana from a researcher who has received a favorable recommendation from HHS. As of December 12, 2019, there were 605 DEA-registered schedule I researchers authorized to conduct research with marijuana, marijuana extracts and/or tetrahydrocannabinols in the United States.

DEA's August 2016 Policy Statement and Subsequent Efforts to Expand the Number of Registrants to Grow Marijuana

In August 2016, after consultations with both FDA and NIDA, and following the denial of two petitions from former Governors to reschedule marijuana,[60] DEA published a policy statement in the Federal Register (81 FR 53846) ("2016 Policy Statement"). The 2016 Policy Statement addressed applications by persons seeking to become registered under the CSA to grow marijuana (i.e., manufacture) in order to supply DEA-registered researchers in the United States for bona fide research.

Since publication of the 2016 Policy Statement, the Department of Justice has subsequently engaged in a review of the Policy Statement and the proposed changes, and determined that adjustments to DEA's policies and procedures may be necessary under applicable U.S. law to be consistent with certain treaty functions. As DEA explained in its August 2019 letter to each of the then-33 pending applicants who sought authority to grow marijuana, given that the size of the applicant pool is unprecedented in DEA's experience, the agency has determined that adjustments to its policies and practices with respect to the marijuana growers program are necessary to fairly evaluate the applicants under the factors outlined in 21 U.S.C. 823(a), including 823(a)(1), which requires that DEA "limit the … bulk manufacture of [Schedule I and II] controlled substances to a number of establishments which can produce an adequate and uninterrupted supply of these substances under adequately

[60] 81 FR 53687.

competitive conditions for legitimate medical, scientific, research and industrial purposes."

In addition, since publication of the 2016 Policy Statement, the Department of Justice, in consultation with other federal agencies, has been engaged in a policy review process to ensure that the marijuana growers program is consistent with applicable laws and treaties. That review process remains ongoing; however, had progressed to the point where DEA was able to issue a notice of applications on August 27, 2019, (84 FR 44920).

In August 2019, DEA acknowledged that the as a result of the AIA, some who applied for a registration pursuant to the 2016 Policy Statement for the purpose of growing cannabis that contains no more than 0.3 percent delta-9-tetrahydrocannabinols on a dry weight basis, including cannabis that contains cannabidiol and falls below the delta-9-tetrahydrocannabinol threshold, no longer need to register for the DEA for that purpose. Accordingly, those applicants were allowed to withdraw their application and were eligible to receive a refund from DEA for fees paid at the time of their application.

In the near future, DEA intends to propose regulations that would govern persons seeking to become registered with DEA to grow marijuana as bulk manufacturers, consistent with applicable law, taking into account recent changes in the Controlled Substances Act. At present, a notice of proposed rulemaking is under review by the Office of Management and Budget.

Throughout this process, DEA and the Department remain committed to supporting research opportunities and these advancements are in effort to register more marijuana manufacturers, and expand the amount and type of marijuana grown for research purposes.

Conclusion

The Diversion Control Division within DEA is charged with preventing the diversion of legitimate sourced controlled substances while ensuring an adequate and uninterrupted supply for legitimate medical, commercial, and scientific needs. We are steadfast in our effort to fulfill that mission, and to work with our partners to improve this process.

DEA is committed, consistent with the CSA, to assisting the health care needs of patients and supporting research involving marijuana. DEA shares the view that medical decisions should be based on science and adherence to the established drug approval process which ensures that only safe and effective drugs are approved to be available in the United States. DEA continues to make the approval of schedule I researchers a top priority and we look forward to continuing our efforts with our interagency partners to expand research efforts for all controlled substances, including marijuana.

Thank you for the opportunity to testify today and we look forward to continuing to work with Congress on this important topic.

* * *

Ms. ESHOO. Thank you, Mr. Strait. Now we have concluded not only the opening statements of members but the testimony of the witnesses. We are going to move to members' questions now, and I recognize myself for 5 minutes.

I would like to ask a few foundational questions of the panel, and I think that the following can be answered with a simple yes or no. Is more medical research needed on the therapeutic effects and the health consequences of cannabis?

Dr. VOLKOW. Yes.

Dr. THROCKMORTON. Yes.

Mr. STRAIT. Yes.

Ms. ESHOO. Is the cannabis from the University of Mississippi, which is the only approved cannabis for Federal research, adequate for medical research?

Dr. VOLKOW. No.

Dr. THROCKMORTON. No.

Mr. STRAIT. We would like additional sources, but we also recognize that importation is allowed in certain circumstances.

Ms. ESHOO. Should legitimate researchers be able to access a wider array of cannabis products for their research?

Dr. VOLKOW. Yes.

Dr. THROCKMORTON. It would help drug development.

Mr. STRAIT. Yes.

Ms. ESHOO. Have there been, in your view, real-life consequences to researchers not being able to conduct research on a variety of cannabis products?

Dr. VOLKOW. Yes.

Dr. THROCKMORTON. Product development has been slow.

Ms. ESHOO. So there has been an effect because of that.

Dr. THROCKMORTON. Uh-huh.

Mr. STRAIT. I don't disagree with what my colleagues have said.

Dr. VOLKOW. I know one point that we haven't discussed enough, which has been hindered, is our ability to actually recognize when drugs may be particularly harmful. So that is another aspect of the limitations.

Ms. ESHOO. The main reason cannabis research is restricted is because cannabis is listed as a schedule I drug. Yet two active compounds in cannabis, THC and CBD, are both approved ingredients for drugs that are scheduled as schedule III and schedule V respectively. So how can cannabis be schedule I and considered to have no accepted medical use because that is part of the schedule I, but both of its major active ingredients can be considered to have medical use?

Dr. VOLKOW. I defer to my colleagues at the FDA for answering that.

Dr. THROCKMORTON. Separately those two compounds are safe and effective for intended uses and so meet the statutory standard for accepted medical use.

Ms. ESHOO. How do you pull them out and separate them?

Dr. THROCKMORTON. That is what the drug development process is meant to encourage. It is to have people——

Ms. ESHOO. So, if FDA decides to pull those out to be applied to and used and be part of a certain drug, you just automatically vanish—schedule I vanishes as a result of that?

Dr. THROCKMORTON. When Congress defined what the schedules were to be, they said that there were tests to be applied for whether you had accepted medical use. There are five that we would be happy to talk in greater detail offline. When you apply those tests to marijuana, at least when the FDA and NIDA have applied those tests to marijuana three times in the recent 20 years or so, our conclusion, our recommendation to the DEA is that it did not meet the test for accepted medical use. It mostly has to do with whether you have identified a therapeutic value for the product and whether you can describe it.

Ms. ESHOO. It is more the trigger than anything else.

Dr. THROCKMORTON. Yes.

Ms. ESHOO. To Dr. Throckmorton, does the FDA have all the authorities it needs to regulate CBD products for consumer safety?

Dr. THROCKMORTON. I believe we do. When I talk to drug——

Ms. ESHOO. Are you sure?

Dr. THROCKMORTON. When I talk to drug developers that come in and talk to me and they say, "We are interested in studying a compound found in cannabis," whether it is CBD or it is one of the other 80 cannabinoids or the terpenes or whatever else, I say: If you can get me a legal source for that compound, a legal source for that compound, I am going to treat you exactly the same way I would treat any other drug in development.

Ms. ESHOO. OK.

Dr. THROCKMORTON. Except I am going to give you some additional resources in the forms of——

Ms. ESHOO. I still have more questions. Now, the FDA has estimated that it will take three to five years to complete rulemaking in relation to CBD products. Is this still accurate?

Dr. THROCKMORTON. We understand the——

Ms. ESHOO. Is it?

Dr. THROCKMORTON. It is unfortunately not a yes-or-no question, ma'am. We know that there is interest in moving quickly. We understand that three to five years is longer than people would like. We are looking——

Ms. ESHOO. What is the estimate today?

Dr. THROCKMORTON. We are looking at a full range of options. We are interested——

Ms. ESHOO. You don't want to tell me. It seems to me that maybe three to five is still in place, but you don't want to say.

In your testimony, you said the FDA knows of CBD products that may not contain the amount of CBD indicated on the label or may contain other potentially dangerous compounds. Has the FDA issued any labeling requirements for CBD? My time is—you may answer.

Dr. THROCKMORTON. The labeling requirements would be imposed on the approved drugs, Epidiolex. That product is well manufactured, possesses—we have no concerns like that that I am aware of. The products that the warning letters are subject to that that comment related to are the unapproved products that have been marketed in the States.

Ms. ESHOO. Thank you.

Well, my time has expired, and I recognize the ranking member now for his 5 minutes of questions.

Mr. BURGESS. Thank you, Madam Chair.

And, Dr. Throckmorton, staying with you for just a minute on the Epidiolex question. When I look at my drug discount app, it is like $1,300 a month for a therapeutic course of that. So, if somebody didn't have $1,300, could they just go buy CBD oil and supplant the use of Epidiolex?

Dr. THROCKMORTON. Well, we always recommend that you use an approved product for a number of really good reasons. But what we learned when we did that sampling of unapproved products is that we don't know what will be in that oil if you choose to take it. It may contain things that would be dangerous to you. We also know it is reasonably likely that it could not contain the amount of CBD that you were looking to take for whatever condition.

Mr. BURGESS. Just along the lines of the timeframe that Chairwoman Eshoo asked you about just, for point of reference, when we did the Cures for 21st Century bill, pretty much standard accepted lengths of time in FDA for approval of a new drug was 14 to 16 years, and about a billion and a half dollars. Do I remember that correctly? So three to five years actually sounds like you are moving with great dispatch, would that be a fair statement?

Dr. THROCKMORTON. The three to five years comes from our general experience with rulemaking rather than any specific——

Mr. BURGESS. So it is not a recent——

Dr. THROCKMORTON. It is not related specifically to drug development or product development. It is just that rulemaking has steps that we have to use.

Mr. BURGESS. We will move forward with the DEA with this. Has DEA ever done an administrative change in a scheduled drug without being prompted by Congress?

Mr. STRAIT. Oh, absolutely, yes. We initiate scheduling actions with some frequency. It could come through a petition received from a public citizen. It could come as a direct result of an approval of a new drug, a new molecular——

Mr. BURGESS. Would that not come through the FDA, though?

Mr. STRAIT. Yes. In that circumstance, yes.

Mr. BURGESS. So you couldn't just do that de novo and say, "We are going to change the schedule of this medication on an administrative basis"?

Mr. STRAIT. The agency retains the ability to initiate its own proposal as well. In that instance, we would put together——

Mr. BURGESS. Initiate, but you can't complete it without input from the FDA.

Mr. STRAIT. No. As you say in your opening remarks quite correctly that we are tethered to the science that we are given by our colleagues over at HHS.

Mr. BURGESS. Yes, I don't know if that is inappropriate; being tethered to science can be a good thing.

Dr. Volkow, you actually mentioned in your written testimony about the risk of addiction with cannabis products. Presumably you are talking about marijuana. That is a thing? That is a real thing?

Dr. VOLKOW. It is a real thing, and it is THC, the active ingredient responsible for the addictiveness of marijuana. And the plants contain higher and higher content of THC.

Mr. BURGESS. So is marijuana a gateway drug? Some people call it that. Is that a fair statement?

Dr. VOLKOW. It decreases the likelihood that you are sensitive to the addictive effects of other drugs, and that is why it has coined the term of "gateway drug"; it makes you more sensitive.

Dr. BURGESS. So yesterday we spent a full hearing in Oversight and Investigations on the scourge of opiate addiction. We do worry that, if we go too far in one direction or another, that ten years from now, we will be having a hearing on perhaps we have gone too far with what we did with liberalizing marijuana laws. But let me just ask you this: You also mentioned the National Highway Traffic Safety Administration, and the effects of driving under the influence. Our traffic laws and our state partners, have they kept up with all of the changes in marijuana policy that have occurred across the country?

Dr. VOLKOW. No. One of the major challenges in doing so is that it is very difficult to quantify whether someone is intoxicated with marijuana or not. With alcohol, you actually measure the alcohol content in plasma, but that measure does not guarantee for marijuana that you are under the influence of the drug or not. So you can have very high levels from having taken it three days ago in a regular user. So that has been a major challenge.

Mr. BURGESS. So you can't really quantitate to the degree of behavioral disruption that may occur.

Dr. VOLKOW. That has been much harder to do.

Mr. BURGESS. And as a consequence for our law enforcement partners and our partners at the State that are writing State traffic laws, that becomes a difficulty. Is that correct?

Dr. VOLKOW. Correct. And that is an area that we are trying to bring up new strategies to identify intoxication with marijuana from NIDA.

Mr. BURGESS. As a practical matter, that actually happened in my district: A pedestrian who was struck by an automobile, the driver of the automobile had under the 0.08 limit in their blood alcohol, but they also had a positive quantitative test for THC. That individual was no billed by the grand jury. I don't know whether that was right or wrong, but it seems to me that the potential for the additive effects should be something that law enforcement would bear in mind when deciding whether or not to bring a case like that. It was clearly a very tragic situation, young high school athlete who got hit. So it was a high-profile case in the community and something I will never forget.

Thank you, Madam Chair. I yield back.

Ms. ESHOO. The gentleman yields back.

It is a pleasure to recognize the gentlewoman from California, Ms. Matsui, for her 5 minutes of questions.

Ms. MATSUI. Thank you very much, Madam Chair.

And I really appreciate the hearing we are having today. This issue really needs to be examined.

And thank you very much for the witnesses for being here today. At the University of California, researchers are doing important work to study the health effects, public safety, and environmental impacts of marijuana. I would like to discuss how our existing Federal regulations may be limiting researchers from fully understanding cannabis' potential risks and benefits.

Now despite the fact that cannabis is being cultivated right in California to sell at local dispensaries, under current law, UC researchers must obtain their study samples through the NIDA contracted site in Mississippi. In order to study what the public is purchasing in dispensaries, UC researchers have applied for a license to cultivate cannabis locally. However, these researchers have not heard back from the DOJ and DEA as to the status of their applications.

Mr. Strait, where is the Department of Justice in its process of granting or denying applications some researchers have put forth at a university to study to cultivate cannabis at a university?

Mr. STRAIT. As I said in my opening, we certainly support all research endeavors.

One of the challenges we see that often leads to this misperception about delays on the DEA side is we look for a complete application before we forward that application to our colleagues at the Department of Health and Human Services. So there are three things that we need: We need a protocol, which most researchers if they are federally funded or even State funded have; a CV for the researcher, which every researcher certainly has; but sometimes the delay is the result of the third piece, which is that institutional review approval. Sometimes, for purposes of timing, the researchers will submit an application, knowing that their state university or their state system, their university has not met to review their application.

Ms. MATSUI. Well, I now the University of California, I think they pretty good about doing this. And so we would like to be able to expedite as much as possible because their research is going to be very important as far as all of this.

From the researcher's perspective I understand there is some ambiguity around the ability to conduct research with synthetic CBD for potential applications in humans. For the panel, what is your agency's position on the current status of CBD? Is there a distinction between marijuana-derived CBD and hemp or synthetically derived CBD when it comes to regulating these products? Dr. Volkow?

Dr. VOLKOW. From our perspective, we are interested in understanding what are the effects of the chemical compound that goes by the name of CBD. With respect to actually its pharmacological actions, but the potential of negative effects and the potential of therapeutic actions. So, for all, the molecule is the one that is of interest. At the same time, though, we are doing research to try to investigate how, when it is mixed with other cannabinoids, that may influence its effects.

Ms. MATSUI. OK.

Dr. Throckmorton, do you agree?

Dr. THROCKMORTON. Yes. One of the things that happened in the results of the farm bill was that cannabidiol was removed from oversight from the Controlled Substances Act. In some sense that allows us to encourage its conduct—studies and things using it without interacting——

Ms. MATSUI. It opens it up.

Dr. THROCKMORTON [continuing]. With DEA. We believe that is a powerful, potentially powerful, in terms of getting new studies done.

Ms. MATSUI. Great. Mr. Strait?

Mr. STRAIT. Yes, and Dr. Throckmorton is 100 percent correct. I think the passage of the farm bill created a little bit of a question mark as to the legal status of synthetic CBD versus that derived from natural sources. Very clearly that which is derived from natural sources, if it contains less than 0.3 percent THC, it is no longer controlled under the CSA.

Ms. MATSUI. Dr. Throckmorton, if a researcher wants to conduct clinical cannabis research that may lead to a new drug, what requirements need to be fulfilled with the FDA?

Dr. THROCKMORTON. When you say "cannabis," are you talking about farm-bill-compliant low-THC cannabis? It is important, when we talk to investigators, we think about it in sort of two tracks, an arrow going one way, and arrow——

Ms. MATSUI. Right. Right. Right.

Dr. THROCKMORTON. One arrow, the farm-bill-compliant cannabidiol and other compounds extracted from hemp, we view as subject to the Food, Drug, and Cosmetics Act. They are able to be used for investigational use. Come in and talk to us; we will treat you as any other drug substance for study.

If it is high-THC cannabis, then that still applies, but in addition, we would want to make certain that they work with the DEA because there are other requirements under those circumstances.

Ms. MATSUI. OK. Fine. Thank you, and I have gone over my time.

I yield back.

Ms. ESHOO. The gentleman yields back.

Mr. Strait, would you respond after you get back to your agency with Congresswoman Matsui on University of California's application, please?

Mr. STRAIT. Absolutely.

Ms. ESHOO. This is the greatest public university in the world. They know how to do applications. They know how to do applications. Well, it is causing a ruckus, but I will stand——

Mr. UPTON. You do not have any right to object.

Ms. ESHOO. I will stand with my statement representing the greatest private university in the world, Stanford.

It is now a pleasure to recognize the gentleman from Michigan, Mr. Upton, for his 5 minutes of questions.

Mr. UPTON. You are just lucky Pete Olson is not here this morning, but I do not have my jersey on.

Thank you, Madam Chair, for this hearing. I do have a couple of questions.

Dr. Throckmorton, you mentioned that Epidiolex is one of the three drugs that have been approved, and two others in addition to that. What are the illnesses or conditions that they were approved for?

Dr. THROCKMORTON. Right. So Epidiolex is approved for two genetic seizure disorders, severe seizure disorders in children, and that contains cannabidiol.

Mr. UPTON. Is it injected? Is it oral? Is it shot? Is it——

Dr. THROCKMORTON. It is oral.

Mr. UPTON. Oral?

Dr. THROCKMORTON. It is given in an oil form. It is fat soluble, and so it is a syringe basically.

The other compounds are all synthetic. They are not extracted from the cannabis plant, and they are approved for wasting diseases. There are nausea and vomiting associated with chemotherapeutics. We can get you a full list of those, but it is more general. Those compounds contain THC. So they have a different active ingredient than the Epidiolex does.

Mr. UPTON. So Greg Walden talked about something. As consumers, 33 States now have approved medical uses. Eleven States—Michigan is one—

that is both medical as well as recreational, or adult use. And I guess consumers are very interested in, you know, how much is in here? I mean, we know, when we drink a beer, different alcohol content, whether it is a craft beer, you know, maybe a State like—that has a smaller threshold like Utah.

But, in addition, you have got the law enforcement issues. I was with one of my sheriffs last week. He, unfortunately, had—we had a situation like Dr. Burgess had in his district with a student returning back to Michigan State, and, sadly, he was involved in a terrible auto accident, and, in fact, afterwards, they—he survived, but they found out that he was—had a high level of THC, as I understand it.

Where are we in terms of some visible standards or some review that folks can look at as it relates to the cookies or the brownies or whatever it is, the cereal that they are going to eat and consume as relates to perhaps the safety of that, and where are we as relates to law enforcement who, as—you know, it is not like the breathalyzer. They have got to do a variety of different cognitive exercises to try and determine whether or not that individual has taken too much, and it is a blood sample, but where are we in terms of trying to help the consumer know the right information if they choose to take, in these States, a legal substance?

Dr. VOLKOW. I can speak on the research perspective. We are interested in understanding what content of THC is associated with specific pharmacological effects, including side effects, and so research has been done to show that, if you consume anywhere between two and eight milligrams, you are going to get high, but, in general, you do not have any adverse effects.

So what we would like to be able to do from the research perspective is to create a unit of marijuana that can be utilized consistently across research to help us understand how exposures of different content THC——

Mr. UPTON. And how long—when is that research going to be completed?

Dr. VOLKOW. The research on doses has been done. The research on creating a unit of THC that can be used consistently is something that we are working on to try to consolidate and get a perspective of what are the differences on the consumption by people——

Mr. UPTON. Are we a year out? How long do you think that will take? What is——

Dr. VOLKOW. I would hope that we will be able to implement the standard dose for research purposes within one year, but that is very different from implementing a unit dose for legal—for products that are not legally accepted federally, and that is the States are trying to come themselves with standard doses, and you mentioned it for the cookies, or—but that varies also between the States.

Mr. UPTON. Yes. Anybody else have a comment?

Dr. THROCKMORTON. I do, Mr. Upton. You raised an incredibly important point that is important to understand about the development of nondrug products containing things like CBD. So, as the FDA thinks about how to develop those products, one thing we remember is that there would be requirements on a product that we approved regarding accurate labeling, regarding dosing.

So, for instance, the cookie that we are discussing, if that packaging was approved, if we found a pathway that enabled us to allow CBD in a cookie, along with that packaging would come labeling that would say it contains ten milligrams or a hundred milligrams or whatever else; could include other conditions of use that could help understand when it would appropriately be used and things like that. So part and parcel with the work we are doing is to think about the consequences, the important consequences, which would include that kind of labeling improvement. We would have more understanding. People would have a better understanding. They would also have more assurance that the product actually contained the CBD——

Mr. UPTON. I know my time has expired, but just a "yes" or "no." Do you have authority for that labeling now?

Dr. THROCKMORTON. It is—absolutely, we have that authority.

What we need is to determine the pathways to take——

Mr. UPTON. Right.

Dr. THROCKMORTON [continuing]. For those nondrug-containing CBD products.

Mr. UPTON. I yield back.

Ms. ESHOO. The gentleman yields back.

It is a pleasure to recognize the Chairman of the full committee, Mr. Pallone, for his 5 minutes of questions.

The CHAIRMAN. Thank you, Chairwoman Eshoo.

As I said in my opening statement, the cannabis policy landscape is evolving across the States and territories. Yet, at the Federal level, the policy has remained largely the same, and one issue that researchers across the Nation have raised with the committee is the fact that they are not able to conduct research on cannabis products available through State cannabis dispensaries.

Dr. Volkow notes in her testimony that the cannabis available in States to consumers is much more potent than what has been available in the past, and that means that Federal researchers cannot adequately study the health potential or adverse health consequences of products that are more readily available.

So this poses a legitimate public health challenge as it impedes the ability for researchers to truly understand the impact of products regularly used by consumers and prevents us from advancing sound science.

So, Dr. Volkow, you noted in your testimony that having only a single domestic source of research of cannabis limits the diversity of products and formulations available to researchers and slows the development of cannabis-based medications, so let me ask, yes or no, Dr. Volkow, do you believe Federal researchers should have access to cannabis has State-authorized dispensaries?

Dr. VOLKOW. Yes.

The CHAIRMAN. And, Dr. Throckmorton, yes or no, would access to cannabis outside of the University of Mississippi be beneficial to drug developers in the U.S.?

Dr. THROCKMORTON. Yes.

The CHAIRMAN. And, Mr. Strait, as you mentioned in your testimony, DEA is actively working to consider applications for additional cannabis growers. What is the status—this is not yes or no— what is the status of this effort, and when can we expect that the agencies would finalize rulemaking?

Mr. STRAIT. So we actually have a draft regulation in place. In August of 2019, we were able to get to the point of our policy review process where we were able to publicly acknowledge, consistent with our regulations, who our pending applicants were as of August 27th, 2019.

We know that we have to probably do notice-and-comment rulemaking to implement regulations on two matters. One is how we are going to evaluate all of our pending applications; and then, two, what additional types of regulations might need to be in place in order to—you know, in order to impose on those that would grow. So that regulation is in a draft form. I cannot talk too much about it, but rest assured we have submitted it to OMB. It has been drafted, and, tomorrow, many of us will be getting on a call to talk through it.

The CHAIRMAN. All right. Thank you.

I want to switch to CBD. A Google search can lead any consumer to Web sites that offer CBD-infused gummies, cereal cookie. This is in addition to personal care products and dietary supplements. One recent estimate by an independent company suggested that the CBD market can bring in as much as $15 billion by 2025.

So, Dr. Throckmorton, I understand your agency is working to regulate CBD products. However, FDA has suggested that it could take three to five years before rulemaking to clarify the regulatory pathway work to be completed.

Can you explain to the committee the scientific and regulatory activities the agency believes are needed to ensure the safety of CBD in other products, such as food and dietary supplements?

Dr. THROCKMORTON. Sure. And I want to start by saying that three to five years was an estimate, that we understand the importance that people have in identifying in a rapid process to a pathway for nondrug CBD products.

Having said that, rulemaking is the one pathway that is identified in statute for an exception to the prohibition against the use of drug substances in foods and dietary supplements. So that prohibition, as I just—you know, as I mentioned in my opening remarks, exists, and, for the agency to change, we need to find a mechanism to allow a path forward for nondrug CBD products to be developed.

We are in the process of doing that. Rulemaking is one thing that is under consideration. As has been mentioned, there are a number of legislative ideas that people have had. We have had other meetings where people have raised other suggestions regarding this as well.

Bottom line is we get it. Bottom line is we understand that we need to identify a path as quickly as we can, but we need to be grounded in science. You mentioned yourself—many of us have mentioned—fundamentally, there are many unknowns about cannabidiol. There are things that we know that it can do, adverse effects that I mentioned in my testimony related to liver jury, related to potential male reproductive injury that we need to know more about.

We need to know more about its uses in vulnerable populations and for long periods of time because, if it is placed in a nondrug product, there will be no learned intermedia. There will not be a doctor or a nurse or anyone that will talk to the patient or to help them make their choices about the use of that product.

You could get up in the morning, take your CBD—to get started—in your coffee, take another dose of CBD for lunch when you have your sandwich, and then end in the late afternoon with an alcoholic beverage containing CBD; and the aggregate amounts of CBD then matter. We need to decide how to do that safely.

Our fundamental focus for foods and dietary supplements is safety, and we need to have more data than we do available at present in order to make that determination, in order to help inform what the right, best steps are.

The CHAIRMAN. All right. Thank you.

Thank you, Madam Chair.

Ms. ESHOO. And, in the appropriations bill that was passed last year, there were moneys that go directly to FDA to move up the work on CBD, correct?

Dr. THROCKMORTON. That is correct.

Ms. ESHOO. Yes. All right.

Dr. THROCKMORTON. And focused, I believe, in the——

Ms. ESHOO. Yes.

Dr. THROCKMORTON [continuing]. Nondrug space——

Ms. ESHOO. Yes. So you have the money, and now you have got to get it going.

It is a pleasure to recognize Mr. Guthrie for his 5 minutes of questioning, the gentleman from Kentucky.

Mr. GUTHRIE. Thank you very much. Thank you for being here.

And, Dr. Volkow, we have heard that it can take up to a year to get a schedule I registration. That process of adding new cannabinoids to an existing registration, and getting approval for protocol modifications is time consuming, and how does the DEA registration processes for modifying a schedule I registration to conduct research of cannabis impact ability to do research? But I also understand, Mr. Strait, you said—oh, actually, I wanted to ask you something first, if that is OK.

Mr. STRAIT. Sure.

Mr. GUTHRIE. Before I get to answer your questions, last October, myself and others sent a letter asking about the implementation and recommendations included in the committee staff report on the opioid distribution. To date, we have not received DEA's response, and I would ask that, after the hearing, that we follow up together to see if we can get DEA's responses to that report.

Mr. STRAIT. I would be happy to follow up with that.

Mr. GUTHRIE. OK. Thank you. So, getting to my other question, just the time-consuming process in ability to do research, and I do believe, Mr. Strait, you said it was like 52 days to get a registration, and it seems like we are hearing different than that. Can both of you, both Dr. Volkow, you talk about the time-consuming process for that?

Dr. VOLKOW. Yes. And there are two issues with it. One of them has to do with the process of how lengthy it is to get an approval to do a human subjects protocol, and, if it is schedule I, that is much longer. And, on average, about 52 days by the DEA actually counts the moment that that protocol has been deemed complete and moves forward, but what we have heard from the researchers is that it is not so straightforward to get the protocol in a way that the DEA can work with it, because it is complex.

And another issue that becomes—makes it harder is that the DEA State local agents interpret the rule differently, and, as a result of that, that further hinders the problem. So those are the issues that we see.

The other aspect where we are also seeing an impact on schedule I is that there are certain scientists that do not even want to go there because they say, "I do not want to go there; it is going to take too much effort to do research on a schedule I," and so we lose potentially-valuable scientists into looking at things that are important.

Mr. GUTHRIE. OK. Mr. Strait, do you have any comment on that, or——

Mr. STRAIT. Yes. Thank you. Thank you for giving me the opportunity.

You know, this is a common refrain we have heard from our partners over at HHS. One of the challenges that they have is that, when we try to get information from them about who the concerns are being raised by, maybe it plays into the fear of DEA, but we are kind of cited with PII, that they cannot disclose information to us, that they are prohibited from doing it. So we struggle to try to understand who the people are that are having these difficulties so that we can give them some special attention, and we are happy to give them that special attention.

The other point I wanted to make is the inconsistent applicability of our DEA regulations across our 23 field divisions or the concerns of that, and, as I mentioned to some staff before we started this call, we are actually getting ready to host a management conference across our entire division from all across the country, and we are going to actually invite Dr. Volkow or her designee to come in and address this because I think that is something that we can solve easily. That is not anything that we need Congress' help on.

Mr. GUTHRIE. OK. Thank you.

And I will yield a minute and a half, my remaining time, to Mr. Griffith.

Mr. GRIFFITH. Thank you very much.

Virginia actually has the oldest medicinal marijuana law on the books. It was passed in 1979 with Chip Woodrum, who is now deceased, as the House patron, and former member of this committee, Rick Boucher, who was then a State senator, as the Senate companion, to say that they would allow the use of medicinal marijuana in the Commonwealth of Virginia. However, the DEA had not allowed it, and so the doctors did not want to risk their license by prescribing it. It required a legitimate prescription. And that is where my bill came from, was that this is what Virginia has stood for, for decades.

In 1998, there was an attempt to repeal it because they thought it was like California's law that just said, you know, "if it makes you feel good, you can try it" kind of thing, which Virginia rejected, but, still, the DEA has not acted. So, when I hear people talking about, you know, "It will take us three to five years; we have to do the research," my question is, why hasn't the research been done?

And, Dr. Throckmorton, I would have to say that it causes me some great concern that apparently the FDA thinks it is OK for opioids and opiates and barbiturates, but somehow marijuana should stay schedule I. That is illogical to me. And so I just—I lay that out.

Marinol, in the case of my two fathers, was available. The problem is they were so sick, they could not swallow it and hold it on their stomachs. That is why their friends were smuggling in—with the doctors turning a blind eye—smuggling in the marijuana so they could smoke it and then eat.

So we need to find a solution, and we should have started working on this back in 1979 or earlier, but we have not done it.

I yield back.

Mr. GUTHRIE. I yield back also.

Ms. ESHOO. The gentleman yields back. Excellent points.

Pleasure to recognize the gentlewoman from Florida, Ms. Castor, for her 5 minutes.

Ms. CASTOR. Well, thank you, Madam Chair, for calling this hearing. Thank you to our witnesses for being here today.

I think it is clear that cannabis research is caught up in conflicting regulations. You cannot remove cannabis from schedule I because it lacks proof for medical and controlled or controlled recreational use, but you can't research to determine if it is safe because it is included on the schedule I.

Dr. Volkow, you ended your testimony by saying that cannabis research is urgently needed, so let's focus on how we can streamline our research process for cannabis and possibly other schedule I substances.

First, what are the requirements and challenges for conducting research on schedule I substances?

Dr. VOLKOW. What I was commenting before, the main difference relates to the fact that you have to get the DEA registration, so that makes the process much more complex than just doing research with any other substance, and that can take time.

Ms. CASTOR. And that clearly deters research——

Dr. VOLKOW. Yes.

Ms. CASTOR [continuing]. On those substances?

Dr. VOLKOW. Correct.

Ms. CASTOR. In thinking about how we reduce those barriers for research with cannabis and possibly other schedule I substances, you did answer to Representative Guthrie—you pointed out a few of the barriers.

What do you recommend should change in the process right now?

Dr. VOLKOW. Well, we have been working among the agencies to come to—to try to come up with a process that will allow it to safeguard the public, but at the same time to facilitate and accelerate research. So those are the two issues that coming up with a category that enables researchers to be able to accelerate the pace at which they are doing research without in any way jeopardizing the public, and that is wherein, again, the DEA, the FDA, and the NIH have been working together.

Ms. CASTOR. There are a number of bills that have been highlighted for the committee's consideration today. Would you point to any of those pieces of legislation that would help streamline the process appropriately?

Dr. VOLKOW. You are putting me in a little difficult position because there are six of them, and we do not legislate; we basically bring science. And what I can tell is that the science tells us that marijuana is a substance that can produce addiction.

Now, we also know from studies that it is likely that there is potential for the therapeutic use of the cannabinoids within marijuana, and, thus, to the extent that we, among the six ones that you are proposing, can accelerate research while protecting the public, then that is what you all have to weigh.

Ms. CASTOR. All right.

Dr. Throckmorton, has FDA seen an uptick or change in the number of applications from researchers to conduct research on hemp or other low-THC cannabis products since these are no longer considered schedule I substances?

Dr. THROCKMORTON. Thank you for that question, and short answer: yes.

Ms. CASTOR. Do you support removing marijuana from the Controlled Substances Act to remove barriers to research?

Dr. THROCKMORTON. At present, my focus is on cannabidiol, and focused on supporting those new INDs, those new investigational studies that we have seen in house.

So your first question is worth going back to for just a moment. We now have almost 40 investigators that have come in to us proposing to use CBD and other substances found in hemp. We believe that represents an important new opportunity for us in terms of investigating CBD and those compounds for drug development, and I want to make sure that we give them every opportunity, every support that we possibly can.

The question about marijuana is more complicated. It has to do with what you mean by "marijuana." Obviously, one street corner sells one kind of marijuana, and another street corner sells a different kind of marijuana. Making a conclusion that both of those marijuanas somehow have medical value is challenging scientifically, and I think Dr. Volkow would agree with me with that, and that is one of the findings that we would be obliged to make were we to try to make a recommendation to the DEA to reschedule marijuana from schedule I. So, from a scientific perspective, there are real challenges to making that conclusion.

We have been asked to look at it three times in the past, and, each time, we have decided, as I had mentioned before, that it was not possible given where we were with the science.

Ms. CASTOR. You know, when it comes to CBD, it is like the cat is already out of the bag. It is amazing, the marketing for CBD. What would you advise the public about the efficacy of the products on the market today? Do they really help? And do we even have a handle on what is truly in all of those products?

Dr. THROCKMORTON. Both questions would be: We don't know. We don't know whether the various claims being made are accurate to the standard that I would expect for a drug product being developed, and we don't know well enough what is found in those products that are being sold under a variety of State initiatives. We need more data in both of those places.

With regards to efficacy, my job is to make sure that those manufacturers, those around 40 that want to study this are able to do that quickly, study what works and study what does not quickly.

With regards to safety, the agency understands that we desperately need to collect all of the available information about the safety of CBD in all of those various uses. That is challenging for us. We have been in the process of a yearlong effort to collect all of those available data. We have identified some gaps. I think I mentioned some in my testimony previously—things we believe we absolutely need to know. We are in the process of figuring out how to close those gaps.

Ms. ESHOO. The gentlewoman's time has expired.

Pleasure to recognize the gentleman from Virginia, Mr. Griffith.

Mr. GRIFFITH. I thank the——

Ms. ESHOO. Looking for another good story here.

Mr. GRIFFITH. Well, I may or may not have one at this point. I have got lots of stories, but we may not have time.

Mr. Strait, I know that you disagreed with the earlier assessment on the University of California, having attended the great university in Blacksburg, Virginia, Virginia Tech, which I am so proud to represent.

That being said, going back to Dr. Burgess' questions, if the FDA recommends that the DEA reschedule a compound, is the DEA required to comply with that rescheduling recommendation?

Mr. STRAIT. If they recommended rescheduling, we are bound to their—the statute actually says that the Attorney General shall be bound by the recommendations of the Secretary as it pertains to scientific and medical matters.

Mr. GRIFFITH. As the Secretary determines?

Mr. STRAIT. Correct.

Mr. GRIFFITH. All right. So you can confirm that the DEA has never refused to reschedule a compound after being given a recommendation to do so by the FDA or the Secretary?

Mr. STRAIT. I am certainly not aware of any instance where that would be the case.

Mr. GRIFFITH. All right. Now, continuing, Mr. Strait, as you know, the U.S. is a party to the United States Single Convention on Narcotic Drugs, which imposes manufacturing and distributing restrictions on marijuana. Some have cited our involvement in that agreement as a potential reason why the Federal Government should not lift restrictions on marijuana.

Regarding American domestic manufacturing of research-grade cannabis, why is it that other countries who have signed the same treaty, such as Canada, Israel, Ireland, New Zealand, Australia, and the Netherlands have several legal manufacturers of research-grade cannabis, and their products are legally imported to the U.S., but the U.S. has only one, the University of Mississippi, as we have heard earlier?

Mr. STRAIT. So you are precisely right; there is a growing number of countries that have implemented laws in their countries that fully effectuate their requirement, their obligations under the Single Convention on Narcotic Drugs. We have, too, and that is the reason why we have the University of Mississippi, or this NIDA drug supply program. What we are trying to do is, as we expand the number of growers, we are trying to take a look at whether or not there are things that need to be changed—altered, I would say; not newly created, but just altered slightly—in order to make sure that we are in compliance with our treaty obligations.

Mr. GRIFFITH. Well, then I hope that you all would work on that quickly. You said earlier applications for research are being approved, but you said regulations and paperwork—and I am paraphrasing—are perceived to be so onerous that people will not do it. Well, connect the dots. The paperwork and the regulations, the perception becomes reality, and, as we have heard from Dr. Volkow, sometimes that becomes a problem, and I think that is why you have not received more applications.

Do you want to say something on that point? And I just have a couple minutes.

Mr. STRAIT. If I may?

Mr. GRIFFITH. Quickly.

Mr. STRAIT. And I am going to be very quick. But I did want to go back to your comment and that of Congresswoman Castor's, which is to say that there is a solution that this interagency group and others worked on all throughout the summer as it relates to some important legislation dealing with the permanent control of fentanyl-related substances in schedule I. We as an administration came out with kind of some commonsense practical solutions to address all of the concerns raised by the research community. We are happy to share that if——

Mr. GRIFFITH. And whatever—and if you could share that, and whatever you can—whatever help you need from us, I think this committee would be willing to help in any way it can.

The DEA's 2016 policy statement said it would be consistent with the 1961 Single Convention on Narcotic Drug Treaty if the DEA were to register research-grade marijuana growers outside of the NIDA contract system so long as the growers agreed to only distribute marijuana with prior written approval from the DEA. However, in your testimony, you said DEA has changed course, saying that, quote, since publication of the 2016 policy statement, the Department of Justice determined that adjustments to the DEA's policies and procedures may be necessary to be consistent with certain treaty functions.

What changes need to be made in order to be consistent with those treaty functions?

Mr. STRAIT. Well, I cannot really get into too many details because, again, it is a deliberative process that we are engaged in right now as we speak with the Office of Management and Budget.

Mr. GRIFFITH. Can you get that to me as quickly as you can?

Mr. STRAIT. I absolutely will.

Mr. GRIFFITH. And I appreciate that. If you would give it to the committee and to me as well, that would be appreciated.

Can you provide any additional rationale that would mandate the DEA to re-evaluate the 2016 policy statement beyond the volume of the applicant pool?

Mr. STRAIT. I am sorry. Can you repeat that? I am not sure I understand.

Mr. GRIFFITH. Yes, sir. Can you provide any additional rationale that would mandate DEA to re-evaluate its 2016 policy statement beyond the volume of the applicant pool?

Mr. STRAIT. I would say the size of the applicant pool is probably one of the single greatest issues that we are trying to contend with, is how to meet the statutory text of the basis by which we are supposed to be evaluating all applications for both manufacturers of schedule I controlled substances.

Mr. GRIFFITH. We will be happy to change that statutory text if need be.

I yield back. Thank you, Madam Chair.

Ms. ESHOO. Gentleman yields back.

Pleasure to recognize the gentleman from Maryland, Mr. Sarbanes, for his 5 minutes of questions.

Mr. SARBANES. Thank you, Madam Chair. I thank the panel for being here today.

Dr. Volkow, first of all, thank you for your work, which I know well, and you have brought a lot of important testimony to this committee in the past.

I have heard from schools in my State, such as University of Maryland-Baltimore, that have communicated to me the difficulty in conducting research due to the current regulations and are nervous that any unintended violation of these strict and arduous restrictions can result in loss of their Federal research grants. Obviously, we have had a lot of discussion about that here today.

Despite these barriers, schools and researchers are eager to advance the understanding of the topic, and, just last year, the University of Maryland School of Pharmacy began offering a master of science in medical cannabis science and therapeutics. They now have this degree and focus opportunity.

I have a letter here, Madam Chair—I would like to submit this for the record—from the University of Maryland-Baltimore on the topic of cannabis research and cannabis training programs for the record. I would ask that this be accepted into the record.

[Material submitted for inclusion in the record follows:]

Mr. SARBANES. Dr. Volkow, would you agree that, as more patients are accessing cannabis products in States where they have been legalized for medical or recreational use in Maryland—of course we have taken that step with medical use—that our provider workforce should be educated on these topics and ready to respond to patients' questions?

Dr. VOLKOW. I agree that we need to have much more education with respect to actually how and that the use of marijuana products can negatively impact or help someone. The problem is that we do not have sufficient evidence that could help us mount those programs in a way that it is actually required. So, at this point, I don't feel that the evidence, like the National Academy of Science concluded, is sufficient to say we are going to recommend that this product be used by this patient.

There are many concerns, and it is not trivial. One of the problems that was noted is many patients—for example, the elderly may be given some of these products; they are on other medications, and they are not told what effects of the combination of THC with these medications, and the clinicians do not even know about it, nor do the patients.

So I do believe in the importance of expanding our knowledge so that we can then develop educational training programs that are based on knowledge, not on anecdote. And that is why I highlight the urgency of doing research on its therapeutic, as well as on its potentially adverse, effects.

Mr. SARBANES. Well, I think you are highlighting the impediment to creating workforce categories that can be a resource of expertise and perspective when it comes to cannabis that is presented by the kind of research issue that we are talking about today because, if you cannot—it is sort of a chicken-and-egg situation. If you cannot open the doors to more effective research, then, obviously, creating specific workforce categories that can take advantage of that and help push it forward and sustain it is made more complicated.

I would note that a survey of health providers from 2015 concluded that the health providers themselves perceive a knowledge gap in areas relating to medical cannabis dosing, development of therapeutic treatment plans, differences between various cannabis products and other areas. So the providers themselves have certainly perceived that there is the need for more research and expertise to be developed in this area, and I assume you would agree that incentivizing research on medical cannabis, for starters, would help address these knowledge gaps and support a more informed and robust provider workforce?

Dr. VOLKOW. Yes. I think we have an obligation to do the research to determine, what are the consequences of the products that people are taking with the expectation that they are going to be beneficial? We owe it to them to give them that knowledge, whether it is true or not. That is why we do research. So I completely agree of the urgency of expanding our understanding of the so-called medical properties of marijuana in diverse patient populations.

Mr. SARBANES. Thank you. I yield back.

Ms. ESHOO. The gentleman yields back.

Pleasure to recognize the gentleman from Oregon, Mr. Walden, for his 5 minutes of questions.

Mr. WALDEN. I walked back in from the other hearing, Madam Chair, so thank you because I know how important this issue is to all of us and especially to Oregonians.

Mr. Strait, I want to shift gears to hemp, as there is a lot of interest in my district from farmers who are growing hemp for CBD, and Oregon State University is working with the USDA's Ag Research Service to launch Federal hemp research. Given that the 2018 farm bill removed hemp from the CSA, is a DEA registration required to conduct research on hemp-derived CBD?

Mr. STRAIT. No.

Mr. WALDEN. No. Relatedly, USDA's interim final rule for hemp production, DEA is supposed to participate in oversight. Is the DEA prepared to handle registration of the private and public labs to handle hemp-compliance sampling?

Mr. STRAIT. The issue of hemp testing, which is actually baked into the U.S. Department of Agriculture——

Mr. WALDEN. So to speak, yes.

Mr. STRAIT [continuing]. Interim final rule—no pun intended.

Sorry about that.

Mr. WALDEN. There you go.

Mr. STRAIT [continuing]. Was predicated on the concept that those who performed testing probably made reasonable sense for them to hold a schedule I license in the event that they ended up procuring a sample that was not hemp; it actually ended up being hot and contained more than 0.3 percent THC. So that is an interim final rule. I know they are soliciting comments on that, and I know that that is an issue of concern that has been raised by some in the public.

Mr. WALDEN. Yes. There are quite a few of these issues. I know somebody that had a commercial driver's license who was using CBD oil to deal with something, or taking it, and then did a drug test, and it triggered the drug test as if he had used marijuana, which of course affected his CDL. So these are issues we are running into in real lives. He was not a marijuana user. You can have your own opinion on that, but he tried CBD.

And I want to go to Dr. Throckmorton. When it comes to CBD, are you able to tell us if FDA is any closer to determining if there are appropriate regulatory frameworks for nondrug uses, including for products marked as food and dietary supplements, and has the lack of research on the substance been an impediment to that process?

Dr. THROCKMORTON. I can tell you that process is a high priority for us. We understand the interest. As I said before, we are committed to working with you to find a path forward on that.

I would also say that the lack of information we have about the safety regarding cannabidiol is a challenge for us that we are looking to fill. We need to understand the use of CBD, the safety of CBD, in order for us to decide how best to place it in nondrug products.

Mr. WALDEN. And so I guess I want to push a little just in terms of the impediments to getting answers because this is playing out in real life. I have friends that swear by CBD. I have friends whose doctors have said, "Do not worry. Go ahead and take it. It does not impact anything else you may be taking." They know that? Have you done the research?

Dr. THROCKMORTON. Well, in fact, we know that is likely not accurate. Based on what we know from the Epidiolex, the approval of the product that contains cannabidiol, cannabidiol does interact with other drugs, and we can get you that list if you are interested, but, in fact, there are interactions that could occur that could be clinically significant, and I think blood thinners are one, for instance.

Mr. WALDEN. Yes.

Dr. THROCKMORTON. And so we would want to make sure that information is available to people.

Mr. WALDEN. Let me suggest they don't know that is available. They are actually being told by medical providers, at least this one case I know, that "don't worry, there is no interaction," and this is a legitimate doctor telling a patient.

This is happening in real—I mean, I have got colleagues that have been on television proclaiming the importance of CBD in food products and drinks and consuming it. That is fine. That is up to them, but I do not think—and if people want to use it, that is their business. I got it. But I just want people to have the facts and the data.

So I think what we are trying to do here is figure out what are the impediments to getting that data, and what does it take to get the agencies to a point where you are leading, not way trailing? Because the States are way ahead of where we are federally. We have got legacy rules we are trying to figure out here. Doctor?

Dr. THROCKMORTON. And we have been fortunate to work with the States. So you are right; the States are further ahead in some ways because they have had to be. You have had to face the use of these products in your own jurisdiction. The States have been very interested in understanding these same things. The State public health officials get that we need to understand the safe uses of cannabidiol and then make it—educate the prescribers, educate the choices that they are making very quickly. Unfortunately, historically, marijuana was used for its THC content.

Mr. WALDEN. Sure.

Dr. THROCKMORTON. And it has only been recently that the cultivars containing large amounts of CBD have sort of come to the floor.

The State data collection has been, historically, largely focused in that other direction.

Mr. WALDEN. Yes.

Dr. THROCKMORTON. And so they are changing course. It is just a matter of time.

Mr. WALDEN. Oh, yes. No, I understand all that. If you could get me that list, if it is readily available.

Dr. THROCKMORTON. Absolutely.

Mr. WALDEN. Is it on the FDA Web site? Is it—I mean——

Dr. THROCKMORTON. Absolutely.

Mr. WALDEN. Please do. Thank you.

And thanks for your indulgence, Madam Chair, and I yield back.

Ms. ESHOO. The gentleman yields back, and I think it is terrific that we have our next member, another gentleman from Oregon, so we have got a set of bookends here, Mr. Schrader, for his 5 minutes of questions.

Mr. SCHRADER. Thank you very much, Madam Chair.

I think it is great that, if we have—all three witnesses agree we need medical research into the effects of the hemp or CBD or marijuana products. The sad part is we are not testing the right stuff.

I fail to understand, with all due respect, Mr. Strait, why we have one bloody facility in an artificial environment, Mississippi, that is the really the sole nexus for research and analysis of CBD products.

Could you explain why that is?

Mr. STRAIT. So that location is actually more—probably better asked of Dr. Volkow because it is pursuant to a contract administered by the National Institutes of Health. DEA is mainly interested in——

Mr. SCHRADER. Well, I guess if I may interrupt briefly here. It is limited time. You know, it seems to me we ought to be testing the products that are on the marketplace. That is where FDA, NIDA, you are most concerned. What is the consumer—what is the American citizen actually being exposed to or hopefully benefiting from?

Mr. STRAIT. Yes.

Mr. SCHRADER. The idea that we are using a specific facility that does not mirror what people are actually ingesting, smoking, whatever, is ludicrous. I am worried—you are talking about more regulations coming out. We should be making less regulations and just say there is a legally approved facility in the State of Oregon, Colorado, District of Columbia. Those are things that people are actually going to be exposed to. We approve that research for that facility. Why are you not doing that?

Mr. STRAIT. And, Dr. Schrader, I cannot agree more in what you are saying, and that is certainly a conversation we have been having internally. The challenge, of course, is that the underlying principles of the CSA, the Controlled Substances Act, require that people who are going to lawfully possess, distribute, conduct research with schedule I controlled substances have to procure those substances from a valid source, and that valid source is—you know, at this point, it is another DEA-registered facility.

Mr. SCHRADER. Well, valid source in the eyes of the Federal Government——

Mr. STRAIT. Correct.

Mr. SCHRADER [continuing]. Not just you, perhaps, is this—you know, is whatever. I am arguing respectfully that the committee should be looking at legislation, if need be. I do not think we need legislation. It just should be something FDA, NIDA, and DEA can say, “Hey, you know, there is all these approved facilities out there in these States. We are not adjudicating whether or not it is a controlled substance or not. They are here. They are being used for certain products that consumers are being exposed to. We need to investigate them and make sure that they are not affecting adolescents adversely, fetal development, male fertility, whatever the deal is,” and get it out there. There is so many benefits.

My colleague from Oregon talked about benefits. I have got a farmer in the State of Oregon, a farm that is very conservative by nature. They had a father that was ailing, facing terminal illness. Pain relief was not getting done. They turned to CBDs. Their father was able to communicate for the first time in weeks with them, and he had a productive quality of life to the very end.

These are the products we need to be starting to get engaged in, or I just do not see that happening.

Talk to me a little bit, Mr. Strait, about approvals by both Tilray and Biopharmaceutical Research. Talk to me a little—these are not from Mississippi. How come they get through and not other products?

Mr. STRAIT. I am not familiar with those two companies in particular, but there are instances where pharmaceutical companies can be manufacturing through synthetic means some of these substances and then making those substances available for research purposes.

Mr. SCHRADER. OK. It concerns me that you are not aware of those being approved by DEA. I guess I would like to get more information after the hearing on that.

And there is an apparent tendency to approve more foreign applications than domestic applications that get held in limbo for years. We have got, what, 12 or 15 different applications that are pending and going through this long, exhaustive regulatory process. That seems incongruent with the fact that these products are out there now. We need the research now. Everyone on the panel has agreed to the research. Let's just get it done. What is the holdup?

Mr. STRAIT. Congressman Schrader, we have the same frustration you do.

Mr. SCHRADER. Very good. Well, Madam Chair, I will yield back. I just appreciate everyone's interest, and we just need to move forward and test the products that people are being exposed to.

Ms. ESHOO. I agree 100 percent. I do not understand—I still do not understand why the agencies, the three that are before us, can't get this done, but we will keep questioning, and the next one to question is the gentleman from Indiana, Dr. Bucshon.

Mr. BUCSHON. Thank you very much, Madam Chairwoman.

This hearing is really very important. I was a physician before I was in Congress. I am still a physician; I just do not practice. And, as a doctor, data is critical. You practice medicine based on facts and data. So I really appreciate this hearing.

And I do support the legitimate medicinal use for THC, but our knowledge on this subject actually is very limited and needs more research.

Dr. Volkow, I am going to go along the lines of the developing brain. Up to what age would you say the brain continues to develop?

Dr. VOLKOW. The fastest growth is during the first two decades and then until probably age 24 and then it slows down, but it never really goes away.

Mr. BUCSHON. Right. So I think people, a lot of times, have a misunderstanding. When we are talking about the developing brain, people think it is little children, but, actually, it really goes up substantially until your mid-20s approximately?

Dr. VOLKOW. Right.

Mr. BUCSHON. Great. Thanks. And you presented this, but we all know THC can have damaging effects on the developing brain, as you mentioned. In fact, the studies you conducted, the National Institute of Drug Abuse, show a direct correlation between persistent cannabis use and cognitive decline from one's childhood to midlife. Epidemiologic studies have further found that youth who regularly use cannabis have lower academic achievements and a higher risk of dropping out of school. Frequent cannabis use during adolescence is associated with changes in the area of the brain involved in attention, memory, emotions, and motivation. And, Madam Chairwoman, I have a slide deck that Dr. Volkow presented to the Doctors Caucus a number of years ago, and I would like to introduce that into the record.

Ms. ESHOO. So ordered.

Mr. BUCSHON. It outlines some of the things that you have been talking about today.

Additionally—and this is where I am going to focus my question on. NIDA recently put out research describing record levels of teens vaping marijuana, vaping THC products. Can you elaborate on that data?

Dr. VOLKOW. Yes. We have seen overall vaping has increased among teenagers, and, in the United States, 40 percent of the teenagers have vaped in their lives, and despite the fact that this is a new technology. Three years ago, most of the vaping was related to flavors. Two years ago, most of the vaping was related to nicotine. And what we saw this last December was there was a significant—a doubling of the number of teenagers vaping for THC.

Now, considering that vaping THC delivers very high content of THC, this is worrisome. It is also worrisome because, as you know, the injuries from—the acute injuries from vaping are predominantly associated with vaping of THC.

Mr. BUCSHON. Right.

Dr. VOLKOW. So this is concerning, and we are seeing also significant increases from in the past two years up on the regular use of cannabis, which we think are driven in part by the vaping.

So it is affecting the pattern of use of marijuana among teenagers.

Mr. BUCSHON. OK. So, then, along those lines, are researchers able to conduct Federal research on the THC and e-liquids and THC vape liquids sold at vape shops in States that have legalized marijuana for recreational use, and, if they can't, why not?

Dr. VOLKOW. The researchers are afraid that, if they use Federal funds to purchase products that are illicit by buying them in dispensaries, they will lose their funding. So, as a result of that, overall, research is not done by investigators that are being funded through the NIH, which is a federal agency.

Mr. BUCSHON. And, based on what you just talked about, about the rapid increase in vaping amongst teenagers, would you say that we need to do something about that?

Dr. VOLKOW. I would completely agree. We need to be able to move rapidly into the field and understand the products that patients or citizens are being exposed to.

Mr. BUCSHON. I think that just confirms what all of us have been saying throughout this hearing.

And I am also concerned that law enforcement is not equipped to address cannabis-impaired driving. I did have also a case in my district where a young lady was sledding and was hit by a car, and the person that hit her was not impaired by alcohol or opioids, failed a field sobriety test, and subsequently we find out it is marijuana, but there is no legal standard. Unlike alcohol, obviously, there is no reliable test.

For that reason, I introduced H.R. 3890, the Combating Impaired Driving Act, in 2019, to direct the Department of Transportation to provide funding for grants and pilot programs to address impaired driving.

Dr. Volkow, according to your organization, marijuana is the illicit drug most frequently found in the blood of drivers who have been involved in vehicle crashes, including fatal ones, and in your testimony, you describe that the risk of being involved in a crash significantly increases after cannabis uses.

Can you describe the difficulties law enforcement may have in testing for marijuana? Do you agree we need more funding to provide advanced measuring testing for cannabis-impaired driving?

Dr. VOLKOW. Yes, and, as I mentioned before, the problem that we have is the content in alcohol, you know a certain level is associated with motor impairment, but, in marijuana, it has a very long half-life, and it accumulates in the fatty tissues in our body. So, if you are a regular marijuana user, you may get high, and, three hours later, you still have very high levels even though you are not intoxicated.

On the other hand, if you are a naive user and you consume marijuana, have very low levels, you may be intoxicated. So there is not a one-to-one correspondence.

Mr. BUCSHON. Right.

Dr. VOLKOW. So we are trying to actually incentivize researchers to come up with innovative ways of determining whether someone is intoxicated or not, and we are funding researchers in that way.

Mr. BUCSHON. My time has expired, but, Madam Chairwoman, I think that again outlines why we need more research. I yield back.

Ms. ESHOO. I think, if there is anything to come out of this hearing is that the research is absolutely essential—absolutely essential. So much of this is two and two equals five. Well, it does not. So the gentleman from Massachusetts, Mr. Kennedy, is recognized for 5 minutes.

And I want to say how much I appreciate his—the input that he gave the Chair, and we will, as he said earlier, have a followup hearing with other stakeholders. Important to start out with our three government agencies, but I think that our subcommittee will benefit from the additional testimony of others. So he is recognized for his 5 minutes of questions.

Mr. KENNEDY. Thank you, Madam Chair. Thanks for holding this hearing, and thanks for adding the weight of the committee behind this conversation. Thank you to our witnesses for being here, for your service, for your work, and for your diligence.

As some of you know, I was initially hesitant to support legalization. My concerns stemmed from my work with the mental health community where many advocates have told me that they are worried about the impact of increased access to another controlled substance on the patients that they serve. But as States have moved forward with legalization, including my own, I tried to understand how we could protect for the public health concerns. I talked to experts. I talked to doctors. I talked to families. I talked to advocates. I talked to regulators. I have talked to some of you.

And that is where I started to get frustrated; frustrated that, as a Federal legislator, my hands were tied because our Federal policies still rested on Richard Nixon's decision to put marijuana in the same category as heroin; frustrated, as constituents told me that marijuana was the only thing that eased their pain. We have heard some of those stories today.

But when I asked regulators and subject agencies how we could ensure that this drug, like all drugs, was subject to the highest patient safety standards, I was told that we could not until we had more research. So I asked, how do we get more research?

Remove marijuana from schedule I, I was told.

How do we do that?

Well, we need more research.

The Federal Government has hid behind that catch-22 for a long, long time, and, meanwhile, millions of Americans, mostly Black and Brown, have been locked up for nonviolent drug offenses.

Meanwhile, desperate parents are forced to turn to a black market with no concern for patient safety to get their children the relief that they need. Meanwhile, our cities and States are trying, at times stumbling, to put in place a thoughtful and thorough regulatory framework with zero support from Federal partners. And, meanwhile, a brand new corporate industry is rising up, rife with predictable economic injustices that spring up whenever government fails to regulate.

Prohibition has clearly failed, and America is not waiting for its government anymore. That is why I decided to co-sponsor Congressman Nadler's MORE Act, which would finally deschedule, not reschedule, cannabis. It would expand critical research, and the reason I think this bill is superior to the policy on the table today, it makes an intentional and aggressive commitment to restorative justice in communities of color.

But, to the witnesses today, I understand and appreciate the deliberative detailed approached that you have outlined. I commend and I share your commitment to public health and safety. Clearly, that is why you are here. But I think it is clear that we are also out of time. States just are not waiting anymore. Incremental adjustments and the long path and a little more research are not enough. If the Federal Government wants to be active and honest and a smart stakeholder in marijuana policy, we have to break free from that catch-22.

So, in your testimony, you each pointed to the restrictions imposed by research because marijuana is a schedule I drug.

Dr. Throckmorton and Dr. Volkow, you have already indicated, and I just wanted to make sure I am clear, in your opinion, would those barriers be eased if marijuana was descheduled. Dr. Volkow?

Dr. VOLKOW. What was the question specifically?

Mr. KENNEDY. Would those restrictions on research be eased if marijuana was descheduled?

Dr. VOLKOW. The scheduling of marijuana—and that is why I want to comment on it because that is not specifically what we do. We have to recognize that marijuana has harmful effects. We know that, and the harmful effects can actually be very consequential, and, at the same time, it is a drug that is addictive.

So my perspective is—that is why I keep on saying it—what is the policy that will protect the public of the adverse effects of marijuana while at the same time accelerate our ability to take advantage of the potentially beneficial effects that the plant has? That is my perspective.

Whether it is descheduled or not, that is not what our agency does.

Mr. KENNEDY. Understood. And so let me just be clear about the question. Would the barriers to research be eased if marijuana was descheduled?

Dr. VOLKOW. If it were descheduled, it would be easier to do research; we know that.

Mr. KENNEDY. Yes. Dr. Throckmorton as well?

Dr. THROCKMORTON. I agree.

Mr. KENNEDY. And, additionally, in your opinion, would your office or agency be unable to continue its regulatory role regarding marijuana if it were to be descheduled, Dr. Volkow?

Dr. VOLKOW. Well, we do not regulate marijuana. We do research. So our agency is not involved. That would be transparent to us.

Mr. KENNEDY. So it would—your agency would not be harmed in any way by continuing to conduct its regulatory authority?

Dr. VOLKOW. It will—I mean, it is—by descheduling a drug, it is not—it is going to accelerate the ability to do research, but at the same time, it may have unintended negative consequences in that more people may be afflicted. So that is, again, why we bring the science, and the policy decisions of what is the optimal way of moving forward takes other factors into consideration, like the ones that the FDA has described.

Mr. KENNEDY. And, Doctor, again, just to clarify, I understand the balance, and I appreciate that balance. I think that is what we are all trying to strike today.

My question was, does the role of your agency change if marijuana is descheduled?

Dr. VOLKOW. No.

Mr. KENNEDY. Yes. Dr. Throckmorton?

Dr. THROCKMORTON. Well, it would matter how it happened obviously. It is, in essence, another system on a subset of drugs under development. So drugs containing compounds for marijuana potentially are used—go through the Controlled Substances Act, as well as the Food, Drug, and Cosmetic Act. To the extent that that step was removed and the authorities of the Food, Drug, and Cosmetic Act were maintained, it would not have an impact.

Mr. KENNEDY. Mr. Strait, I assume that the answer for you would be, yes, it would change from DEA?

Mr. STRAIT. Yes.

Mr. KENNEDY. Yes.

Mr. STRAIT. Since our obligation is to enforce the Controlled Substances Act, yes.

Mr. KENNEDY. Understood.

I yield back. Thank you.

Ms. ESHOO. Gentleman yields back.

Pleasure to recognize the gentleman from Florida, Mr. Bilirakis, for his 5 minutes of questions.

Mr. BILIRAKIS. Thank you, Madam Chair.

And I really thank the witnesses for testifying today. It has been very informative. Unfortunately, I was at Telecommunications for a while, but I am back now.

Dr. Volkow, do you think that the process for conducting research on schedule I substances coupled with the limitation on the supply of research-grade cannabis have discouraged some researchers from investigating the compound?

Dr. VOLKOW. The answer is yes, and it has slowed it down, yes.

Mr. BILIRAKIS. OK. Let's see. I have a couple of questions here that I want to go over.

Mr. BILIRAKIS. Mr. Strait, would you agree that scientists studying cannabis and its effects, either bad or good, is it a fundamentally different question than legalizing, decriminalizing, or even discussing medical or recreational cannabis?

Mr. STRAIT. Absolutely. We want DEA just like our colleagues at HHS want to be tethered to science as it pertains to research with marijuana Mr. BILIRAKIS. Very good.

Next question is for Mr. Throckmorton—Dr. Throckmorton, excuse me. Are products available in State-regulated markets like edibles, concentrates, oils, wax, tropicals, for example, et cetera? I mean, those particular products, are they commonly available to clinical investigators through Federal sources? And if not, how might that pose a risk to the public health?

Dr. THROCKMORTON. So I wouldn't be able to comment on their availability to the nondrug centers because that isn't part of what I regulate. I focus on the drug side.

On the drug side, with the passage of the farm bill, hemp-derived compounds are now available for research. And we are eager to support that any way that we possibly can. We think that is an exciting new avenue to get some of the questions we really desperately need answered.

Mr. BILIRAKIS. Doctor, one more question. With the recent spate of lung illnesses related to illicit THC vaping products, what were some of the key takeaway lessons learned regarding the Federal state of oversight and research into current products and consumption methods?

Dr. VOLKOW. Sorry. I thought you were asking——

Mr. BILIRAKIS. Yes. No, this is for——

Dr. VOLKOW. You are bringing up an example about why——

Mr. BILIRAKIS. And I would like——

Dr. VOLKOW. We need so much more knowledge. We did not know about hyperemesis until 2006. And as a result of that, we didn't know how to diagnose it. Now we are seeing it in the medical emergency rooms, and it is associated with high content THC and chronic use. But we are just assuming based on what the patients are telling us, since we are unable to actually sample from the sources that they are consuming. And that is just one example about why we need to understand the consequences of consumption of different products of marijuana, because we are seeing adverse effects.

And so if we want to proclaim, well, there are medical qualities to it and we need to have evidence to show that it is the case, we also need to understand how to optimally dose it and what product characteristics are safe, and we don't have that data.

Mr. BILIRAKIS. Thank you.

Dr. Throckmorton?

Dr. THROCKMORTON. I just want to say Dr. Volkow is raising an incredibly important point. Patterns of use, how these substances are being used are changing year to year. The new use of cannabidiol vaping, things like that. Just the ways these are being consumed, the doses they are being consumed, the populations, the perceived benefits are all changing. We as a Federal architecture need to find some way to track that, to understand it, to identify new risks as they emerge quickly, ideally find new ways to assess efficacy and things like it that are identified. But it is a central challenge, I think, for all of us working in this area.

Mr. BILIRAKIS. Thank you very much. And I agree.

I am going to yield the rest of my time to Mr. Griffith, please.

Mr. GRIFFITH. Thank you very much.

Mr. Strait, several studies found that research-grade marijuana from the University of Mississippi is genetically distinct from the marijuana coming from State dispensaries, such as we heard of earlier in the testimony from Oregon. Four years ago, DEA announced that it would accept applications for the manufacture of research-grade marijuana in order to increase the diversity of products for scientists to study. Thus far, the agency has not acted. And as we heard earlier today, DEA intends to propose new regulations that will govern the marijuana growers program for scientific and medical research.

Can we have your assurance publicly and on the record that the DEA will work expeditiously to review legitimate applications to produce marijuana for federally approved scientific research? And will current applicants be permitted to amend their applications to conform to the new rules so they are not caught in a catch-22 or a vortex of time?

Mr. STRAIT. On your first comment, yes, we definitely will move expeditiously. We are moving expeditiously, although I know it is not acceptable for anyone here in public office. So we appreciate your patience on that.

And your second question?

Mr. GRIFFITH. The second question was, if you already have an application pending and the rules change, instead of having to start back at go, you know, proceed directly to go and do not collect your $200, can they just amend so they can move forward? And a yes or no, because my time is up.

Mr. STRAIT. On that point, when we announced the notices of application in August of 2019, some of those applicants had been— had applied two years ago. We gave them the opportunity then to get a full refund. And, of course, we would do that.

Ms. ESHOO. The gentleman's time has expired.

The Chair now recognizes the gentlewoman from Michigan, Ms. Dingell, for her 5 minutes of questions.

Mrs. DINGELL. Thank you, Madam Chair.

I want to associate my comments today with everybody at this podium. And I think there is bipartisan frustration on this issue. I think my colleague, Mr. Kennedy, probably summarized where I am very deeply. I—Michigan is one of the States that is now one of the legal States that this is being traded in. I was—I will be very blunt, I did not support it when it was on the ballot. I come from a family that has seen what drug addiction does to people. But like my colleague, Mr. Griffith, Mr. Schrader, my husband, who many know in this room, suffered from great pain, and many people said that marijuana would be the only thing. Though would he try it, and he would not try it—can you see John Dingell smoking marijuana—because it was not legal, you didn't know the side effects, and it might have given him relief in the end.

But I was the keynote speaker at Hash Bash this past year. Yes, you should laugh. My staff told me—I don't even know how it got scheduled, if you want to know the truth. I am still trying to figure that out.

Ms. ESHOO. It wasn't schedule I.

Mrs. DINGELL. But I got up and said, I have never smoked marijuana, and don't think I ever will smoke marijuana, but I was getting a lot of indirect smoke that day. But I made the point—I talked to a lot of the scientists, and there were very clearly three things that need to happen. And I am as committed as anybody at this—we need to get more research on this issue. And we all keep asking you the same questions because we are not—we don't understand what the answers are or why if we all agree we need more research and we need it for medicinal purposes, we need it for automobile. I am working on impaired driving legislation right now too. Every one of us has got a story from our districts somehow, some way that there is a problem. And we are in the biggest catch-22 that you can ever see or imagine. So you have got to help us figure out how we are going it to get out of this catch-22.

It is one of the reasons I introduced, with my colleague, Representative Blumenauer, the Medical Marijuana Research Act, because just in case you can't tell, I am pretty passionate about it now. Even though it is legal for recreational use in 11 States, Michigan being one, we have just started it, it has gone recreational marijuana the last couple of weeks. The National Academy of Sciences has done a study, which I have right here, that found that the research of the health effects of cannabis and cannabidiol has been limited in the United States. And this lack of knowledge poses a public health risk.

I would like to make sure it is submitted for the record, Madam Chair.

Ms. ESHOO. So ordered.

[Material submitted for inclusion in the record follows:]

Mrs. DINGELL. So having agreed with all of my colleagues here, having the three of you already establish we have got problems, can we go back and look at some of these questions that everybody keeps asking?

Dr. Volkow, you talked about the administrative burden that current Federal rules mandate. We keep asking you why it takes months to navigate, but we are looking for those details. How would simplifying Federal guidance surrounding schedule I registration improve NIDA's ability to conduct this research? What do we need to do? And why is it only one kind of marijuana that is OK at the University of Mississippi? Can you give us more detail and highlight, you know, why Federal research is done only a single source of cannabis? How does this reliance on a single source limit our understanding of the health impacts?

Dr. VOLKOW. We agree, and we are also, of course, frustrated by the challenges of advancing the science and at the same time recognizing that we have a problem. I wish marijuana had no untoward effect; it would be quite remarkable. But unfortunately, high content THC can have, as I mentioned, pretty adverse effects.

Now, there is, as the national academy mentioned, there is evidence, though it is not solid enough for FDA approval, that there are some benefits clinically for some effects of the active ingredients of marijuana. So how could it—what is one of the things that we have been proposing? And again, we are not legislators. And it is the FDA and the DEA that regulate. But what we wanted to achieve is can there be a subcategory for schedule I that allows researchers to do research with the proper regulations but expedited. That is one of the things that we have been working with our colleagues on.

Mrs. DINGELL. How do we keep you from working and getting it done?

Dr. VOLKOW. We need to actually solve the problem, and I—and I agree. And I also think that we need to figure out a way to be able to also take advantage of some of the new producers of different cannabis plants in order to evaluate the diversity of problems that are out there, as opposed to limiting us with a Mississippi farm. These are regulations. This is not us wanting to say territorially we are the only place that can provide it. It is impeding research and knowledge.

Mrs. DINGELL. I am unfortunately out of time, but I could have asked a lot more questions.

Thank you, Madam Chair.

Ms. ESHOO. The gentlewoman yields back.

A pleasure to recognize the gentlewoman from Indiana, Ms. Brooks, for her 5 minutes of questions.

Mrs. BROOKS. Thank you, Madam Chairwoman.

And I apologize to the panel, there is another hearing going on, so I have been going back and forth a bit, but your testimony is critically important to us. And I think from my colleague across the aisle there has been frustration, because I think we are trying, as Members of Congress, to figure out what specifically we need to be doing to help to accelerate medical research. I think that is the top priority of this committee, I believe, and the purpose in having this hearing.

And so—and with that, you know, hearing testimony and knowing friends who have suffered from tremendous pain, particularly from cancer, I want to focus a little bit on pain therapy. We have talked a little bit about it and, Dr. Volkow, thank—and thank all of you for your work. I have very mixed feelings about the issues around marijuana, having long ago been a criminal defense attorney and seeing so many of my clients have substance abuse problems and many of them starting at a young age with marijuana, and then later as a former United States attorney working with the DEA and involved in, you know, disrupting trafficking organizations, drug trafficking organizations that ruined neighborhoods and communities and caused a lot of significant problems. I—but yet I also have a number of friends and people I know who have suffered tremendously, whether it is with cancer or other things, where marijuana has helped them with their pain, or those at end of life, as we have heard those stories. So we are really conflicted here.

We as a Congress, I think, have a lot of issues around we are trying to figure out how to break through and move the ball forward because it is taking years, and we just don't have the answers and we are so behind.

So what barriers, Dr. Volkow, remain at NIH to study the new therapies around pain and where cannabis can particularly help with pain? And even addiction therapies we are hearing. Can you share with us what are the barriers around the research specifically relative to pain?

Dr. VOLKOW. We are prioritizing as it relates to cannabis research, its potential value for the treatment of pain, for addiction, and also for HIV, and as an anti-inflammatory drug. So researchers are being funded both for THC as well as for CBD. We would like to have more investigators involved, and that is where the whole discussion has been going back and forth. Many investigators that don't have the infrastructure support that is necessary shy away because they feel it is too much of an obstacle to try to go through a schedule I. But we are funding research.

Mrs. BROOKS. Dr. Volkow, would these be private sector investigators or these university investigators or hos-—what type of investigators do we—what kind of investigators do we need?

Dr. VOLKOW. We want both of them. And one of the areas that we are very interested is actually pairing academic investigators with industry so that the products that are being developed then can go into the market. So we fund different mechanisms to try to facilitate those interactions. So you don't want to limit it just to the academicians. You want to also facilitate research by the private sectors.

Mrs. BROOKS. Are there any significant pieces of research that have been completed? I know you talked about 11 year—or studies over long periods of time of adolescents and of children that you are following, and I appreciate. What are the numbers of years that you are typically looking for relative to research?

Dr. VOLKOW. Well, it depends on what you are aiming for. For example, to try to understand how marijuana affects the developing brain, you need to follow it up doingbrain development. So that will take 10, 15 years. If you are trying to determine, for example, to what extent THC can have analgesic effects for, say, in a patient suffering from low back pain, I am just—that may be a study that you can complete in three or four years. So it depends very much what the aim is, what the study is going to be doing.

Mrs. BROOKS. And approximately how many studies are we funding now, you know, focused specifically on pain management?

Dr. VOLKOW. On pain management we are funding $39 million for therapeutics of cannabis. And of them, I would sort of say probably 35 to 40 percent may be pain, but I have to check the figures, but I just guesstimate.

Mrs. BROOKS. Off the top of your head, are there any significant negative results that have shown in your current research?

Dr. VOLKOW. Too early to say, from the ones that are ongoing.

Mrs. BROOKS. Thank you so much. Thank you all for your work. I yield back.

Ms. ESHOO. The gentlewoman yields back.

Pleasure to recognize the gentlewoman from Illinois, Ms. Kelly, for her 5 minutes of questions.

Ms. KELLY. Thank you, Madam Chair. And thank you to the witnesses for being here today.

My State of Illinois was the 11th State to approve adult use cannabis. But with that said, I am interested in hearing about the research that exists about cannabis, particularly for vulnerable populations. I am the chair of the Congressional Black Caucus Health Brain Trust and have worked with my colleagues to create legislative and policy solutions to reduce health disparity and promote good health in all communities.

So, Dr. Volkow, your testimony discusses the adverse health effects of cannabis when it comes to prenatal and adolescent development. What is the state of the science in this area? And are there studies that focus on minority populations?

Dr. VOLKOW. Yes. And based on the science, we do know that the use of THC during pregnancy is associated with significantly negative outcomes for the newborn and the mother. There are cannabinoid receptors in the placenta, and the cannabinoid receptors emerge very early on in fetal development and they guide, tell the brain actually how neurons in the brain are moving and connecting. So it is something that needs to be taken with caution.

We know that in adolescents, as has been mentioned, in all, every single story has shown overall independently that it leads to worse educational outcomes. And what we are now using is more sophisticated technology, larger samples, to understand how factors differs between one individual and the other. For example, through the ABCD study, we have shown that adverse social environments have a very negative effect in amplifying the consequences of insults into the brain. So if you come from a deprived environment, your brain is actually going to have a much slower development than if you are in an environment that enriches your experience. And in those circumstances, drugs have a greater negative effect.

So we—I mean, these are stories that are ongoing, but it is clear drug and marijuana is not a good thing for the developing brain.

Ms. KELLY. Well, I am glad to hear that you have a more diverse sample than it sounds like you did from the beginning. You said you are bringing more diversity.

Dr. VOLKOW. Absolutely. We need to understand diversity. Diversity in terms of ethnic background, diversity in terms of economic opportunities, because those are influencing multiple factors on the development of a child.

Ms. KELLY. And, Dr. Throckmorton, in your testimony, you mention that the FDA is actively working to learn more about the safety of CBD and CBD products. Among the list is work to understand the effects of CBD on special populations, such as the elderly, children, adolescents, and pregnant and lactating women. Can you elaborate more on this?

Dr. THROCKMORTON. The best data we have available comes from the control trials that were used to approve Epidiolex, which is the product for procedure disorders. It was conducted largely in young children. And so we simply don't have any extensive randomized controlled trials in those populations. We all sort of acknowledge they are terribly important.

When we approved Epidiolex, we also posted on the web what we do know about the demographics of response to the drug. So you can go on to what we call our drug trial snapshot page, and it will show you the safety and effectiveness of Epidiolex broken down by sex, gender, age, ethnicity. And you can look and see for yourself what we know about Epidiolex, but we need to have a lot more information to expand that to understand the impact on the elderly, for instance, and on pregnant and lactating women, because they just simply weren't in the trials and so we haven't had that opportunity yet. But it is something we recognize, and we are working to try to fill as quickly as we can.

Ms. KELLY. Assuming you are working to get more diversity in the trials.

Dr. THROCKMORTON. Absolutely, yes.

Ms. KELLY. I, like my colleague, I go back and forth about how I feel about recreational marijuana. I don't know if that is because I went to college in the 1970s, if that is the reason why. But I just read in the paper, you know, Chicago allowed it starting January 1. And the paper talked about how the emergency room visits have gone up because of this. And even places that treat dogs, because people are, I guess, careless with the edibles. I don't know. And they found more dogs are getting sick too. So it just seems like we need to educate the public more too about the effects. And I don't know if it is just an early overexuberance because it just became legal or will we continue to see increased emergency room visits.

Dr. VOLKOW. And I am just going to comment on that because, actually, one of the aspects that have been coming back and back, marijuana is not a safe drug. It has negative effects. And among the ones that we are more concerned is that is what affects young people. And one of the ones of greatest concern has been the association of the use of marijuana with psychosis. And stories across the world, for example, as a psychiatrist, I was trained that the prevalence of schizophrenia is the same across the world, it is one percent. Well, it so happens that that is not the case. And in some places, it is six to eightfold higher. And in those places, it is associated with the consumption of very high content THC.

So in the Netherlands, for example, which has the highest rate of schizophrenia linked with the consumption of THC, you can have plants that have 38 percent THC. And this is not just explained by having the genetic risks. There is something about high-content THC that is triggering psychosis, and we need to recognize it.

Ms. KELLY. I know my name time is up. Thank you, Madam Chair.

Ms. ESHOO. The gentlewoman's time has expired.

Pleasure to recognize the gentleman from Montana, Mr. Gianforte.

Mr. GIANFORTE. Thank you, Madam Chair. And thank you for the panel being here today.

Understanding the full consequences of readily available marijuana on public health and individuals is imperative. We have heard that today. We should be concerned about the lack of Federal research on marijuana because, when we consider such a drastic change, we must ensure that that policy is based on sound science. So the focus today on research is very appropriate.

In November, I joined with 16 other Members of Congress in asking Attorney General Barr to study the societal impacts of legalizing marijuana for recreational purposes. As we start to see preliminary data from States like Colorado and Oregon, it is important to fully evaluate their experiments before making Federal policy. I appreciate that Mr. Walden and Mr. Burgess have asked for a hearing on this research, and we should continue to investigate.

We should know how best to help people who need medical marijuana and how greater access to recreational marijuana will impact our communities, families, and users. However, expanding access to marijuana without the benefit and guidance of the facts and sound science is of grave concern. This is incredibly concerning because we have an addiction crisis in my home State of Montana. Methamphetamines and now opioids devastate our communities and tear up too many families.

Meth accounted for 86 percent of drugs trafficked in Montana in the past five years. Montana has worked hard to support people fighting addiction through drug treatment courts. These courts help people get clean and get back on their feet while staying engaged in their communities, all at a fraction of the cost of incarceration.

To consider making any schedule I drug legal and more readily available without adequate research is a misplaced priority when addiction continues to ravage our country. Instead, we should support focusing on combating addiction, building on this committee's bipartisan work and the success of the SUPPORT Act from last Congress. We need to continue to support those who face addiction and need the help the most, rather than making marijuana easier to access when we don't know the full effects on our communities.

Dr. Volkow, ensuring access to mental health services is a top priority of mine. Unfortunately, Montana has the highest suicide rate in the country. I have introduced the National Suicide Hotline Designation Act, which makes 988 the national suicide hotline number. This important bill will protect emergency access to care for those facing a mental health crisis, especially those in rural areas who lack access to mental health professionals.

In your testimony, you state that serious mental illness and suicides are on the rise in our country. And while multiple factors very likely contribute to this rise, it is imperative to understand if exposure to cannabis in adolescents is one of them. Does current research draw a connection between marijuana use and increased risk for suicide or mental health problems?

Dr. VOLKOW. There have been some large epidemiological studies that have noted an increased risk for suicide among regular users of THC, but the evidence is not as extensive as associated with psychosis. And so we cannot ignore it, but we need to determine if it is reproducible and understand the extent to which it is contributing indeed to suicidally. So it is something that has been noted by large epidemiological studies.

Mr. GIANFORTE. OK. And from your experience as a researcher in this area, do we fully understand the connection between marijuana and mental health and suicide?

Dr. VOLKOW. Marijuana, if you take high-content THC, in almost any one of us, if the content of THC is high enough, it is going to make us paranoid, extremely anxious, and very, very afraid, if not fully psychotic. And that can explain and one could conceive why in those circumstances someone, if they feel threatened, may actually attack someone else or attack themselves.

So in some people, that results in a chronic syndrome, and that is where we don't have sufficient knowledge of understanding why is it that in most cases it is just a very short limited psychotic episode and why is it that use of marijuana in some results in longlasting effects; that we do not know yet.

Mr. GIANFORTE. OK. So just to summarize—I appreciate your expert opinion—it is possible that cannabis could increase suicide rates. Is that correct?

Dr. VOLKOW. The epidemiological data has given some evidence that it may. But I want to be cautious again. I think that one of the issues that we have been criticizing the whole field of marijuana is that people say you are exaggerating. How do you know that a person to start with was depressed and was suicidal thinking that put them at risk to take marijuana to auto-medicate? So how do you now it is really a causal as opposed to an auto-medication? That is what I want to——

Mr. GIANFORTE. But it brings us back to the fact we just have to do the research.

And with that, Madam Chair, I yield back.

Ms. ESHOO. The gentleman yields back.

A pleasure to recognize the gentlewoman from Delaware, Ms. Blunt Rochester, for her 5 minutes of questions.

Ms. BLUNT ROCHESTER. Thank you, Madam Chairwoman, for this important hearing. And thank you to the witnesses.

As you can tell, many of my colleagues, we are going over time on the time we have because there are so many questions that we have. And as I thought about this, it really is a multitude of issues that we are dealing with in this one hearing, both protecting and enhancing public health, providing economic opportunities but in a just way, restorative and criminal justice as well as public safety.

I am encouraged at the inclusion of comprehensive legislation that addresses some of the social justice aspects of cannabis reform. Even a minor criminal record can lead to barriers in employment, housing, and education. It is also a significant drain on our national economy. That is why I have introduced bipartisan legislation, the Clean Slate Act, which would seal an individual's Federal record, criminal record for nonviolent or simple possession offenses involving cannabis.

As Congress continues to evaluate our Nation's approach to cannabis, let us continue to include criminal justice reform as a critical part of the conversation.

Dr. Throckmorton, as you mentioned in your testimony, the FDA has approved one cannabis derived product for medical treatment, Epidiolex, which is used to treat rare pediatric seizures. Can you walk us briefly, very briefly through how the FDA came to approve it?

Dr. THROCKMORTON. Happy to very shortly. So we have a process that we have laid out in a variety of different ways, including small business assistance and things that basically gives a roadmap to drug developers, beginning with conversations with us, coming in and just basically saying I want to develop a drug to do the following and this is where I think I might get my drug, my active pharmaceutical ingredient so called. We walk them through a series of meetings leading to, if successful, a drug approval of the kind that we were able to do for Epidiolex.

Ms. BLUNT ROCHESTER. So you have a roadmap that we can actually get a copy of?

Dr. THROCKMORTON. Absolutely.

Ms. BLUNT ROCHESTER. OK. So we will we request a copy of that roadmap. And also, what I would like to follow up on is what you have learned through the clinical trials from that as well.

Since the 2018 farm bill, we have seen a massive expansion in commercially available CBD products, everything from CBD active wear to CBD toothpaste. Many of these products assert that they contain various wellness benefits like reduced levels of anxiety or better sleep. I want to continue on. The FDA has stated that many of these products are marketed with unsubstantiated therapeutic claims.

Doctor, could you talk about what the FDA does to—what actions do you take for these bad actors? What are you currently doing?

Dr. THROCKMORTON. Sure, thank you. And we would be happy to follow up with details too there. So, fundamentally, if someone makes a claim that their product treats, diagnoses, mitigates, or prevents a disease, they are a drug. And if they are doing that without approval from the Food and Drug Administration, they are an unapproved drug, the subject to our enforcement actions. You know, they are making claims that they don't have any substantiated evidence for, we take an enforcement strategy that focuses on the high-risk things, the really egregious claims.

Ms. BLUNT ROCHESTER. So can you just give us some examples of what you did, who you targeted, what you did?

Dr. THROCKMORTON. So the egregious claims that we have—recently we took an action, we sent 15 warning letters out, identifying specific products that made those kinds of claims or in some other way violated the Food, Drug, and Cosmetics Act. We called on them to stop whatever the violation was that they were committing. Most of them had to do with labeling, and gave them steps that they needed to take in order to come back into compliance.

Ms. BLUNT ROCHESTER. Just so I am clear, the warning letter went to the person who is the bad actor.

Dr. THROCKMORTON. Manufacturer.

Ms. BLUNT ROCHESTER. The manufacturer. How is the public informed of that to be aware?

Dr. THROCKMORTON. So those letters are public. You can go on to our Web site and see the series of warning letters. This is actually I think the third time we have done this that we put out. And then we obviously have a follow-up plan for each of those companies to make sure that they come into compliance.

Ms. BLUNT ROCHESTER. One of the areas I didn't, when I ran through all of those intersections, I didn't run through consumer protection, and I think that is another big area. I know if I go into a store, I am not likely to then go on your Web site to figure out, is this dangerous for me or not. And so I think this is something else that we need to follow up, as we look at research and other issues, how to best protect the consumer.

Thank you so much, Madam Chairwoman, for this very important hearing, and I look forward to the next one. And I yield back the balance of my time.

Ms. ESHOO. And thank you for your important work as well. The gentlewoman yields back.

A pleasure to recognize the only pharmacist in the Congress, Mr. Carter of Georgia, you are recognized.

Mr. CARTER. Thank you, Madam Chair.

Mr. Strait, I am going to start with you. Dr. Burgess asked you earlier in this hearing about changing a drug from one schedule to another. And I wanted to expound upon that and ask you, you mentioned that it can be initiated a number of different ways. When was—what initiated the change from hydrocodone from a C– III to a C–II? Do you know?

Mr. STRAIT. Yes, that was a petition from a doctor.

Mr. CARTER. From a doctor. Why did it take so long? The opioid epidemic started in the early 1990s, lasted—and arguably the epitome of it was in 2006 to 2010, and yet it took you until 2014 to initiate that—or to complete it. Excuse me.

Mr. STRAIT. Yes, to complete it. So I believe that petition came in——

Mr. CARTER. Why did you have to wait on a petition?

Mr. STRAIT. I am sorry?

Mr. CARTER. Why did you have to wait on the petition?

Mr. STRAIT. We don't have to wait on a petition.

Mr. CARTER. Then why, with the opioid epidemic being as bad as it is, did it take the DEA until 2014 to reschedule hydrocodone from a C–III to a C–II?

Mr. STRAIT. Well, actually, back when that petition came in, I would argue that a lot of folks in the medical community were actually concerned about access to opioids. And so a petition to reschedule marijuana, despite its potential for abuse and its actual abuse, kind of ran contrary to some of those other broader concerns by the medical community.

Mr. CARTER. I—OK. Dr. Volkow, you and I have worked together for many years now, and I have great admiration for your work and great respect. You were asked earlier, I believe it was from Representative Castro, if marijuana is a gateway drug. And I have to be quite honest with you, you gave a very scientific response, something about sensitivity.

Is marijuana a gateway drug, in your opinion? And I ask you that as a psychiatrist. You understand we have had, in this subcommittee here, we have had panels of parents, of loved ones who have lost loved ones to opioid addiction, who have all said that it started with experimenting with marijuana.

Dr. VOLKOW. Indeed, they all—most of the epidemiological studies show that the first drug of initiation is marijuana. And because of that, that is another big argument for saying why it is a gateway drug. The counter argument and why it is not so simple is that it states that if you have the vulnerability for drug taking, it is much more likely as you are a teenager that you will encounter marijuana, then heroin. And, ergo, you start with marijuana and then you go into other drugs.

That is why it is not such a simple and that is why I basically say, overall, I would state, based on stories, not just in epidemiology or in laboratory animals, that if you expose them early on, they are more sensitive to other drugs that it——

Mr. CARTER. Wouldn't you agree that the psychological effects of experimenting with marijuana lead to experimenting with other drugs, which leads to more addiction? No question about it. That has been proven time and time again.

Dr. VOLKOW. But the same thing pertains to nicotine. So nicotine is another one——

Mr. CARTER. And what have we done with nicotine? We put limitations on it.

And I want to cut to the chase. If you want to see time fly, wait until you get up here for 5 minutes, but I want to cut to the chase. Everyone up here has expressed the same concern: We need more research. Tell us what we need to do.

Mr. Strait, what do you need? Do you need a schedule I–A that is not going to have anything in it except for marijuana? That is fine with me. I will create it.I will legislate that. But tell me what it is going to take. I don't—please.

Mr. STRAIT. Two things. We have seen a 150 percent increase in the number of schedule I marijuana—manufacture—researchers in the United States in the last five years. We are making progress. We want to do more, for sure.

What do we need in terms of improving access to research? I feel as if this interagency group of folks here have worked collaboratively on a proposal that would actually do just that.

Mr. CARTER. And is that the proposal you mentioned earlier about Fentanyl?

Mr. STRAIT. Correct. Absolutely. Yes. It is within the context of fentanyl——

Mr. CARTER. Can you make sure we get a copy of that? Because I want to see it, because we invite your input. We want to do the right thing.

You know, I saw an article just here recently that said that there is actually the—the use of new research found opioids were prescribed less often in States where marijuana had been legalized for medicinal or recreational use. You know, as a practicing pharmacist for many years, I have always said that the only thing worse for me than filling a prescription for someone who doesn't need it is not filling a prescription for someone who does need it.

If marijuana truly does have medicinal benefit, I want to use it. I am adamantly opposed to the recreational use of it. I think it is a gateway drug, and it should not be used recreationally. But if there are benefits to it, I want it to be used. All we want here, everyone has expressed the same thing throughout this whole hearing. Tell us how we can get this research done. Tell us how we can find out.

It is the epitome of ineptitude that the Federal Government has this scheduled as a schedule I drug and 11 States have approved it recreationally. Embarrassing.

Thank you, and I yield back.

Ms. ESHOO. So there.

OK. The gentleman from California is recognized, Mr. Cárdenas, for his 5 minutes of questioning.

Mr. CÁRDENAS. Thank you very much, Chairwoman Eshoo and also Ranking Member Burgess, for having this important hearing in this committee, in this committee where it belongs, the Health Subcommittee of the Energy and Commerce Committee.

Too often we either talk about cannabis as either a criminal justice issue or a medical issue. The reality is that we cannot pull them apart. Research has shown that for youth, in particular, incarceration is tied to poor physical and mental health outcomes later on in life. Compared to those not incarcerated, children and adolescents in the system for more than a year were three times more likely to have functional limitations, over four times more likely to have symptoms of depression, and over two times more likely to have suicidal effects into adulthood.

Now, I am not talking about the use of cannabis. I am talking about incarceration. Let me make that clear.

Nearly 75 percent of all of the people arrested for cannabis-related offenses are under the age of 30, and one in four—one-fourth are under the age of 18. That is almost a quarter of a million teenagers arrested for these types of offenses each year in the United States of America.

Given that we know being arrested for possession, growing or selling cannabis, can lead to incarceration, and we know that incarceration has adverse health consequences, we can establish that, at a minimum, cannabis criminalization causes some negative public health consequences. So the question then turns to balancing these public health concerns. We also know that a conviction for a controlled substance can lead to difficulty with job prospects, which could lead to both unemployment and underemployment, which has potentially adverse public health consequences. Similarly, a drug conviction means a currently enrolled college student receiving Federal student loan money would have their financial assistance terminated. This can harm the future employment, earnings, and ultimately, health prospects of that youth.

Examining the public health harms created by criminalization of cannabis is the type of research that could be conducted without having to expand the research supply.

I think it is really important for us to understand that calling cannabis a gateway drug in an anecdotal fashion is unfair to the American people and it is really not the proper dialogue that policymakers and/or researchers and/or medical experts should be having. And the reason why I say that is because, if we are going to have that discussion, we should have the discussion and the question, is alcohol a gateway product or substance? Is nicotine a gateway product or substance?

So to think that cannabis is in and of itself a category I, an evildoer to all that touch it, is something that should not be the subject of dialogue when it comes to true policymaking and also when it comes to real honest research, not anecdotal answers and questions.

What I have—I think one of the main things that we need to understand as policymakers is that the inception of the United States Congress calling cannabis a class I drug, I would encourage everybody in this room and everybody in this country to look at the footage on the floor of the United States Congress and the nonresearched derogatory statements that were being made specifically about a certain community and how using cannabis would lead to rape and murder of women and citizens of this country. I am cleaning it up a little bit because I think it is unfortunate that we have that stain on the United States Congress. And so far, we haven't had the will to actually correct it.

The United States Congress made a mistake, and every Congress since has not had honest hearings and honest dialogue and has not allowed, truly allowed, the researchers in this great country to do the true research that needs to be done for us to properly categorize cannabis in this country. And as a result of that, we have millions of individuals in this country, as I outlined earlier, who have been subjected to incarceration and a criminal record that otherwise they would have a much more productive and better life, and that society would be much better off, including the taxpayers, if we were to actually get this right.

So hopefully we will have the opportunity to do that in future hearings of the United States Congress so we can get it right and we can get the research done and we can end this anecdotal discussion and have a real, real discussion about the facts.

With that, I yield back.

Ms. ESHOO. The gentleman yields back.

The gentleman from Illinois, Mr. Shimkus.

Mr. SHIMKUS. Thank you, Madam Chairman.

Ms. ESHOO. My partner in all things 911.

Mr. SHIMKUS. Oh, yes, that is right.

Thank you all for being here. It is been a long day for you all. And I didn't have to sit through all of it, at least in the hearing room. So I appreciate that you have had to do that. And so I am going to try to be fairly brief.

And this one is to Dr. Volkow first. Are you familiar with the most recent article that came out of The Lancet Psychiatry about the risk of drug-induced psychosis converting to full schizophrenia?

Dr. VOLKOW. That is correct.

Mr. SHIMKUS. Can you comment on—I mean, I have got the stats and stuff. Can you tell me—I mean, summarize that report and maybe comment on your observations of that.

Dr. VOLKOW. This report is consistent with a concern that the use of marijuana, particularly high THC, can produce chronic psychosis. Overall, the statement, as I have made, is that most cases are of the use of marijuana trigger an acute psychosis that by itself will go away. What this study does is it shows that those individuals that went into an emergency department for an acute psychotic episode associated with the use of cannabis were much more likely to subsequently go into a chronic psychosis.

So this study links the use of marijuana, not just with acute psychosis, but provides evidence that it increases your risk of transitioning into a chronic psychotic episode, as is the case of schizophrenia.

Mr. SHIMKUS. OK, thank you. Let me—because I have been— mental illness, mental health, early use, what we call when they— a lot of people self-medicate through drugs based upon psychosis. And I think a lot of us may have had personal experiences with family members or friends and neighbors that have kind of fallen into this trap. And I think part of it is early drug use at an early age.

Let me go to this other subject that we have been dealing with. And this will be back to you, Dr. Volkow, and to I think Mr. Strait, and it really deals with this vaping and the THC and also the vitamin E acetate issue. So the question is, first of all, is it possible for scientists with a schedule I license to conduct federally funded research on THC oil in these vaping products?

Mr. STRAIT. Are we talking about the stuff that is actually being consumed illegally, I presume, as opposed to——

Mr. SHIMKUS. Right.

Mr. STRAIT [continuing]. Creating a THC extract that could then somehow be tested?

Mr. SHIMKUS. Yes. I think part of—that is the direction, yes, sir.

Mr. STRAIT. Yes. So as we had said earlier, the challenge, of course, with that is we certainly understand that researchers want access to that material. Under the Controlled Substances Act, researchers generally or have to obtain a controlled substance from another DEA registrant. This is something that Dr. Volkow has mentioned it. A failure to do so might impact their ability to keep their Federal funding for their program. So some of them have expressed some concerns about that.

Mr. SHIMKUS. And then let me just follow up. Would you agree that, with the CDC, that the scheduling status for cannabis makes it challenging for the epidemiological testing of these vaping products?

Dr. Volkow, you are shaking your head yes. Do you want to elaborate?

Dr. VOLKOW. Yes. Yes, it is, because you want to, when you start to see, for example, these emergency room admissions occurring in different States or communities, you would like to be able for researchers to go in and try to understand what is it in those products that is accounting for the rise in these cases, and that is not— currently not possible, if you want to use funding from Federal agencies like ours.

Mr. SHIMKUS. Great. Thank you. And I want to yield my last minute to Morgan.

Mr. GRIFFITH. I appreciate the gentleman very much.

Earlier, Mr. Strait, we were talking about the applicants that are already in place. So 33 applicants who grow marijuana for research are out there. Y' all are changing the rules. I asked if they would be able to amend their petition. You said, well, yes, we did this before. We refunded their money. I don't think they want their money refunded. They want to be able to not have to go back and start all over again with their application.

So can they just amend their application? Wouldn't that make sense?

Mr. STRAIT. Thanks for giving me the opportunity to clarify. What I meant and what I said and meant was for—because the applications had come in prior to passage of the farm bill and that some of these applicants may have actually applied to produce things that now are no longer controlled under the CSA, we gave them the opportunity to withdraw their application for purposes of no longer needing it. Those that have applied, they are in the queue and they will not have to reapply. We will be adjudicating every single application.

Mr. GRIFFITH. I appreciate that. Thank you. That makes more sense than what I thought I heard. I appreciate the clarification.

Mr. STRAIT. You bet.

Mr. GRIFFITH. I yield back.

Ms. ESHOO. The gentleman yields back.

The Chair recognizes the gentleman from Illinois, Mr. Rush, for his 5 minutes of questions.

And we have—we don't have very many members left, and it is my understanding that votes are going to be called shortly, so I think that we will be on time.

Mr. Rush, you are recognized.

Mr. RUSH. I want to thank you, Madam Chair, for holding this hearing.

And this hearing is particularly timely and more and more States are loosening their restrictions around marijuana, including my home State of Illinois, which just legalized recreational marijuana beginning the first of January of this year. As such, I believe more than ever that it is important that we prioritize the research upon, not only the benefits, but also on the risk of marijuana.

I worry, Madam Chairman, that too little is known about when and how marijuana can be harmful, particularly after frequent and long-term use. And that said, it seems to me that many States, including mine, are stampeding to legalize both medicinal and recreational use of cannabis, particularly because there is a budgetary crisis that these States are confronting. And the revenues from increased marijuana sales and legalized marijuana, particularly at the recreational level, is meant to help correct the budgetary issues that they are facing.

And I want to ask Dr. Volkow a question. Would you please expand on the possible health risk and implication for citizens, both on adults and adolescents of these States, which are exhibiting what I call a mob marijuana mentality and who are engaged in what I would refer to as a marijuana mania, that really exists in my State and in some of the situated States across the Nation?

Dr. VOLKOW. Yes. And I like you way you call it the marijuana mania, because it is actually a change in belief without the fact that there hasn't been any evidence to make us think that it is safe. And I don't want to negate the possibility that, in some instances, cannabis can have therapeutic benefits, but we cannot deny the fact it has some very untoward effects. That does not negate the possibility that we can come up with indications that can—where marijuana can be used safely for therapeutic purposes. These things are not exclusive.

But it is clear, the evidence is clear that use of marijuana is associated with negative effects. And we are already seeing it by the significant increase in emergency department admissions that are being observed in the States that are legalizing marijuana, as well as hospital admissions. This is happening.

By changing the culture, by legalizing it, by creating a sense that it is a safe drug, more people are being exposed to it. And as a result of that, that otherwise they wouldn't have because they wouldn't want to do something illicit. The more people get exposed to it, the greater the likelihood that we are going to see adverse effects, which is what we are observing.

So the data is clear that it can have adverse effects and why— I mean, and at the same time where we are leading as a country, which is quite amazing, is how rapidly the perception of risks disappear among the public. And we need to actually create the balance that brings evidence of really what marijuana can do, so that the individuals that want to take it know the positives and the negatives and they don't do it blindly, which is what we are observing happening.

Mr. RUSH. Another area that I am really concerned about, along with this mania that exists is this empty excuse of—or this expungement of records. It is OK, all right, but the cause of those records is being ignored.

Is there a nexus between marijuana—the offense of marijuana, smoking marijuana or ingesting marijuana, and abhorrent social behavior which creates a law enforcement issue which, in my theory, is that led to mass incarceration? I don't know whether or not you can make the connection, but can you make that connection?

Dr. VOLKOW. Well, I think at the point of incarceration and incarceration of individuals with a substance use disorder, when you do the studies, it has clearly showed that not only it does not in any way benefit or protect anyone; it actually makes them much more vulnerable to relapsing and drug taking and other adverse mental consequences. So incarceration has an adverse effect on those that are suffering.

Mr. RUSH. I want to thank you, Madam Chair. I yield back.

Ms. ESHOO. The gentleman's time has expired.

It is a pleasure to recognize the gentlewoman from—so we are going to go to Ms. Barraga´n for her 5 minutes of questioning. And we have two members that are waiving on to the committee. And I sure hope we will be able to take your 5 minutes of questions as well.

Ms. Barragán, you are at bat.

Ms. BARRAGÁN. Thank you.

Ms. ESHOO. Five minutes.

Ms. BARRAGÁN. Great. Thank you.

And thank you all for being here today and providing informative information. I thought it was pretty powerful, and the most powerful was to hear from Congressman Griffith and his story. It is the personal stories that are the most impactful.

When I was very young, my father had Parkinson's disease, and he had it pretty much all of my life. And I remember when I would see him in pain, I would just ask is there anything that could be done for him. I don't care if it is legal or not. And it was more of the sense of, you know, you are a child and seeing your parent suffer and you want to give them something to make that pain go away. And so I am firmly in the same boat of supporting efforts to make sure that we are providing things like marijuana for medical purposes to make sure patients are having access to what they need to help give them some comfort, especially when they are near the end of their life. There is no reason that people need to be suffering. And so his story was pretty compelling for me.

I am wondering if anybody on the panel today supports any of the bills, any of the legislation that is before us today. Does anybody want to comment on any support on any of the bills?

Dr. VOLKOW. We have been asked that question, and I actually was asked more specifically which one I favor, and I said I favor actually the advancing of science and the ability to do things in a way that can help us accelerate research. But specifically which is the best bill, I think that that is more on the side of you who are actually the ones that are creating them. But my colleagues may— I may put them on the spot.

Ms. BARRAGÁN. And I am not asking for the best bill. I am asking for, you know, these are the three bills I would support that I think would be helpful or that I think would be beneficial.

Dr. VOLKOW. And the one that I had—have gone on the record for these that are basically—and we have been working with my colleagues at the FDA and the DEA that are favored is the creation of a subcategory for schedule I substances that would allow us to do research expeditiously. And it is not just for marijuana, it is in general schedule I substances, so that researchers don't—don't have to go through all of the obstacles and the delay process. That is what we have been—actually one of the things that we are very specifically tried to achieve.

Ms. BARRAGÁN. Gentlemen, any——

Dr. THROCKMORTON. I would be happy to provide comment on any particular bill that you wanted us to help you with, obviously. I think Dr.

Volkow said it very well before. The goal needs to be kept in mind. So whatever the vehicle, decontrol or other approaches that are suggested and that are included in some of those legislations, we need to think about the goals in mind. And in particular, from the FDA's perspective, the outcome needs to keep in mind the need for continued drug development and appropriate scientific study.

Mr. STRAIT. And from the Department of Justice side, none of these bills have actually been reviewed by the administration, so there is actually no official position in terms of any of the proposals. But as we are all talking about today and as I think we all have kind of mutually agreed upon, the key is science and having the access to the data to support sound decisionmaking, whether that be legislative or within the executive branch absent legislation.

Ms. BARRAGÁN. Right. So I want to shift for a moment on the issue of sickle cell and the impact it has had on African Americans. I think in some States they have a list of medical marijuana uses, and I have talked to patients—I have seen what sickle cell has done to patients and the pain that they have suffered, and many sickle cell patients use marijuana to address acute pain that is a symptom of the disease. And some of the States currently have medical marijuana laws but have chosen not to include sickle cell disease on the list of conditions that would qualify a patient to receive the medication.

Dr. Throckmorton, is there a way we can assure that States that allow for medical marijuana have a comprehensive list of conditions that would qualify for the medication so that those who would potentially benefit from its effects are not excluded?RPTR GIORDANOEDTR SECKMAN[12:59 p.m.]

Dr. THROCKMORTON. So which medications are you talking about? So——

Ms. BARRAGÁN. We are talking about the use of marijuana for sickle cell.

Dr. THROCKMORTON. OK. Yes. So the medications for sickle cell disease that I would advocate for are the ones that we have had the good fortune to be able to approve in recent years.

Ms. BARRAGÁN. Well, no. I am asking——

Dr. THROCKMORTON. They are not for pains. And those medications, we can and do work with providers to make certain that they understand they are available. We hope to include them—make them available——

Ms. BARRAGÁN. Right. That was not the question. The question was that the States that provide the lists where people can use medical marijuana, like how do we ensure that some of these diseases are included. So——

Dr. THROCKMORTON. I am happy to talk with you offline.

Ms. BARRAGÁN. OK.

Dr. THROCKMORTON. Those States are making those choices without Federal input, so——

Ms. BARRAGÁN. OK. Thank you. I yield back.

Ms. ESHOO. The gentlewoman yields back.

Pleasure to recognize the gentleman from California, Dr. Ruiz, for his 5 minutes of questions.

Mr. RUIZ. Thank you, and thank you all for being here. Dr. Volkow, you say in your written testimony that, quote, CBD is ubiquitous, and it is possible to purchase CBD extracts as well as food, drinks, cosmetics, and other CBD-containing products which are sometimes marketed with health and wellness claims that are not backed by science, unquote.

It is also worth noting that, while more than 30 States allow for comprehensive medical use of cannabis and the FDA has approved some derived and cannabis-related drug products, cannabis does not have the FDA approval for any indication.

We have seen that cannabis can be used to treat certain ailments, such as for children with particular seizure disorders that are refractory to other treatments; as an appetite stimulant for patients suffering from AIDS or receiving chemotherapy; as an adjunct to other therapies in the treatment of chronic pain syndromes, which is of particular interest during the current opioid epidemic. Pain and spasticity in multiple sclerosis is another use. However, there is evidence show that chronic use is not without its consequence: for example, cannabinoid hyperemesis syndrome, a syndrome of cyclic intractable vomiting and chronic abdominal pain; disadvantaged attention, learning, and processing speed among teens who use marijuana regularly.

These neurobehavioral changes can even be seen on brain MRIs of these patients. These changes can be permanent. Earlier onset, as you had mentioned earlier, of schizophrenia and bipolar disorders in young users of marijuana.

So it is clear that more research need to be done to better understand the risks and benefits.

Dr. Throckmorton, it seems the FDA has found therapeutic value in marijuana-related compounds, but for limited and specific uses. Can you discuss what factors went into approving these drugs for medical use for these specific populations?

Dr. THROCKMORTON. Sure. It began with the basic science work that groups like NIDA does, so it began with supporting the kinds of research that NIDA supports to identify compounds and targets—therapeutic targets of interest; so suggesting from animal models or other places that the drugs had use in those areas.

And then something called translational science needs to happen, which is a drug manufacturer or a drug developer picks up that idea and comes and talks to us and says: We believe this is a product that we can turn into a drug. What are the pathways—what do we need to do? What are the next steps?

Typically that includes additional clinical studies, sometimes additional non-clinical studies, and the result is something called the new drug application, chosen—the therapeutic area then is chosen by the individual company. They are choosing to invest in pain, or they are choosing to invest in—you know—I do not know—infectious diseases, or whatever else it is, with a particular product. Our job is to make sure that that assessment occurs, occurs quickly and efficiently, and is scientifically driven, and results—you know, if the data are what they need to be, and then approval of a drug for a specific condition with an understanding of its safety and effectiveness.

Mr. RUIZ. And, based on this approval process, can FDA extrapolate the safety of CBD for other products?

Dr. THROCKMORTON. Extrapolation for effectiveness is very hard to do, and we have done it in very limited spaces. It is probably something we could talk about in more detail offline.

Safety is something that we are sometimes able to do more readily. A drug in a class that has an adverse effect, we will worry about does that same adverse effect occur in other drugs in the class? We have discovered over the years that very small differences in molecules have very large impacts in terms of effectiveness.

THC and CBD are very close to one another at a molecular level and yet have extraordinarily different patterns of use.

Mr. RUIZ. So your comments earlier said that CBD does not come without its risks. That is what we have all been talking about here. Your testimony outlines some of these risks. Can you elaborate more about what you know about CBD so far and what questions the agency may still have related to other uses?

Dr. THROCKMORTON. And now you are talking about safety, or are you talking about effectiveness?

Mr. RUIZ. Safety in other uses.

Dr. THROCKMORTON. So safety, I think, as you said, my testimony outlines, I would say, several buckets: one, adverse effects that we have observed in the clinical trials leading to the approval of Epidiolex; two, unknowns, things that we believe we need to have additional information about. I would put in that category particularly things like——

Mr. RUIZ. Right.

Dr. THROCKMORTON [continuing]. The liver injury and testicular injury.

Mr. RUIZ. I only have seven minutes, and I just want to make a very important statement here, that, as you conduct your data collections, you have got to ensure that you have a diverse sample of populations. Too many research is done on men and non-Hispanics and non-African-Americans in the medical world, and I believe that, in all categories of research, you need more women, and you need more people of color. OK?

Dr. THROCKMORTON. Agreed.

Mr. RUIZ. All right. Thank you. I yield back.

Ms. ESHOO. The gentleman yields back.

The Chair now recognizes Ms. Schakowsky of Illinois, waiving onto the subcommittee, for her 5 minutes.

Ms. SCHAKOWSKY. Thank you, Madam Chair, and I appreciate being able to waive onto the committee.

I am a proud original cosponsor of Representative Jeffries' Marijuana Freedom and Opportunity Act and a cosponsor of Representative Nadler's MORE Act, which would both remove cannabis from regulatory Controlled Substances Act and add the criminal justice and mass incarceration address-it issue that we have been perpetually backing, and so that would get rid of that.

Here is what—I want to focus on research, too. Everybody has, it seems, or most people. On January 1st, Illinois legalized recreational cannabis across our State, and dispensaries sold more than $19.7 million in cannabis over the first 12 days.

However, research at Northwestern University, which is in my district and is a leading research institution, have no way of accessing the cannabis that is sold in these dispensaries. And instead Northwestern scientists often face extreme difficulty in securing and maintaining cannabis and Federal funding for the research.

So I am glad that there is strong bipartisan support, at least for most of H.R. 3797, Representative Blumenauer's Medical Marijuana Research Act of 2019. The bill would streamline the cannabis research process to ensure that our academic institutions remain at the cutting edge, et cetera.

Dr. Volkow and Dr. Throckmorton, how can we establish a process by which researchers in a State like Illinois, where recreational marijuana has been legalized and several different strains of cannabis are now widely available—how could Illinois acquire the research supply through local dispensaries?

Ms. VOLKOW. And this is a question that we have been discussing it, and DEA is the one that is actually on the process of identifying additional sources of marijuana so that researchers can investigate marijuana from different dispensaries. So that is ongoing, and so—but that is regulated by the DEA.

Ms. SCHAKOWSKY. And can we look forward to some change there?

Mr. STRAIT. As we have previously discussed, I think one of the challenges is unfortunately the fact that, for your purposes, a researcher who is procuring a controlled substance for research purposes is obligated under the Controlled Substances Act to procure that substance from another Federal DEA register——

Ms. SCHAKOWSKY. Right.

Mr. STRAIT [continuing]. To research it.

Ms. SCHAKOWSKY. Right.

Mr. STRAIT. So none of these dispensaries are applying for a registration. None of them are registered with the DEA, and, therefore, they are unable to distribute to researchers.

Ms. SCHAKOWSKY. So we would have to get marijuana off the Controlled Substances Act—out of it in order to do the research that we absolutely need to do on what is being sold right now, and millions and millions of dollars being spent on it, and many, many users?

Mr. STRAIT. Well, certainly that is your discretion and Congress' discretion as one way to solve that issue. I do not know at the end of the day where this administration would come down on that approach.

Ms. SCHAKOWSKY. Is that the only way?

Mr. STRAIT. No. I think there are other legislative means by which Congress could propose to change that specific requirement, but I do believe that it would require some legislative changes to the Controlled Substances Act.

Ms. SCHAKOWSKY. I did want to say about that piece of legislation, H.R. 3797, that I do have a concern that DOJ would have the ability to deny medical marijuana licenses based on even minor past drug convictions, and I hope that we can also remedy that. Though I know that we do not all agree on deregulation and descheduling, we, I think, at the very least, should be able to work together to ensure adequate research is able to be conducted so that we know the consequences of what people are using right this very minute in the State of Illinois and many other States.

And I yield back.

Ms. ESHOO. The gentlewoman yields back. Votes have been called, and I recognize the gentlewoman from the State of Washington, Ms. McMorris-Rodgers, for 5 minutes.

Mrs. RODGERS. Thank you.

Thank you, Madam Chair, and I also want to recognize the ranking member and all the committee members. I appreciate this committee being engaged on this public health and consumer safety topic around cannabis. I get asked about this a lot in Washington State. We legalized both recreational and medicinal marijuana the same year as Colorado. I believe we were the first two States.

I am a cosponsor of Blumenauer's Research Act because I do think that we need more research. I also represent Washington State University, and it is in the same situation as Ms. Schakowsky's university around wanting to do more research around the issue.

Since we have legalized marijuana, the number of cannabis products available on the marketplace has exploded over the years, and so have the marketing tactics that promise cannabis is a miracle for your health. A quick search promises you cannabis products will help you sleep, relieve your pain, calm your anxiety, shrink tumors, cure diseases, and a whole lot more.

The concern is that these claims are not yet backed by scientific research or clinical trials. I am concerned about manufacturers who are ignoring all the unknowns of cannabis and spending health promises to fuel an industry that is projected to be nearly $2 billion by 2022.

I do believe that this industry, like with the FDA-approved CBD oral solution for epilepsy—and others have mentioned this—is on the verge of major breakthroughs that can improve people's lives, and we should be encouraging these developments. Like other cures and treatments, cannabis products should be held to a standard that people can trust so that the bad actors cannot spin to make a quick buck.

Bottom line: this is a public health and a consumer safety issue. Those priorities should be at the forefront as we unlock the mysteries of cannabis.

Dr. Throckmorton, I wanted to ask—and others have been on this topic also, but, as I mentioned earlier, the FDA has approved only one CBD product, a prescription drug product to treat epilepsy.

That being said, all sorts of CBD products are being marketed and sold throughout the country. We have no idea what the health implications may be.

So what is the solution to this? How should it be handled?

Dr. THROCKMORTON. So not one solution; that shouldn't be a surprise, right? I personally believed one really important element is to encourage the development of a mature industry using these products—an industry used to manufacturing standards; industry used to packaging standards, labeling standards; an industry of the kind that you see when you go into Walmart and Costco and places like that. Those products are being manufactured to a standard, as you said, which I think is very valuable.

I hope that, by the recent increase in interest in doing research using these products, behind that will be a growth of an industry that wants to do the right thing, that wants to be science-driven, appropriately labeled, manufacturing to a high-quality standard. I think that is one important element, among other things.

I also think it is terribly important that we lay out a pathway for nondrug products containing compounds from hemp so that there is a clear path that developers can follow to find a way forward as far as developing those products and making them appropriately available.

Mrs. RODGERS. Do you see that happening at the State level in any of the States where marijuana has been legalized?

Dr. THROCKMORTON. Yes, I do.

Mrs. RODGERS. Either for the industry or the nondrug products?

Dr. THROCKMORTON. We have really benefited from talking with the states. I would say your State has been particularly helpful to us as we talked to them about their experiences because you have had to deal with all of these things.

The States are all taking different approaches, but many of them—and I would say including your state—I know are grappling with these issues around labeling and dosing and manufacturing quality and things like that, and we are trying to learn from those experiences as we try to formulate a policy at the Federal level.

Mrs. RODGERS. Another big concern is the increase in traffic accidents and traffic fatalities around the use of these products, and we have seen some pretty dramatic increase in numbers around accidents, at the very time that we are working here diligently to make our roads safer, and now also the number of fatality accidents that involve one of these products.

What needs to happen in that regard to make sure that we are safe on the roads?

Dr. THROCKMORTON. So it is one of the unknowns we have identified for cannabidiol. We have studied it in children. We never did those kinds of studies because children don't drive, but we understand we need to understand the effects of CBD on driving impairment. We need to have that—those data as soon as we can.

Mrs. RODGERS. OK. Well, there is a lot more to explore here. Thank you all for being here.

Thank you, Madam Chair.

Ms. ESHOO. The gentlewoman yields back, and we thank her for participating in our hearing.

So let me, on behalf of all of the members of the subcommittee, thank our witnesses. This is a long hearing. I might add it is the very first hearing on cannabis in the history of the Energy and Commerce Committee, which is the oldest committee in the Congress.

So it has been a long hearing, but I think a highly—excuse the expression—instructive one because of the participation of all of the members, and we will have another hearing from other stakeholders that are not agency stakeholders. So thank you again to each one of the witnesses.

Where you weren't instructive, it was instructive to us, and so much of your testimony was. We learned from you. And we have, I believe, the vehicles to develop a roadmap to address this lack of really substantive research that is absolutely needed. That is foundational to what—you know, so many of our undertakings.

So I want to submit the following statements for the record, and I also want to remind members—of course they are not here—that, pursuant to committee rules, they have ten business days to submit additional questions for the record to be answered by the witnesses or to whomever questions are submitted. We count on our witnesses to respond promptly to any of the questions that you may receive, and I trust that you will do that.

So I request anonymous consent to enter into the record the following documents: the statement from the Greenwich—from Greenwich Biosciences; a statement from the American College of Occupational and Environmental Medicine; a statement from the National Safety Council; a letter from the National Consumers League; a statement from Doctors for Cannabis Regulation; testimony of Aaron Smith, executive director of the National Cannabis Industry Association; a letter from over 100 organizations in support of H.R. 3884; a letter from five organizations representing State legal cannabis businesses; a statement from the California Cannabis Industry Association; the testimony of Congressman Hakeem Jeffries in support of H.R. 2843; a statement from Kris Krane, president of 4—the number 4 and the word "Front"—Ventures; a statement from Americans for Safe Access; a report from the National Cannabis Industry Association entitled "Adapting a

Regulatory Framework for the Emerging Cannabis Industry"; a statement from the American Property Casualty Insurance Association; the testimony of Paul Armentano, deputy director of the National Organization for the Reform of Marijuana Laws; a response letter from FDA/NIH to Senator Schatz; a letter from the minority requesting a hearing on cannabis, and here we are, and I said yes; a letter from the American Academy of Neurology in support of H.R. 171; a letter from the American Academy of Neurology in support of H.R. 601; a Bloomberg News article entitled "Pot Imports Grow as U.S. Stalls on Medical Research"—quite timely; a collection of six letters from organizational supporters of H.R. 3797; a statement from the Biopharmaceutical Research Company; a letter from Smart Approaches to Marijuana; a letter from the Michael J. Fox Foundation in support of H.R. 601; a statement from the Consumer Brands Association; a letter from the DEA in reply to an application to grow marijuana for research purposes; and slides created by NIH entitled "Effects of Cannabis on the Human Brain."

Without objection, so ordered.

[Material submitted for inclusion in the record follows:]

Ms. ESHOO. Does the ranking member have anything he wishes to submit?

Mr. BURGESS. I would not do anything to prolong the hearing.

Ms. ESHOO. All right. So, on that happy note, thank you to each one of our witnesses again.

To everyone that remained in the hearing room, thank you for your attentiveness.

And, to the reporters, the press, thank you for your interest.

At this time, the subcommittee is adjourned.

[Whereupon, at 1:22 p.m., the subcommittee was adjourned.]

Prepared Statement of Hon. Eliot L. Engel

Thank you Chairwoman Eshoo and Chairman Pallone for holding today's important hearing on legislative proposals to modernize federal policies on cannabis.

As an advocate for legalizing cannabis, I have been supportive of state laws to legalize cannabis, including marijuana. As this sea change has occurred, federal laws have begun to catch up. In 2018, I served as a Conferee to the Agriculture Improvement Act, better known as the Farm Bill, which took a step forward in legalizing cannabis by allowing the cultivation of hemp. This past June, I voted for an appropriations amendment that would prohibit the Department of Justice from interfering in state cannabis programs, including those involving marijuana.

Many of the proposals under consideration today would help us move closer to the complete legalization of cannabis. The Marijuana Freedom and Opportunity Act, introduced by New York Congressman Hakeem Jeffries, would decriminalize marijuana and THC by removing it from the list of Schedule I substances. It would also provide states with the necessary resources to expunge marijuana convictions, which have had a disproportionate impact on minority communities. Congressman Jeffries' legislation, which I have cosponsored, would provide commonsense reforms to our nation's antiquated cannabis laws.

It is also critical that we streamline the federal process for medical research on cannabis. Currently, a number of regulatory and legal barriers dissuade promising research into cannabis. The bipartisan Medical Marijuana Research Act would alleviate many of these barriers and open the door into cannabis research.

I look forward to working with my colleagues, on both sides of the aisle, on advancing cannabis policies that are in tune with this new decade.

116th Congress, 1st Session, H.R. 171

To provide for the legitimate use of medicinal marijuana in accordance with the laws of the various States.

In the House of Representatives

January 3, 2019

Mr. GRIFFITH introduced the following bill; which was referred to the Committee on Energy and Commerce

A BILL

To provide for the legitimate use of medicinal marijuana in accordance with the laws of the various States.

Be it enacted by the Senate and House of Representatives of the United States of America in Congress assembled,

Section 1. Short Title

This Act may be cited as the "Legitimate Use of Medicinal Marijuana Act" or the "LUMMA."

Sec. 2. Scheduling of Marijuana; Prescriptions

(a) SCHEDULE.—Marijuana is moved from schedule I of the Controlled Substances Act to schedule II of such Act.

(b) PRESCRIPTION.—

(1) IN GENERAL.—In a State in which marijuana may be prescribed by a physician for medical use under applicable State law, no provision of the Controlled Substances Act (21 U.S.C. 801 et seq.) or of the Federal Food, Drug, and Cosmetic Act (21 U.S.C. 301 et seq.) shall prohibit or otherwise restrict—

(A) the prescription of marijuana by a physician for medical use;

(B) an individual who is an authorized patient from obtaining, possessing, transporting within the individual's State, or using marijuana for that individual's medical use;

(C) an individual authorized under State law to obtain, possess, transport within their State, or manufacture marijuana, from obtaining, possessing, transporting within that State, or manufacturing marijuana pursuant to that authorization; or

(D) a pharmacy or other entity authorized under State law to distribute medical marijuana to an authorized patient, from obtaining or possessing marijuana for that purpose, or from distributing marijuana to an authorized patient for medical use.

(2) PRODUCTION.—No provision of the Controlled Substances Act (21 U.S.C. 801 et. seq.) or of the Federal Food, Drug, and Cosmetic Act (21 U.S.C. 301 et seq.) shall prohibit or otherwise restrict an entity authorized by a State, in which marijuana may be prescribed by a physician for medical use, for the purpose of producing marijuana for prescription by a physician for medical use, from producing, processing, or distributing marijuana for such purpose.

Sec. 3. Definitions

In this Act—

(1) the term "authorized patient" means an individual using marijuana in accordance with a prescription of marijuana by a physician for medical use;

(2) the term "physician" means a practitioner of medicine, who—

(A) graduated from a college of medicine or osteopathy; and

(B) is licensed by the appropriate State board;

(3) the term "prescription" means an instruction written by a medical physician in accordance with applicable State law that authorizes a patient to be issued with a medicine or treatment; and

(4) the term "State" includes the District of Columbia, Puerto Rico, and any other territory or possession of the United States.

Sec. 4. Relation of Act to Certain Prohibitions Relating to Smoking

This Act does not affect any Federal, State, or local law regulating or prohibiting smoking in public.

116th Congress, 1st Session, H. R. 601

To increase the number of manufacturers registered under the Controlled Substances Act to manufacture cannabis for legitimate research purposes, to authorize health care providers of the Department of Veterans Affairs to provide recommendations to veterans regarding participation in federally approved cannabis clinical trials, and for other purposes.

In the House of Representatives

January 16, 2019

Mr. GAETZ (for himself, Mr. SOTO, Mr. PANETTA, Mr. BUCK, and Ms. DEGETTE) introduced the following bill; which was referred to the Committee on Energy and Commerce, and in addition to the Committees on the Judiciary, and Veterans' Affairs, for a period to be subsequently determined by the Speaker, in each case for consideration of such provisions as fall within the jurisdiction of the committee concerned

A BILL

To increase the number of manufacturers registered under the Controlled Substances Act to manufacture cannabis for legitimate research purposes, to authorize health care providers of the Department of Veterans Affairs to provide recommendations to veterans regarding participation in federally approved cannabis clinical trials, and for other purposes.

Be it enacted by the Senate and House of Representatives of the United States of America in Congress assembled,

Section 1. Short Title

This Act may be cited as the "Medical Cannabis Research Act of 2019."

Sec. 2. Increasing the Number of Federally Registered Manufacturers of Cannabis for Legitimate Research Purposes

(a) IN GENERAL.—Section 303 of the Controlled Substances Act (21 U.S.C. 823) is amended—

(1) by redesignating subsection (k) as subsection (l); and

(2) by inserting after subsection (j) the following:

"(k) REGISTRATION OF MANUFACTURERS OF CANNABIS FOR LEGITIMATE RESEARCH PURPOSES.—

"(1) IN GENERAL.—Any manufacturer of cannabis for research shall obtain a separate registration under this subsection for that purpose—

"(A) annually; or

"(B) for a longer period as determined necessary by the Attorney General to supply cannabis for the full duration of a particular multi-year study for legitimate research purposes.

"(2) ADEQUATE AND UNINTERRUPTED SUPPLY.—

"(A) ANNUAL ASSESSMENT.—On an annual basis, the Attorney General shall assess whether there is an adequate and uninterrupted supply of cannabis for legitimate research purposes.

"(B) INITIAL YEAR.—Not later than 1 year after the date of enactment of the Medical Cannabis Research Act of 2019, of the applicants meeting the requirements of this Act, the Attorney General shall register under subsection (a) and this subsection at least 3 applicants to manufacture cannabis for legitimate research purposes in addition to any manufacturers that are registered under subsection (a) to manufacture cannabis as of the date of enactment of the Medical Cannabis Research Act of 2019.

"(C) SUBSEQUENT YEARS.—For calendar year 2019 and each subsequent calendar year, of the applicants meeting the requirements of this Act, the Attorney General shall register (including any registration renewal) under subsection (a) and this subsection at least 4 applicants to manufacture cannabis for legitimate research purposes.

"(3) REQUIREMENTS.—A manufacturer registered under this subsection shall—

"(A) comply with all applicable requirements of this Act;

"(B) limit the transfer and sale of any cannabis manufactured pursuant to this section—

"(i) to researchers who are registered under this Act to conduct research with controlled substances in schedule I; and

"(ii) for purposes of use in preclinical research or in a clinical investigation pursuant to an investigational new drug exemption under 505(i) of the Federal Food, Drug, and Cosmetic Act;

"(C) have completed the application and review process under subsection (a) for the bulk manufacture of controlled substances in schedule I;

"(D) have established and begun operation of a process for storage and handling of controlled substances in schedule I, including for inventory control and monitoring security;

"(E) have the ability to provide at least 10 unique plant cultivars to ensure plant diversity and scale up to produce bulk plant material on an uninterrupted basis sufficient to supply forecasted demand;

"(F) be licensed, by each State in which the manufacturer conducts its operations pursuant to this subsection, to manufacture cannabis;

"(G) have completed a criminal background check for all personnel involved in the operations of the manufacturer pursuant to this subsection to confirm that such personnel have no conviction for a violent felony; and

"(H) have the ability to test for and isolate at least 12 cannabinoids for the purposes of producing specific products for specific studies by compounding pharmacists or others, labeling, and chemical consistency.

"(4) APPLICATION CONTENTS.—As part of an application to be registered under this subsection, an applicant shall include a written explanation of how the applicant's proposed manufacture of cannabis would augment the Nation's supply of cannabis for legitimate research purposes.

"(5) PROCESS.—Not later than 1 year after the date on which the Attorney General receives an application to be registered under this section to manufacture cannabis for research, the Attorney General shall—

"(A) grant, or initiate proceedings under
section 304(c) to deny, the application; or

"(B) request supplemental information from the applicant.

"(6) RULE OF CONSTRUCTION ON REGISTRATION FOR PURPOSES OTHER THAN RESEARCH.— Nothing in this subsection shall be construed to affect the provisions of this section prohibiting or otherwise pertaining to registration of manufacturers of cannabis for purposes other than research, including for purposes of strictly commercial endeavors funded by the private sector and aimed at drug product development.

"(7) NO DISCRIMINATORY TREATMENT BY FEDERAL GOVERNMENT.—Notwithstanding any other provision of law, no Federal department or agency shall deny or limit any funding, other assistance, licensing, or other privilege with respect to any person on the basis that such person is, or is legally receiving cannabis from, a manufacturer of cannabis that is—

"(A) registered under this subsection; and

"(B) in compliance with the requirements of this Act.

"(8) SPECIAL RULE.—If cannabis, or any component thereof, is placed in a schedule other than schedule I, the Attorney General may, as the Attorney General determines appropriate—

"(A) treat the reference to 'subsection (a)' in paragraph (2)(C) of this subsection as a reference to subsection (d); and

"(B) treat the references to schedule I in paragraph (3) as references to the appropriate schedule.

"(9) DEFINITION.—In this subsection, the term 'legitimate research purposes' has the meaning given to such term for purposes of subsection (a)(1)."

(b) TRANSITIONAL PROVISIONS.—

(1) CURRENT REGISTRANTS.—Notwithstanding paragraph (1) of section 303(k) of the Controlled Substances Act, as added by subsection (a), any manufacturer that is registered under section 303(a) of the Controlled Substances Act (21 U.S.C. 823(a)) to manufacture cannabis as of the date of enactment of this Act shall not be required to obtain a separate registration under such section 303(k) for the 1-year period following the date of enactment of this Act.

(2) PENDING APPLICATIONS.—Except as provided in paragraph (1), the Attorney General of the United States shall grant or deny, in accordance with section 303 of the Controlled Substances Act (21 U.S.C. 823), as amended by subsection (a), each application to manufacture cannabis to supply researchers in the United States that was submitted—

(A) pursuant to the policy statement entitled "Applications To Become Registered Under the Controlled Substances Act To Manufacture Marijuana To Supply Researchers in the United States" published by the Drug Enforcement Administration in the Federal Register on August 12, 2016 (81 Fed. Reg. 53846); and

(B) before the date of enactment of this Act.

(c) TECHNICAL AMENDMENT.—Section 102(16) of the Controlled Substances Act (21 U.S.C. 802(16)) is amended by inserting after "The term 'marijuana '" the following: "or 'marijuana' or 'cannabis.'"

Sec. 3. Provision by Department of Veterans Affairs Health Care Providers of Information Regarding Veteran Participation in Federally Approved Cannabis Clinical Trials

(a) PROVISION OF INFORMATION AND FORMS.—Notwithstanding any other provision of law, health care providers of the Department of Veterans Affairs may—

(1) provide information to veterans regarding participation in federally approved cannabis clinical trials; and

(2) complete forms relating to such participation.

(b) RECEIPT OF INFORMATION.—Health care providers and other employees of the Department may accept information regarding federally approved cannabis clinical trials provided by individuals who are not employed by the Department who are researchers registered under the Controlled Substances Act (21 U.S.C. 801 et seq.) to conduct research with controlled substances in schedule I of section 202(c) of such Act (21 U.S.C. 812(c)).

(c) RESEARCH.—The Secretary of Veterans Affairs 23 may conduct research on cannabis if the employees of the Department who are conducting such research are researchers registered under the Controlled Substances Act (21 U.S.C. 801 et seq.) to conduct research with controlled substances in schedule I of section 202(c) of such 2 Act (21 U.S.C. 812(c)).

116th Congress, 1st Session, H. R. 1151

To allow veterans to use, possess, or transport medical marijuana and to discuss the use of medical marijuana with a physician of the Department of Veterans Affairs as authorized by a State or Indian Tribe, and for other purposes.

In the House of Representatives

February 12, 2019

Ms. LEE of California introduced the following bill; which was referred to the Committee on Energy and Commerce, and in addition to the Committees on the Judiciary, and Veterans' Affairs, for a period to be subsequently determined by the Speaker, in each case for consideration of such provisions as fall within the jurisdiction of the committee concerned

A BILL

To allow veterans to use, possess, or transport medical marijuana and to discuss the use of medical marijuana with a physician of the Department of Veterans Affairs as authorized by a State or Indian Tribe, and for other purposes.

Be it enacted by the Senate and House of Representatives of the United States of America in Congress assembled,

Section 1. Short Title

This Act may be cited as the "Veterans Medical Marijuana Safe Harbor Act."

Sec. 2. Findings

Congress finds the following:

(1) Chronic pain affects the veteran population, with almost 60 percent of veterans returning from serving in the Armed Forces in the Middle East, and more than 50 percent of older veterans, who are using the health care system of the Department of Veterans Affairs living with some form of chronic pain.
(2) Opioids account for approximately 63 percent of all drug deaths in the United States.
(3) In 2011, veterans were twice as likely to die from accidental opioid overdoses as nonveterans.
(4) States with medical cannabis laws have a 24.8 percent lower mean annual opioid overdose mortality rate compared with States without medical cannabis laws.
(5) Marijuana and its compounds show promise for treating a wide-range of diseases and disorders, including pain management.
(6) Medical marijuana in States where it is legal may serve as a less harmful alternative to opioids in treating veterans.

Sec. 3. Safe Harbor for Use by Veterans of Medical Marijuana

(a) SAFE HARBOR.—Notwithstanding the Controlled Substances Act (21 U.S.C. 801 et seq.), the Controlled Substances Import and Export Act (21 U.S.C. 951 et seq.), or any other Federal law, it shall not be unlawful for—
  (1) a veteran to use, possess, or transport medical marijuana in a State or on Indian land if the use, possession, or transport is authorized and in accordance with the law of the applicable State or Indian Tribe;
  (2) a physician to discuss with a veteran the use of medical marijuana as a treatment if the physician is in a State or on Indian land where the law of the applicable State or Indian Tribe authorizes the use, possession, distribution, dispensation, administration, delivery, and transport of medical marijuana; or
  (3) a physician to recommend, complete forms for, or register veterans for participation in a treatment program involving medical marijuana that is approved by the law of the applicable State or Indian Tribe.

(b) DEFINITIONS.—In this section:
  (1) INDIAN LAND.—The term "Indian land" means any of the Indian lands, as such term is defined in section 824(b) of the Indian Health Care Improvement Act (25 U.S.C. 1680n).
  (2) INDIAN TRIBE.—The term "Indian Tribe" has the meaning given the term "Indian tribe" in section 4 of the Indian Self-Determination and Education Assistance Act (25 U.S.C. 5304).
  (3) PHYSICIAN.—The term "physician" means a physician appointed by the Secretary of Veterans Affairs under section 7401(1) of title 38, United States Code.
  (4) STATE.—The term "State" has the meaning given that term in section 102 of the Controlled Substances Act (21 U.S.C. 802).
  (5) VETERAN.—The term "veteran" has the meaning given that term in section 101 of title 38, United States Code.

(c) SUNSET.—This section shall cease to have force or effect on the date that is five years after the date of the enactment of this Act.

Sec. 4. Studies on Use of Medical Marijuana by Veterans

(a) STUDY ON EFFECTS OF MEDICAL MARIJUANA ON VETERANS IN PAIN.—

(1) IN GENERAL.—Not later than two years after the date of the enactment of this Act, the Secretary of Veterans Affairs shall conduct a study on the effects of medical marijuana on veterans in pain.

(2) REPORT.—Not later than 180 days after the date on which the study required under paragraph (1) is completed, the Secretary shall submit to Congress a report on the study, which shall include such recommendations for legislative or administrative action as the Secretary considers appropriate.

(b) STUDY ON USE BY VETERANS OF STATE MEDICAL MARIJUANA PROGRAMS.—

(1) IN GENERAL.—Not later than two years after the date of the enactment of this Act, the Secretary shall conduct a study on the relationship between treatment programs involving medical marijuana that are approved by States, the access of veterans to such programs, and a reduction in opioid abuse among veterans.

(2) REPORT.—Not later than 180 days after the date on which the study required under paragraph (1) is completed, the Secretary shall submit to Congress a report on the study, which shall include such recommendations for legislative or administrative action as the Secretary considers appropriate.

(c) VETERAN DEFINED.—In this section, the term “veteran” has the meaning given that term in section 101 of title 38, United States Code.

(d) USE OF AMOUNTS.—For fiscal years 2020 and 2021, of the amounts appropriated to the Department of Veterans Affairs—

(1) $10,000,000 shall be used to carry out subsection (a); and (2) $5,000,000 shall be used to carry out subsection (b).

116th Congress, 1st Session, H. R. 2843

To decriminalize marijuana, and for other purposes.

In the House of Representatives,

May 20, 2019

Mr. JEFFRIES (for himself, Ms. LEE of California, Mr. BLUMENAUER, Ms. NORTON, Ms. SCHAKOWSKY, Mr. COHEN, Miss RICE of New York, Mr. CA′RDENAS, Mr. HUFFMAN, Mr. ESPAILLAT, Ms. CLARKE of New York, Mr. RUSH, Mr. POCAN, Ms. GABBARD, Ms. TLAIB, Mr. JOHNSON of Georgia, Mr. HASTINGS, Mr. SERRANO, Mr.

PERLMUTTER, Mr. TRONE, Mr. LOWENTHAL, Ms. HAALAND, Mr. RASKIN, Ms. JAYAPAL, Mr. MCGOVERN, Ms. CLARK of Massachusetts, Mr. CRIST, Mr. NEGUSE, Mr. CORREA, Mr. ENGEL, Mr. SOTO, Mr. GRIJALVA, and Mr. TED LIEU of California) introduced the following bill; which was referred to the Committee on Energy and Commerce, and in addition to the Committees on the Judiciary, Natural Resources, Agriculture, Transportation and Infrastructure, and Small Business, for a period to be subsequently determined by the Speaker, in each case for consideration of such provisions as fall within the jurisdiction of the committee concerned

A BILL

To decriminalize marijuana, and for other purposes.

Be it enacted by the Senate and House of Representatives of the United States of America in Congress assembled,

Section 1. Short Title

This Act may be cited as the "Marijuana Freedom and Opportunity Act."

Sec. 2. Decriminalization of Marijuana

(a) MARIJUANA REMOVED FROM SCHEDULE OF CONTROLLED SUBSTANCES.—Subsection (c) of schedule I of section 202(c) of the Controlled Substances Act (21 U.S.C. 812) is amended—
  (1) by striking "marijuana"; and
  (2) by striking "tetrahydrocannabinols."

(b) REMOVAL OF PROHIBITION ON IMPORT AND EXPORT.—Section 1010(b) of the Controlled Substances Import and Export Act (21 U.S.C. 960) is amended—
  (1) in paragraph (1)—
    (A) in subparagraph (F), by inserting "or" after the semicolon;
    (B) by striking subparagraph (G); and
    (C) by redesignating subparagraph (H) as subparagraph (G);
  (2) in paragraph (2)—
    (A) in subparagraph (F), by inserting "or" after the semicolon;

(B) by striking subparagraph (G); and

(C) by redesignating subparagraph (H) as subparagraph (G);

(3) in paragraph (3), by striking "paragraphs (1), (2), and (4)" and inserting "paragraphs (1) and 25 (2)";

(4) by striking paragraph (4); and

(5) by redesignating paragraphs (5), (6), and (7) as paragraphs (4), (5), and (6), respectively.

(c) CONFORMING AMENDMENTS TO CONTROLLED SUBSTANCES ACT.—The Controlled Substances Act (21 U.S.C. 801 et seq.) is amended—

(1) in section 102(44) (21 U.S.C. 802(44)), by striking "marijuana,";

(2) in section 401(b) (21 U.S.C. 841(b))—

(A) in paragraph (1)—

(i) in subparagraph (A)—

(I) in clause (vi), by inserting "or" after the semicolon;

(II) by striking (vii); and

(III) by redesignating clause (viii) as clause (vii);

(ii) in subparagraph (B)—

(I) by striking clause (vii); and

(II) by redesignating clause (viii) as clause (vii);

(iii) in subparagraph (C), in the first sentence, by striking "subparagraphs (A), (B), and (D)" and inserting "subparagraphs (A) and (B)";

(iv) by striking subparagraph (D);

(v) by redesignating subparagraph (E) as subparagraph (D); and

(vi) in subparagraph (D)(i), as so redesignated, by striking "subparagraphs (C) and (D)" and inserting "subparagraph 6 (C)";

(B) by striking paragraph (4); and

(C) by redesignating paragraphs (5), (6), and (7) as paragraphs (4), (5), and (6), respectively;

(3) in section 402(c)(2)(B) (21 U.S.C. 842(c)(2)(B)), by striking ", marijuana,";

(4) in section 403(d)(1) (21 U.S.C. 843(d)(1)), by striking ", marijuana,";

(5) in section 418(a) (21 U.S.C. 859(a)), by striking the last sentence;

(6) in section 419(a) (21 U.S.C. 860(a)), by striking the last sentence;

(7) in section 422(d) (21 U.S.C. 863(d))—

(A) in the matter preceding paragraph (1), by striking "marijuana,"; and

(B) in paragraph (5), by striking ", such as a marijuana cigarette,"; and 1

(8) in section 516(d) (21 U.S.C. 886(d)), by striking "section 401(b)(6)" each place the term appears and inserting "section 401(b)(5)."

(d) OTHER CONFORMING AMENDMENTS.—

(1) NATIONAL FOREST SYSTEM DRUG CONTROL ACT OF 1986.—The National Forest System Drug Control Act of 1986 (16 U.S.C. 559b et seq.) is amended—

(A) in section 15002(a) (16 U.S.C. 559b(a)) by striking "marijuana and other";

(B) in section 15003(2) (16 U.S.C. 559c(2)) by striking "marijuana and other"; and

(C) in section 15004(2) (16 U.S.C. 559d(2)) by striking "marijuana and other."

(2) INTERCEPTION OF COMMUNICATIONS.—Section 2516 of title 18, United States Code, is amended—

(A) in subsection (1)(e), by striking "marijuana"; and

(B) in subsection (2) by striking "marijuana."

Sec. 3. Level the Economic Playing Field

(a) ESTIMATE.—On an annual basis, the Secretary of the Treasury shall make a reasonable estimate of total tax revenue generated by the marijuana industry for the previous 12-month period.

(b) TRANSFER.—The Secretary of the Treasury shall transfer from the general fund of the Treasury to the trust fund established under subsection (c) the greater of—

(1) an amount equal to 10 percent of the amount estimated under subsection (a); and 8

(2) $10,000,000.

(c) TRUST FUND.—

(1) IN GENERAL.—There is established in the Treasury of the United States a trust fund to be known as the Marijuana Opportunity Trust Fund, which shall consist of amounts transferred under subsection (b).

(2) USE OF AMOUNTS.—Amounts in the trust fund established under paragraph (1) shall be made available to the Administrator of the Small Business Administration to provide loans under section 7(m) of the Small Business Act (15 U.S.C. 636(m)) to assist—

(A) small business concerns owned and controlled by women, as defined in section 3 of that Act (15 U.S.C. 632), that operate in the marijuana industry; and

(B) small business concerns owned and controlled by socially and economically disadvantaged individuals, as defined in section 8(d)(3)(C) of that Act (15 U.S.C. 637(d)(3)(C)), that operate in the marijuana industry.

Sec. 4. Highway Safety Research

(a) STUDY; DEVELOPMENT.—The Administrator of the National Highway Traffic Safety Administration (referred to in this section as the "Administrator") shall—

(1) carry out a study of the impact of driving under the influence of tetrahydrocannabinol on highway safety; and

(2) develop enhanced strategies and procedures to reliably determine the impairment of a driver under the influence of tetrahydrocannabinol.

(b) AUTHORIZATION OF APPROPRIATIONS.—There is authorized to be appropriated to the Administrator to carry out this section $50,000,000 for each of fiscal years 20 2020 through 2024.

Sec. 5. Public Health Research

(a) IN GENERAL.—The Secretary of Health and Human Services, in consultation with the Director of the National Institutes of Health and the Commissioner of Food and Drugs, shall conduct research on the impacts of marijuana, including—

(1) effects of tetrahydrocannabinol on the human brain;

(2) efficacy of medicinal marijuana as a treatment for specific diseases and conditions; and

(3) identification of additional medical benefits and uses of cannabis.

(b) AUTHORIZATION OF APPROPRIATIONS.—There are authorized to be appropriated to the Secretary of Health and Human Services,

$100,000,000 for each of fiscal years 2020 through 2024, for purposes of carrying out the activities described in subsection (a).

Sec. 6. Protect Kids

The Alcohol and Tobacco Tax and Trade Bureau of the Department of the Treasury shall promulgate regulations that—

(1) require restrictions on the advertising and promotion of products related to marijuana, if the Secretary determines that such regulation would be appropriate for the protection of the public health, taking into account—
   (A) the risks and benefits to the population of individuals age 18 and under, including users and nonusers of marijuana products;
   (B) the increased or decreased likelihood that existing users of marijuana products who are age 18 and under will stop using such products; and
   (C) the increased or decreased likelihood that those age 18 and under who do not use marijuana products will start using such products; and
(2) impose restrictions on the advertising and promotion of products related to marijuana consistent with and to the full extent permitted by the First Amendment to the Constitution of the United States.

Sec. 7. Grants for Expungement of Marijuana Convictions

There is authorized to be appropriated to the Attorney General to award grants to States and units of local government for the purpose of administering, expanding, or developing expungement or sealing programs for convictions of possession of marijuana $20,000,000 for each of fiscal years 2020 through 2024 with not less than 50 percent of those funds being directed to cover the cost of public defenders or legal aid providers.

Sec. 8. Rule of Construction

Nothing in this Act, or an amendment made by this Act, may be construed to modify the authority of the Federal Government to prevent marijuana trafficking from States that have legalized marijuana to those that have not.

Greenwich Biosciences Statement for the Record

Chairwoman Eshoo, Ranking Member Burgess, and Members of the Committee, we thank you for the opportunity to submit this statement regarding the importance of FDA regulation of cannabis-derived products.

Since our founding in 1998, GW Pharmaceuticals has been singularly focused on unlocking the potential of cannabinoids as medicines for development through the FDA pathway. Our drug, Epidiolex®, treats seizures associated with Dravet syndrome (DS) and Lennox Gastaut syndrome (LGS) in patients two years of age and older. DS and LGS are two rare, pediatric-onset, life-threatening and intractable epilepsies. With the approval of Epidiolex in 2018, we became the only company to have brought an FDA-approved cannabis-derived therapy to patients in need.

We have accumulated the most comprehensive body of scientific research on cannabinoids, including cannabidiol (CBD), and fully support FDA's thoughtful consideration of new regulatory pathways for consumer-focused CBD products. We will draw on our scientific research to assist this process.

FDA and Congress should take steps to encourage development of more FDA-approved cannabis drugs. As a result of GW's long-term involvement in cannabinoid research, we have a deep understanding of the promise that patients and their families see in cannabis-based products to treat intractable illnesses. The needs of patients motivated our efforts to research and bring Epidiolex through the FDA process.

In opening the door for consumer-market CBD products, FDA risks further diminishing the likelihood that more cannabis-derived products will be developed into proven medicines. The exclusionary rule embodied in the Dietary Supplement Health and Education Act (DSHEA) – which FDA would have to waive for the first time ever before authorizing CBD consumer goods – was intended by Congress to protect medical innovation. Jeopardizing innovation incentives is a serious concern in any circumstances, but it is particularly concerning for cannabis products.

Congress and FDA need to create a regulatory framework that encourages development of cannabis-derived drugs in a highly unique and saturated consumer market. Congress and FDA should support a comprehensive framework for cannabis-derived medicines that: (1) incentivizes the development of FDA-approved cannabis-derived medicines, (2) ensures the safety of consumer products containing cannabis derivatives, and (3) establishes a clear differentiation between FDA-approved cannabis-derived medicines and foods and dietary supplements containing CBD.

Implement New Policies that Encourage Development of More FDA-approved Cannabis-derived Therapies

Congress and FDA should incentivize the development of FDA-approved cannabis-derived medicines. Cannabis holds promise to treat intractable illnesses, but existing incentives are insufficient. Due to a variety of factors, including competition from unapproved products, incentives to develop and drive competition among FDA-approved cannabis medicines are weakened to begin with.

Patients are self-medicating serious diseases with unapproved cannabis products and allowing CBD in supplements will further jeopardize innovation. It has been estimated that over 3,500,000 Americans use unapproved medical cannabis products.[61] And while for some, these products may offer symptom relief, there are risks to patients from self-directed treatment with unapproved products. A recent case study in Epilepsy and Behavior (2018) describes deaths in two patients who had discontinued conventional therapies in favor of self-directed care with unapproved cannabis-derived products.[62]

Quality deficiencies in unapproved cannabis products also pose safety risks for patients. Recent analyses show that unapproved CBD products frequently go to market containing either significantly higher or lower concentrations of CBD than indicated on the product label.[63] Because these manufacturers do not subject themselves to FDA oversight, there is no robust system in place to ensure product quality, identity, purity, or stability among unapproved cannabis preparations. A 2017 analysis found that after 14 days of storage, CBD content in commercial products is reduced by 15%–20% of initial concentrations, depending on method of oil preparation.[64]

---

[61] Pro Con, Number of Legal Medical Marijuana Patients, May 17, 2018 https://medicalmarijuana.procon.org/view.resource.php?resourceID=005889.

[62] Kollmyer D.M., Wright K.E., Warner N.M., & Doherty M.J. (2019). Are There Mortality Risks for Patients with Epilepsy Who Use Cannabis Treatments as Monotherapy, *Epilepsy Behav Case Rep* 11: 52-53.

[63] Bonn-Miller M.O., et al. (2017). Labeling Accuracy of Cannabidiol Extracts Sold Online, *JAMA* 318(17): 1708-1709 (finding nearly 70 percent of artisanal CBD products tested were mislabeled with respect to CBD content); FDA, Warning Letters and Test Results for Cannabidiol-Related Products, https://www.fda.gov/news-events/public-health-focus/warning-letters-and-test-results-cannabidiol-related-products.

[64] Pacifici R., Marchei E., Salvatore F., et al. (2017). Evaluation of Cannabinoids Concentration and Stability in Standardized Preparations of Cannabis Tea and Cannabis Oil by Ultra-High Performance Liquid Chromatography Tandem Mass Spectrometry, *Clin Chem Lab Med* 55(10): 1555-1563.

Gaps in quality assurance practices for unapproved cannabis preparations allow products to reach the market that are contaminated with a variety of harmful substances, including synthetic cannabinoids, molds, and bacteria.[65] In some cases, such quality deficiencies have serious consequences for patients. A recent case report described an eight-year-old boy who was admitted to the emergency room after consuming a commercial CBD product contaminated with synthetic cannabinoids. The child experienced heightened tonic-clonic episodes, intermittent agitation, delirium, depressed mental status, tachycardia, and mydriasis.[66]

The result is a public health challenge on a nation-wide scale. Not since before 1962 has there been such widespread, uncontrolled use of non-FDA approved products in vulnerable populations and for serious medical conditions. Families and patients see hope in cannabis-based products to treat intractable illnesses, but outside of Dravet and LGS, have no choice but to resort to unapproved drugs.

Ensure the Safety of Consumer Products Containing Cannabis Derivatives

FDA and Congress should work together to ensure consumer products containing CBD are safe. CBD is not a benign substance—it can present real safety risks, including liver toxicity if not used under the supervision and monitoring of a healthcare professional. The available data cannot provide complete assurance of safety in the environment of explosive demand for CBD-based consumer products.

FDA should seek to determine levels of CBD where there is sound data and benchmark safety margins. Liver injury occurs at the lowest dose systematically tested in clinical trials—5mg/kg—which presents an unacceptable safety signal for consumption outside a doctor-patient setting. Liver toxicity is unknown below that level, but benchmark safety margins can be applied to arrive at a dose with reasonable assurance of safety. Benchmarks

---

[65] Horth R.Z., Crouch B., Horowitz B.Z., et al. (2018). Notes from the Field: Acute Poisoning from a Synthetic Cannabinoid Sold as Cannabidiol—Utah, 2017-2018. *Morb Mortal Weekly Rep* 67(20): 587-588; Thompson G.R., Tuscano J.M., et al. (2017). Letter to the Editor: A Microbiome Assessment of Medical Marijuana. *Clin Microbiol Infec* 23.

[66] Rianprakaisang, T., Gerona, R., & Hendrickson, R.G. (2019). Commercial Cannabidiol Oil Contaminated with the Synthetic Cannabinoid AB-FUBINACA Given to a Pediatric Patient. *Clin Toxicol* 24, DOI: 10.1080/15563650.2019.1619758.

suggest safety margins to account for: chronic use (10-fold), person-to-person variability (10-fold), and absence of data establishing levels with no-adverse effects (three-to 10-fold). A safe level should account for risk of cumulative exposure; demand is so explosive that consumers may ingest CBD from multiple sources per day. Rulemaking should also account for the potential presence of THC in finished products—it is a myth that CBD consumer products on the market today are free of THC.

Ensure That Consumer-Market Products Containing Cannabis Derivatives are Clearly Differentiated from FDA-Approved Prescription Medications

FDA and Congress should take measures to differentiate between cannabis-derived medicines and CBD products. FDA should use its broad authority to ensure clear differentiation of medicines from consumer products, both for the sake of safety and to preserve the DSHEA principle that prescription drug ingredients should not later be introduced in consumer products. FDA should also close loopholes (e.g., "hemp extracts") that might allow circumvention of CBD rulemaking.

GW Envisions a Clear Path Forward for the Development and Regulation of Cannabis-derived Products

GW envisions a clear path forward for the development of cannabis-derived products through FDA's esteemed regulatory review pathway. Epidiolex has proven that cannabis-derived medicines can be successfully developed through the FDA pathway. For patients living with DS and LGS, their cannabis medicine meets the same "gold standard" applicable to every other approved prescription drug in the United States since 1962. As FDA undertakes rulemaking to create pathways for consumer-market CBD products, its focus should be directed equally toward other patient populations who could benefit from safe and effective cannabis-derived treatments that have yet to be developed.

GW supports a comprehensive approach to the regulation of cannabis-derived products because we believe that such an approach can create conditions that support development of new FDA-approved medicines from the cannabis plant while, in parallel, protecting consumers from unsafe products, bringing much-needed regulation to the existing marketplace, satisfying consumer demand, and creating new economic and agricultural opportunities.

Letter of January 14, 2020, from Stephen A. Frangos, M.D., President, American College of Occupational and Environmental Medicine, to Ms. Eshoo and Mr. Burgess, submitted by Ms. Eshoo

January 14, 2020
The Honorable Anna G. Eshoo
Chair
Subcommittee on Health
U.S. House of Representatives
Washington, DC 20515

The Honorable Michael Burgess
Ranking Member
Subcommittee on Health
U.S. House of Representatives
Washington, D.C. 20515

Dear Chairman Eshoo and Ranking Member Burgess:

The American College of Occupational and Environmental Medicine (ACOEM) requests that this letter be included in the record of the January 15 hearing of thel Subcommittee on Health.

ACOEM recognizes the strong Congressional interest in moving forward on cannabis policies. However, before doing so, federal policy must consider the implications of cannabis use on workplace and public safety.

ACOEM is the pre-eminent physician-led organization that champions the health of and safety of workers and workplaces. The College is dedicated to improving the care and wellbeing of workers through science and the sharing of knowledge. From this perspective, ACOEM offers the following insights for the Subcommittee's consideration.

Employers have a legal responsibility to protect employees from workplace illness or injury under the Occupational Safety and Health

Administration's (OSHA's) general duty clause. Employers also have an ethical responsibility to prevent impaired workers from endangering themselves, their co-workers, and/or the general public.

Regardless of marijuana's legal status in a jurisdiction, Congress should ensure national uniformity in policies with respect to jobs where marijuana use could adversely affect the employee's safety or that of others. This includes allowing employers to establish policies that prohibit the use of cannabis products for all employees due to the inability to test for impairment.

Without measurable concentrations of psychoactive ingredients in marijuana-containing products or known potency of the active ingredient, it is currently impossible to use evidence-based methods to evaluate marijuana impairment in the workplace. While there is much we do not know about marijuana, we know enough to raise concern and caution with regard to federal action:

- Cannabis can significantly impair judgment, motor coordination, and reaction time. Studies have found a direct relationship between blood (usually serum) THC concentrations and impaired driving ability, although the degree of impairment cannot be defined by the level, especially at lower levels.
- It is well documented that persons experiencing impairment from any drug or medication tend to underestimate the severity of their impairment.
- States with legal recreational or medical marijuana are reporting an increase in fatal motor vehicle crashes involving THC (the main psychoactive ingredient in marijuana).
- Those in jobs where marijuana use could adversely affect the safety of others should be held to a higher standard until a scientifically valid method to identify impairment has been developed.

ACOEM recommends that the following be part the process when considering federal legislation:

- Allow employers the latitude to manage risk. In an area where knowledge of risk and impairment is falling far behind the rapidly expanding use of marijuana and other cannabinoids, employers must be able to manage risk in the workplace.

- Reconcile the differences between state and federal laws and establish uniformity regarding marijuana use and the impact on workplace and public safety.
- Assess the impact of cannabis on workplace safety through research.
- Define the correlation of THC concentrations and impairment.
- Identify a reliable, practical mechanism for employers to assess fitness for duty. This is especially important in those states where medical and/or recreational use of marijuana is legal.
- As previously stated, except where specified by law, allow the employer to have primary responsibility to ensure the safety of both employees and the general public. Employers are the ones best suited to determine if a job is safety sensitive and, until the science of marijuana impairment is resolved, an employer should not be expected to manage a risk until that risk can be measured.

In short, marijuana is an impairing substance, and its legalization has huge public and workplace safety implications. Before Congress passes any legislation regarding marijuana, the ACOEM urges legislators to consider carefully the impact of such legislation on workplace safety.

Sincerely,

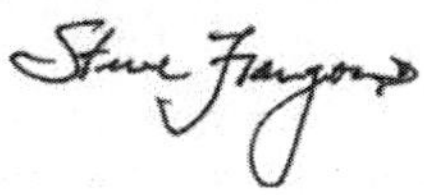

Stephen A. Frangos, MD, MPH, FACOEM
President

Statement of the National Safety Council

Thank you for holding this important hearing, "Cannabis Policies for the New Decade," and for allowing the National Safety Council (NSC) to submit comments for the record.

NSC is a 100-year-old nonprofit organization with the mission of eliminating preventable deaths at work, in homes and communities, and on the road through leadership, research, education, and advocacy. Its more than 16,000 member companies represent employees at more than 50,000 U.S. worksites.

Cannabis laws are changing rapidly, and NSC is concerned that safety is being left behind in policy discussions. The fact that cannabis is an impairing substance is rarely mentioned. NSC encourages this committee to prioritize the safety, health and wellbeing of your constituents as you consider effective federal cannabis policies. It is imperative that this committee keep public safety at the forefront of policy decisions.

We would like to add information to the hearing record on the following topics:

1) Employers should be able to maintain a substance-free workplace.
2) Workers in safety sensitive positions should not be allowed to use cannabis.
3) More research needs to be conducted on cannabis effects, especially regarding safety.
4) Greater funding is needed for drug recognition experts.
5) The developing brain is especially susceptible to damage from drug exposure.
6) Cannabis and cannabis-derived products need robust and accurate labeling.

As you know, state laws vary, but cannabis and cannabidiol (CBD) containing more than 0.3% tetrahydrocannabinol (THC) remain federally illegal.[67] Despite this, cannabis is the most widely consumed illicit substance worldwide, and nearly 55 million Americans 18 or older currently use cannabis.[68] This use affects safety on the roadways, in workplaces and elsewhere. Even in some occupations governed by federal oversight, cannabis use has increased recently as state laws have changed. In other occupations, cannabis positivity has increased in states with recreational use.

As seen from the following charts, state legal treatment of cannabis impacts usage rates. Currently, 11 states have decriminalized cannabis for adult recreational use and 33 permit medical cannabis use. As state legislators return to work, these numbers could increase in the coming months. Changes in state laws have created uncertainty and concern about impairment in workplaces, on the roadways and in other locations. Given the increased use of cannabis among the workforce, especially in states that have legalized and

[67] https://www.who.int/substance_abuse/facts/cannabis/en/.

[68] http://maristpoll.marist.edu/wp-content/misc/Yahoo%20News/20170417_Summary%20Yahoo%20News-Marist%20Poll_Weed%20and%20The%20American%20Family.pdf.

decriminalized cannabis, employer drug testing should be allowed so employers can make decisions that are right for their organizations.

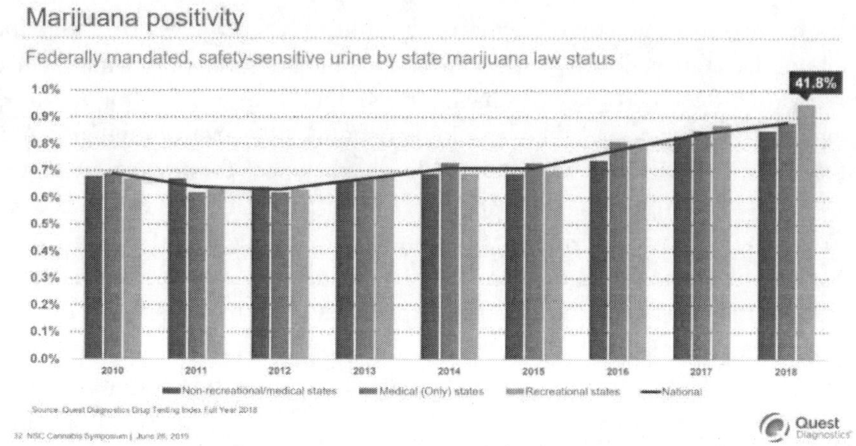

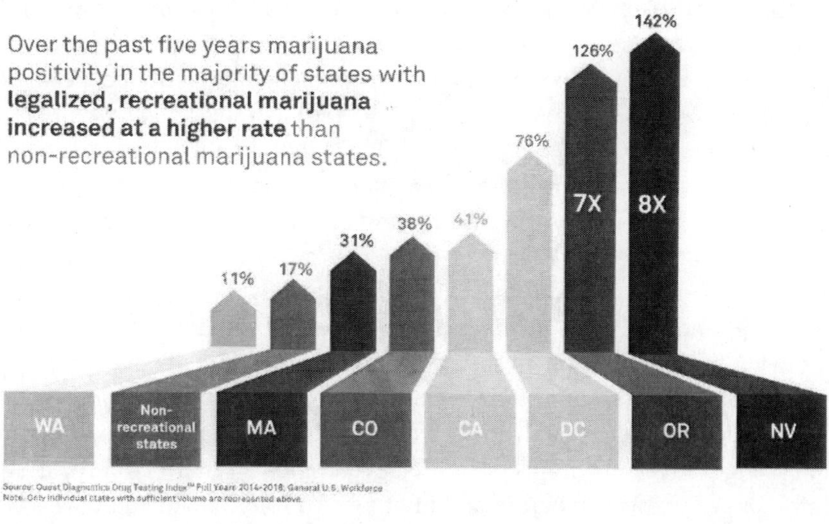

NSC believes that all forms of impairment present a serious threat to safety at work by increasing the risk of preventable injury and death. Workers who are under the influence of alcohol and/or other impairing drugs (legal or illegal) endanger themselves and those around them. NSC supports employer efforts to maintain a substance-free workplace to help ensure the safety of workers.[69]

NSC also believes it is unsafe to be under the influence of cannabis while working in safety sensitive positions.[70] With no scientific test for cannabis impairment, there is no way to determine if someone is impaired with the drug tests available today. If workers have a prescription for cannabis or any other impairing drug, they and their employers should talk about moving to non-safety sensitive positions while taking those substances for medical treatment.

Impairment from cannabis use is not only a concern in the workplace, but also on the roadway. Driving while under the influence of an impairing substance like cannabis endangers all roadway users. However, because there is no scientific test for cannabis impairment, law enforcement relies on drug recognition experts (DREs) to evaluate the signs of impairment from drugs. The U.S. needs more DREs, and Congress should support funding for more DRE training.

The lack of an impairment test and more meaningful data on effects of cannabis are problems we can solve, and NSC urges this committee to evaluate methods to increase research on cannabis. NSC is concerned about the secondary effects of moving cannabis from Schedule 1 of the *Controlled Substances Act*; therefore, NSC supports the bipartisan *Cannabidiol and Marijuana Research Expansion Act* (S. 2032) that would expand the number of institutions conducting research without changing the scheduling of cannabis. NSC encourages the introduction of similar legislation in the House.

Additional issues are arising as the legal status of cannabis is debated. As previously shown, cannabis use in states that have changed their laws is increasing, and this trend includes adolescents.[71] The human brain continues to develop through the mid-twenties, and during this time of development, the brain is sensitive to damage from drug exposure.[72] In 2015, more than 11 million individuals ages 18 to 25 used cannabis.[73] Exposure to cannabis during adolescence adversely impacts brain development.[74] Furthermore, a study comparing cannabis use before and after age 16 found that people who use it

[69] https://www.nsc.org/Portals/0/Documents/NSCDocuments_Corporate/Policy-Positions/Workplace/W-Substance-Free%20Workplace-140.pdf.

[70] "Safety Sensitive" refers to jobs that impact safety of the employee and the safety of others as a result of performing that job. For example, 49 CFR §382.107 defines safety sensitive for commercial motor vehicle operators.

[71] https://jamanetwork.com/journals/jamapediatrics/fullarticle/2593707.

[72] https://www.ncbi.nlm.nih.gov/pmc/articles/PMC3621648/.

[73] https://www.drugabuse.gov/publications/drugfacts/cannabis.

[74] https://www.ncbi.nlm.nih.gov/pmc/articles/PMC4033190/.

before age 16 made twice as many mistakes on tests of executive function including planning, flexibility, abstract thinking and inhibition of inappropriate responses.[75] Congress should be aware of these impacts as you evaluate cannabis policies.

Additionally, labeling requirements for cannabis and cannabis-derived products is unclear, and in some cases unsubstantiated claims are being made. NSC applauds the oversight that has been utilized by some of the agencies here today and encourages more oversight. NSC believes all cannabis and cannabis-derived products being sold and distributed must have child-resistant packaging that specifies serving sizes and concentration of THC, packaging not appealing to children and inclusion of appropriate warning labels. Additional labeling should be considered to prioritize safety and prevent unintended consequences.

There is a great deal to consider as we evaluate changing federal and state laws dealing with cannabis. NSC appreciates the thoughtful time and effort of the Committee in evaluating proposed policy changes and the attention on safety impacts. NSC looks forward to working with you to prioritize safety.

* * *

Letter of January 14, 2020, from the National Consumers League, to Members of the Energy and Commerce Health Subcommittee, submitted by Ms. Eshoo

TO: Members of the Energy and Commerce Health Subcommittee
FROM: Consumers for Safe CBD
DATE: January 14, 2020

RE: Tomorrow's hearing on **"Cannabis Policies for the New Decade"**

The National Consumers League (NCL) recently launched Consumers for Safe CBD in partnership with Consumer Federation of America (CFA) and Community Anti-Drug Coalitions of America (CADCA) to encourage FDA to take strong, effective, and prompt action to protect the public from the potential harms posed by unregulated cannabidiol (CBD). In advance of this

[75] https://www.apa.org/monitor/2015/11/marijuana-brain.

week's hearing on "Cannabis Policies for the New Decade," we wanted to provide you with helpful materials on the rapidly growing and yet, to date, unregulated CBD market.

There are many misconceptions related to CBD and CBD products. Consumers assume the products sold in stores and online are regulated by the FDA, are "pure" CBD as they are often marketed, and pose no threat to their health. In reality, CBD products are often mislabeled and untested, and clinical trials show CBD is associated with potentially dangerous drug interactions and liver damage, or might be injurious to men's reproductive health.

Late last year, the FDA announced it "cannot conclude" that CBD is generally recognized as safe (GRAS) for its use in human or animal food "based on the lack of scientific information supporting the safety of CBD in food." While this determination by the FDA is critically important, we feel strongly that the agency must take additional steps to regulate consumers' cumulative daily consumption of CBD.

This sentiment has broad support. Consumers for Safe CBD recently released public opinion research conducted by Greenberg Quinlan Rosner finding that voters overwhelmingly – an 83 percent majority – support allowing the FDA to test and regulate CBD products. The research found that ensuring the safety and effectiveness of CBD grows even stronger among those who have used CBD products or describe themselves as very familiar with them.

As you discuss cannabis policies this week and in the coming months, we encourage you to consider FDA's recent actions and their impact on consumer decision-making and provide guidance to the FDA on what Congress believes needs to be done to protect consumers in a rapidly expanding yet unregulated CBD marketplace. Below are sample questions that we recommend should be addressed.

- Are you concerned consumers are buying approximately $500 million annually worth of CBD products that may or may not be safe?
- What regulatory actions is the FDA considering to provide consumers with better information about the safety and efficacy of CBD products?
- Does the FDA need more Congressional authority to regulate this burgeoning marketplace where the long-term effects of CBD is largely unknown?

- Do you believe the FDA should enforce current laws against CBD and other products that make untested/unproven medical claims that pose a high risk to consumers?
- Do you believe the FDA should define safe concentration levels of CBD?
- Do you support further research for FDA-approved CBD treatments so that consumers can have more options and more trust in the marketplace?

Thank you for your interest in this consumer health issue. We are available as a resource on CBD and the impact on consumers at any time. Please do not hesitate to reach out to National Consumers League Executive Director Sally Greenberg at Sallyg@nclnet.org at any time.

Written Testimony of David L. Nathan, MD, DFAPA

Doctors for Cannabis Regulation (DFCR) writes today in support of cannabis regulation as an alternative to the failed policy of prohibition – a prohibition that is rooted in the federal Controlled Substances Act (CSA).

DFCR is the nation's premier physicians' association dedicated to the legalization, taxation and – above all – the effective regulation of cannabis for adults. DFCR has hundreds of respected physician members in nearly every US state and territory. DFCR physicians include integrative medicine pioneer Andrew Weil, former Surgeon General Joycelyn Elders, renowned public health physician and Johns Hopkins professor Chris Beyrer, and retired clinical director of SAMHSA, H. Westley Clark.

While we are disappointed that this hearing has included only government witnesses who support the continued illegality of cannabis, we appreciate the committee's willingness to accept this written testimony into the record. We would like to share the scientific and historical evidence that contradicts frequently repeated myths about cannabis, its inclusion in the Controlled Substances Act, and its resultant prohibition.

History

In 1937, the American Medical Association sent Dr. William Woodward to the House of Representatives to testify against the proposed prohibition of cannabis.[76] Refuting hyperbolic tabloid claims, he testified that cannabis is not highly addictive, does not cause violence in users, and does not cause fatal overdoses. He reasoned that cannabis should, therefore, be regulated rather than prohibited. Scientific evidence now confirms that Dr. Woodward was correct.[77,78,79]

In 1969, when the US Supreme Court declared the 1937 law against cannabis to be unconstitutional, the Federal Government was faced with a choice between legalization or another means of continuing the drug's prohibition. President Nixon appointed the Shafer Commission to study the health effects of cannabis and recommend a course of action. To the surprise of many, this blue-ribbon commission concluded that cannabis should *not* be included in new controlled substance legislation, but rather should be regulated like alcohol, which is not scheduled at all.

The commission's findings were ultimately rejected by the Federal Government, which was eager to include cannabis in its nascent "War on Drugs." Fear, not science, was the motivation for cannabis' inclusion in the Controlled Substances Act (CSA), where it was placed in the most restrictive category, along with heroin and PCP.

Cannabis, the Controlled Substances Act, and Obstacles to Research

According to the CSA, a Schedule I drug must meet three specific criteria: "high potential for abuse," "no currently accepted medical use," and "lack of

---

[76] *Taxation of Marihuana, hearings before the House Committee on Ways and Means*, 75th Congress, lst Session, May 4, 1937, cited in "The Prescience of William C. Woodward." Doctors for Cannabis Regulation, 2015. https://dfcr.org/the-prescience-of-william-c-woodward/.

[77] National Academies of Sciences, Engineering, and Medicine. *The health effects of cannabis and cannabinoids: The current state of evidence and recommendations for research.* Washington, DC: The National Academies Press, 2017. https://www.nap.edu/catalog/24625/the-health-effects-of-cannabis-and-cannabinoids-the-current-state.

[78] "Learn About Marijuana: Marijuana and Aggression," Alcohol and Drug Abuse Institute, University of Washington, 3/2015. http://learnaboutmarijuanawa.org/factsheets/aggression.htm.

[79] Collen, Mark. "Prescribing cannabis for harm reduction." *Harm Reduct J.* 2012; 9:1. http://www.ncbi.nlm.nih.gov/pmc/articles/PMC3295721/.

accepted safety." Cannabis does not meet any of these criteria. Cannabis does not share the high abuse potential associated with other Schedule I drugs or other legal recreational substances. According to a comprehensive review by the National Academy of Medicine, cannabis's dependence liability is similar to that of caffeine (9 percent), and it is far lower than dependence associated with alcohol (15 percent) and tobacco (32 percent).[80] Cannabis has a well-researched safety profile, and it possesses no documented risk of lethal overdose.[81] According to a United Nations Report, "There are no confirmed cases of human deaths from cannabis poisoning in the world medical literature."[82] FDA-approved trials[83] and a comprehensive 2017 review by the National Academies of Science, Engineering, and Medicine[84] support the safety and efficacy of cannabis in various patient populations. Today, most states and a majority of physicians recognize the therapeutic value and relative safety of cannabis.[85]

But even if it had no medical value, a free society does not punish competent adults for the personal use of a non-lethal plant. The Federal Government must stop using a sledgehammer to kill a weed.

For years, DFCR has urged the FDA to remove cannabis from the CSA. They have repeatedly refused to do so, citing support for their position from the DEA and NIDA. These groups have claimed that they support more research on cannabis, yet they have continued to block most research.

They have also refused to allow facilities other than the University of Mississippi to cultivate strains for research, despite several years of court

---

[80] National Academies of Science, Engineering and Medicine. *Marijuana and Medicine: Assessing the Science Base*. Washington, DC: The National Academies Press, 1999. Page 95: Table 3.4: Prevalence of Drug Use and Dependence in the General Population. https://www.nap.edu/catalog/6376/marijuana-and-medicine-assessing-the-science-base.

[81] Calabria B, et al. (2010) "Does cannabis use increase the risk of death? A systematic review of epidemiological evidence on adverse effects of cannabis use." *Drug Alcohol Rev* 2010 May;29(3):318-30. https://www.ncbi.nlm.nih.gov/pubmed/20565525.

[82] Martin, B.R. and Hall, W. "The health effects of cannabis: key issues of policy relevance." United Nations Office on Drugs and Crime, December 1, 1999 https://www.unodc.org/unodc/en/data-and-analysis/bulletin/bulletin_1997-01-01_1_page005.html.

[83] Grant, I., Atkinson, J. H., Gouaux, B., & Wilsey, B. (2012). "Medical marijuana: clearing away the smoke." *The Open Neurology Journal*, 6, 18–25. https://www.ncbi.nlm.nih.gov/pmc/articles/PMC3358713/.

[84] National Academies of Sciences, Engineering, and Medicine. *The health effects of cannabis and cannabinoids: The current state of evidence and recommendations for research*. Washington, DC: The National Academies Press, 2017. https://www.nap.edu/catalog/24625/the-health-effects-of-cannabis-and-cannabinoids-the-current-state.

[85] Rappold, R. Scott. "Legalize Medical Marijuana, Doctors Say in Survey." WebMD, 2014. http://www.webmd.com/news/breaking-news/marijuana-on-main-street/20140225/webmd-marijuana-survey-web.

orders to do so. This is a major impediment to research that they have cynically claimed to support, because cannabis grown at the University of Mississippi has THC levels that are closer to those of non-psychoactive hemp than they are to today's psychoactive cannabis strains.

The Folly of Cannabis Prohibition

As physicians, we believe that cannabis should never have been made illegal for consenting adults. It is less harmful to adults than alcohol and tobacco, and the prohibition has done far more damage to our society than the adult use of cannabis itself.

Of course, cannabis is not harmless. People who are predisposed to psychotic disorders should avoid any cannabis use. Also, as with alcohol and other drugs, heavy cannabis use may adversely affect brain development in minors.[86] But cannabis prohibition for adults doesn't prevent underage use nor limit its availability. The government's own statistics show that 80-90% of eighteen-year-olds have consistently reported easy access to the drug since the 1970s.[87] For decades, preventive education has reduced the rates of alcohol and tobacco use by minors,[88] At the same time, underage cannabis use rose steadily despite its prohibition. In the past several years – as more states legalize cannabis for adults – the rate of underage cannabis use has stopped increasing.

Some have argued that if cannabis is legal for adults, then minors will think it's safe for them. But when cannabis is against the law for everyone, the government sends the message that cannabis is dangerous for everyone. Teenagers know that's not true. By creating a legal distinction between cannabis use by adults and minors, we teach our children a respect for

---

[86] Schweinsburg, et al. "The Influence of Marijuana Use on Neurocognitive Functioning in Adolescents." *Curr Drug Abuse Rev.* 2008 Jan; 1(1): 99–111. http://www.ncbi.nlm.nih.gov/pmc/articles/PMC2825218/.

[87] Johnston, Lloyd. *Monitoring the Future: National Survey Results on Drug Use, 1975-2008: Volume II: College Students and Adults Ages 19-50.* Bethesda, MD: National Institute on Drug Abuse, 2009. http://monitoringthefuture.org/pubs/monographs/vol2_2008.pdf.

[88] U.S. Department of Health and Human Services. *The Health Consequences of Smoking—50 Years of Progress: A Report of the Surgeon General.* Atlanta, GA: U.S. Department of Health and Human Services, Centers for Disease Control and Prevention, National Center for Chronic Disease Prevention and Health Promotion, Office on Smoking and Health, 2014. http://www.cdc.gov/tobacco/data_statistics/sgr/50th-anniversary/index.htm.

scientific evidence – and the sanctity of the law. This may be why teen use has remained level or decreased in legalized states.[89,90]

There is a persistent misconception that cannabis is a "gateway" drug. While users of hard drugs often try cannabis first, they're even more likely to try alcohol and tobacco. People generally try less dangerous drugs before trying more dangerous drugs, but the vast majority of those who try cannabis, alcohol and tobacco never go on to use harder drugs. The risk of drug misuse and addiction is now known to be largely due to pre-existing genetic and environmental risk factors,[91] not the use of cannabis, alcohol, or other so-called "soft" drugs. As we learned in high school, correlation does not imply causation.

In 2020, even those who oppose legalization generally believe that cannabis should be decriminalized. But decriminalization is an inadequate substitute for legalization. In legalized states, government licensed retailers scrupulously check IDs and only sell cannabis products to adults.[92] But where cannabis is merely decriminalized, the point-of-sale remains in the hands of drug dealers who sell cannabis – along with more dangerous drugs – to children.

Conclusion

Cannabis should never have been included in the Controlled Substances Act, and today the science is clearer than ever that cannabis – like alcohol – is best controlled when it is regulated rather than criminally prohibited.

Informed physicians may disagree about the specifics of good regulation, but we can no longer support a prohibition that has done so much damage to

[89] Hasin et al. 2015. "Medical marijuana laws and adolescent marijuana use in the USA from 1991 to 2014: results from annual, repeated cross-sectional surveys." *Lancet Psychiatry* 2: 601-608. http://www.ncbi.nlm.nih.gov/pubmed/26303557.

[90] Colorado Department of Public Safety. Impacts of marijuana legalization to Colorado. 2018. https://www.colorado.gov/pacific/publicsafety/news/colorado-division-criminal-justice-publishes-report-impacts-marijuana-legalization-colorado.

[91] Quenqua, Douglas. "A Comeback for the Gateway Drug Theory?" *The New York Times*, December 7, 2017. https://www.nytimes.com/2017/12/07/well/live/a-comeback-for-the-gateway-drug-theory.html?_r=0. See also: Valdez, Avelardo et al. "Aggressive Crime, Alcohol and Drug Use, and Concentrated Poverty in 24 U.S. Urban Areas." *Am J Drug Alcohol Abuse*. 2007; 33(4): 595–603. http://www.tandfonline.com/doi/full/10.1080/00952990701407637.

[92] Buller DB, Woodall WG, Saltz R, Buller MK. "Compliance With Personal ID Regulations by Recreational Marijuana Stores in Two U.S. States." *J Stud Alcohol Drugs* 2019; 80 (6), 679-686. https://www.ncbi.nlm.nih.gov/pubmed/31829920.

public health and personal liberty. Members of the House Energy and Commerce Committee, please work with us to advance public health and protect our children by supporting effective, evidence-based regulation that pending legislation – including the MORE Act – would make possible.

We thank you for your attention to this timely issue.

Respectfully submitted on behalf of the DFCR Board of Directors,

David L. Nathan, MD, DFAPA
Board President, Doctors for Cannabis Regulation
dnathan@dfcr.org 609-688-0400
601 Ewing Street, Suite C-10, Princeton NJ 08540

Testimony of Aaron Smith, Executive Director, National Cannabis Industry Association

Introduction

Chairwoman Eshoo, Ranking Member Burgess, and members of the subcommittee, good morning. I am Aaron Smith, Executive Director and Co-Founder of the National Cannabis Industry Association (NCIA). NCIA is the largest national trade association dedicated to protecting state-regulated cannabis businesses and advancing policy reforms needed to harmonize federal marijuana law with the successful medical and adult-use state cannabis programs that exist throughout the country. Founded in 2010, NCIA represents nearly 2,000 cannabis-related member businesses and tens of thousands of cannabis professionals across the United States.

For almost a century, the United States government has criminalized the production, distribution, and sale of cannabis. However, this era of prohibition has been crumbling in the face of voter and, increasingly, legislative revolt. Even as these federal laws remain unchanged, most states have legalized some form of medical cannabis, and eleven states and the District of Columbia have changed their laws to regulate adult-use cannabis in a manner similar to alcohol. Moreover, Congress recently removed hemp (and any cannabinoids derived therefrom) from the Controlled Substances Act (CSA), legalizing a subset of cannabis plants and derivatives that contain less than 0.3% THC. A recent Gallup poll indicated that 90% of the population supports the legalization of cannabis for medical purposes, and 66% favor allowing recreational use. It is undeniable that the American people are in favor of the legalization of cannabis. It is time for Congress to reflect the will of their constituents. For these, and a multitude of other reasons, I applaud the subcommittee for holding this incredibly important hearing.

As the leading advocate for the state-regulated cannabis industry, NCIA has offered reasoned and responsible approaches that the federal government could adopt to regulate cannabis products after the last vestiges of federal prohibition are removed. Our plan begins with removing cannabis from the Controlled Substances Act – the only way to address the myriad problems caused by our nation's outdated cannabis policies, including the proliferation of unregulated and sometimes unsafe – cannabis products produced in the criminal marijuana market, loss of potential tax revenue, a lack of transparency in the banking system, and misappropriation of scarce law enforcement resources. For more than two decades, states have moved away from the prohibition approach and over two-thirds of Americans now live in a state with laws allowing for the regulated production and sale of cannabis for either medical or adult-use purposes.

NCIA Supports Comprehensive Reform: Descheduling & Regulating Cannabis

There have been scores of cannabis-related bills introduced over the past few years, including the Marijuana Justice Act, the Strengthening The Tenth Amendment Through Entrusting States (STATES) Act, the Secure And Fair Enforcement (SAFE) Banking Act, the Small Business Tax Equity Act, and most recently, the Marijuana Opportunity Reinvestment and Expungement (MORE) Act, which passed out of the House Judiciary Committee on November 20, 2019. NCIA has been at the forefront, advocating in support of each and every one of these bills on behalf of our broad membership base. We commend Speaker Pelosi for bringing the SAFE Banking Act to the Floor. The end result - a vote in favor of cannabis banking - passed by a bipartisan vote of 321-103. This historic vote was not only extremely consequential, but also marks the first step toward recognizing this burgeoning American industry. The state-legal cannabis industry employs more than 200,000 people (with annual growth of 34%) and is estimated to have generated roughly $12 billion in retail sales in 2019. Longer term projections see annual retail sales in the United States surpassing $28 billion by 2023. The cannabis industry delivered an estimated $40 billion economic impact on the United States in 2019. By 2023, it is estimated that the economic impact could exceed $100 billion. The industry is projected to add roughly 235,000 new jobs by 2023. By 2023, the cannabis industry could provide the equivalent of 475,000 full time jobs.[93] There is no other American industry seeing this type of growth and it is time for our federal government to start fully supporting it.

It is therefore our sincere hope that Congress will take a more comprehensive, end-of-prohibition approach in the coming months. Our member-businesses, consumers, the banking industry, and even the federal government would benefit most from more comprehensive reforms that remove marijuana from the Controlled Substances Act and begin the process of regulating the substance at the federal level. It will be through regulation and testing that we are able to displace the illicit market and bring safe and reliable products to adult consumers. De-scheduling and regulating is the responsible approach for the sake of public safety, public health, and public opinion.

It is crucial to remember that what Congress does today will shape the American cannabis industry for decades to come. Outdated and ineffective prohibition policies have caused pain for many, particularly for communities of color. While a new system is being considered, policy makers should strive to create a legal cannabis market accessible to patients and responsible adults that is designed and implemented with equity and fairness in mind. Legislation under consideration during this hearing today would do just that.

H.R. 3884, the Marijuana Opportunity Reinvestment and Expungement (MORE) Act, would federally decriminalize cannabis by removing it from the Controlled Substances Act, and would require the expungement of past federal cannabis convictions. The bill would establish a Cannabis Justice Office to administer a program to reinvest resources in the communities that have been most heavily impacted by prohibition, funded by a 5% tax on state-legal cannabis commerce. It would also allow the Small Business Administration to provide loans and grants to cannabis-related businesses and support state and local equity licensing programs, and would permit doctors within the Veterans Affairs system to recommend medical cannabis to patients in accordance with applicable state laws. NCIA supports all of these efforts, however, we urge Congress to amend the bill by including a regulatory structure to safeguard the public and provide clear direction to the cannabis industry. The federalism

[93] Marijuana Business Daily, Annual Marijuana Business Factbook, 7th Edition (2019).

clash that exists in current law is untenable and is not working for businesses, consumers, or policymakers, among others.

NCIA will continue to advocate for cannabis to be removed from the Controlled Substances Act, commonly referred to as "de-scheduling." De-scheduling is the best approach in order to immediately solve myriad problems related to banking, payment processing, tax parity, as well as public health issues that will be critical to address in a post-legalization world. But, merely de-scheduling is not enough. We need to remove cannabis from the Controlled Substances Act and provide for reasonable social equity reforms that create opportunities for new entrepreneurs and repair some of the damage done by prohibition.

Along with de-scheduling, NCIA recommends that cannabis products, like other highly-regulated consumables, to be regulated by the government agencies that currently regulate most food and drugs, primarily the Food and Drug Administration (FDA) and the Alcohol and Tobacco Tax and Trade Bureau (TTB) within the U.S. Department of the Treasury. NCIA recently issued a comprehensive regulatory plan entitled, "Adapting a Proven Regulatory Framework for the Cannabis Industry" that Congress could adopt.[94] To best address both market and public health concerns, NCIA recommends that cannabis products be divided into four categories, based on chemical components, safety, intended use, and consumption method. Each of these groups would be regulated through a separate regulatory "lane" tailored to the public policy issues raised by that particular classification. The four lanes are: (1) Pharmaceutical drugs; (2) Ingested, inhaled, or topically applied products with more than de minimis amounts of THC; (3) Ingested and inhaled products with de minimis amounts of THC; and (4) Topically applied products with de minimis amounts of THC. This four-lane structure would allow for adequate controls and retail restrictions over products that have psychoactive effects, while allowing greater consumer access to non-psychoactive cannabinoid products.

Public Health & Product Safety

Successful development of a regulatory lane for cannabis products is essential to achieving key policy goals: promoting public health, improving public

---

[94] https://thecannabisindustry.org/reports/adapting-a-regulatory-framework-for-the-emerging-cannabis-industry/.

safety, eliminating the illicit market, creating regulatory certainty and efficiency in the legal market, and generating public revenues, both direct and indirect. As with other products with potentially intoxicating properties, appropriate warning labels should be developed and retail locations should be licensed by the state.

NCIA believes that the FDA should play the same role for cannabis products that it performs in alcohol regulation: protecting public health by registering production facilities, performing inspections in accord with standards most directly applicable to the product, evaluating the safety of non-cannabis-derived ingredients, and monitoring for any adulterants. States would continue to regulate the composition and potency of cannabis-derived ingredients.

A common concern that lawmakers have expressed when considering cannabis reform proposals is what impact legalization would have on crime. While there is no greater calling in public service than public safety, and lawmakers should always consider the health and safety of Americans in everything that they do, data shows that legal marijuana businesses do not present a threat to public safety and may even have a dampening effect on crime. A number of studies, including studies from Preventative Medicine and the Journal of Urban Economics from 2017, found that the presence of dispensaries actually reduces property crimes in the neighborhood. Data from Colorado and Washington, two early adopters of legalized cannabis, showed drops in property and violent crimes post-legalization.

Notwithstanding this encouraging data, NCIA remains committed to finding solutions to some of the important public safety issues facing the industry, like youth use, impaired driving, and diversion. People should not be violating state law, they should not be selling cannabis to minors, they should not be consuming cannabis and driving, and they should not be transporting cannabis across state lines into states that have not legalized cannabis.

NCIA remains committed to working through these public policy issues that affect the health and safety of consumers and non-consumers alike. We are hopeful that with the end of prohibition will come a renewed sense of common purpose with the law enforcement community and that collaboration on public health and safety will be the norm. NCIA stands ready to work with the Fraternal Order of Police, the National Sheriffs Association, the International Association of Chiefs of Police, and any other law enforcement groups interested in finding public policy solutions to any public health and safety issues related to federal legalization of cannabis.

Highway Safety

One thing that both supporters and opponents of cannabis reform agree on is that policies should be adopted to prevent impaired driving and that these policies should be based on science. Several states have adopted per se limits on THC concentration in the blood.[95] While this method is less inaccurate than urinalysis testing for determining relatively recent use, it remains highly unreliable for testing actual impairment. According to the American Automobile Association, there is "no science showing that drivers reliably become impaired at a specific level of marijuana in the blood."

In 2017, NHTSA reported on the unreliability of per se THC/blood concentration and concluded that Washington State's "per se limit appears to have been based on something other than scientific evidence."[96] Instead, NHTSA recommends expanding training for law enforcement drug recognition experts and improved data collection at the state level to help guide future policies.

NCIA stands ready to work with Congress, law enforcement, and other interested parties to find appropriate methods for discouraging driving while under the influence of marijuana. We are supportive of education campaigns and other methods to convey to drivers the inherent dangers and consequences of driving under the influence. We should be exploring solutions to this, as well as other public safety issues. Prohibition will not and has not solved the issue of driving under the influence and people will continue to find a way to purchase what they desire from the illicit market. A more effective strategy would be to engage the consumer, educate them, and make certain that the products that they are consuming are safe for consumption through regulation and testing.

---

[95] "Findings from Four AAA Foundation for Traffic Safety" AAA Foundation for Traffic Safety. Available at: http://publicaffairsresources.aaa.biz/wp-content/uploads/2016/04/Cannabis-Research-Fact-Sheet-FINAL.docx, accessed May 8, 2018.

[96] U.S. Department of Transportation, National Highway Traffic Safety Administration, "Marijuana-Impaired Driving, A Report to Congress," July 2017, https://www.nhtsa.gov/sites/nhtsa.dot.gov/files/documents/812440-marijuana-impaired-driving-report-to-congress.pdf.

Reducing Access to Minors

The National Minimum Drinking Age Act of 1984 required all states to prohibit the purchase and public possession of alcohol by individuals under the age of 21. Failure to impose this standard would result in a state losing federal highway funds. As part of an overall scheme to end cannabis prohibition at the federal level, NCIA supports a similar federal incentive for states to establish a consistent age of 21 for the legal purchase of cannabis. Such a federal law, however, must be crafted so that it does not impair the ability of state-legal medical cannabis patients to possess and use medical cannabis on advice of their physician. Currently, all states with legal adult cannabis markets have instituted age limits, including uniformly setting the legal, non-medical possession of cannabis age at 21, and industry compliance is outperforming that of other age-restricted products.

The cannabis industry is doing its part to prevent teen use by rigorously adhering to age identification laws and regulations. Unlike liquor stores, adult-use marijuana stores are required to deny even mere entry to premises for underaged persons. In fact, age check compliance rates for adult-use marijuana stores are comparable and often exceed those of liquor stores. A 2016 article in the Journal of Studies on Alcohol and Drugs examining identification checks in Colorado adult-use stores found that compliance was extremely high and possibly higher than compliance with restrictions on alcohol sales.

NCIA will continue to work with state regulatory agencies to make certain that cannabis products are not being marketed to children and that young adults have the information that they need to make good decisions.

Research

As an association with a broad membership base, NCIA supports myriad of cannabis related bills that address a multitude of issues, such as research, legalizing cannabis, and social equity. Today, the subcommittee is considering six different bills that seek to address these issue areas. NCIA supports all of these pieces of legislation, with the exception of H.R. 171, the Legitimate Use of Medicinal Marijuana Act (LUMMA).

H.R. 171 seeks to move cannabis from Schedule I to Schedule II of the Controlled Substances Act, meaning that the drug has some medicinal benefit but also a high potential for abuse. According to the National Institute for Drug Abuse (NIDA), about 9% of cannabis consumers will become dependent –

about the same rate as caffeine addiction. As stated earlier in my testimony, NCIA supports removing marijuana from the Controlled Substances Act, not moving it to another schedule. NCIA and our members believe that by re-scheduling marijuana, successful marijuana programs operating in 33 states would be upended across the country. Re-scheduling would also likely require that a pharmacist dispense cannabis only if prescribed by a medical doctor, which would not align federal law with the state laws that are already allowing thousands of state-licensed cannabis businesses to safely serve patients and adult consumers.

Vaping

As reports began to appear of a potential linkage between lung injuries and use of nicotine and/or cannabis vaping products (with the source of those products uncertain at the time), NCIA's Policy Council established a Safe Vaping Task Force. Today, it appears that public health experts have concluded that additives from the illicit market appear to be the primary cause of this outbreak (though the Center for Disease Control has not yet conclusively opined on the proximate cause for all cases). Ultimately, one thing is clear: we must stop the flow of unregulated and untested products to consumers from the illicit market.

The answer to the outbreak of vaping-related health issues is to offer products that have been tested and are regulated by the state. The most effective way to ensure that consumers have access to tested and regulated products is by de-scheduling cannabis. If we de-schedule, test, and regulate these products, then we have a much greater chance at displacing the illicit market. Of course, these regulated products must be able to compete with the illicit market on price, therefore we recommend that states keep taxes low so that the regulated market is not directly competing with the illicit market in terms of cost.

Gateway Theory & Opioids

The theory that cannabis use leads to an increased likelihood of using other controlled substances is not supported by the available science. In fact, even the Drug Enforcement Administration (DEA) has said, "little evidence supports the hypothesis that initiation of marijuana use leads to an abuse disorder with other illicit substances." Cannabis has long been the most frequently used federally illicit drug, which is why its use commonly occurs before use of other substances, but there is no evidence that cannabis consumption is the reason why people move on to other substance use. Moreover, use of other substances, such as caffeine, nicotine, and alcohol often predate initial use of cannabis.[97]

On the contrary, there is some evidence to support the notion that cannabis has the potential to be an "exit drug" for individuals engaging in abuse of other substances, such as opioids. A 2017 study found that 97% of subjects reported decreasing the amount of opiates they consumed when they also use cannabis. That study also found that 81% of subjects ultimately preferred cannabis by itself rather than using it concurrently with opioids, demonstrating the possible exit effect. Another 2017 study observed a "growing body of research supporting the medical use of cannabis as an adjunct or substitute for opioids," and urged policymakers to incorporate cannabis in any opioid response strategy.[98] In fact some states (including Colorado) are allowing the reasons for prescribing medicinal cannabis to supplant the reasons that a doctor is authorized to prescribe opiods.

Perhaps the most striking data comes from a 2014 study of fatal opioid overdoses between 1999 and 2010. That survey found that the 13 states with medical cannabis laws during that period had 24.8% fewer opioid deaths than other states.[99] What's more, the effect of medical cannabis appeared to strengthen over time – overdose death reductions grew from roughly 20% the first year after medical marijuana implementation to nearly 34% five years after implementation.

Similarly, a 2017 study published by the American Journal of Public Health found that the legalization of adult-use marijuana in Colorado was associated with a decline in opioid deaths.[100] While it cannot be concluded that legal access to cannabis is directly responsible for the reduced fatalities, it demonstrates that marijuana does not lead to increased use of opioids in line

---

[97] Reiman, A, et al. "Cannabis as a Substitute for Opioid-Based Pain Medication: Patient Self-Report." Cannabis and Cannabinoid Research., U.S. National Library of Medicine, 1 June 2017, www.ncbi.nlm.nih.gov/pubmed/28861516.

[98] Lucas, Philippe. "Rationale for Cannabis-Based Interventions in the Opioid Overdose Crisis." Harm Reduction Journal, vol. 14, no. 1, 18 June 2017, doi:10.1186/s12954-017-0183-9.

[99] Bachhuber, Marcus A., et al. "Medical Cannabis Laws and Opioid Analgesic Overdose Mortality in the United States, 1999-2010." JAMA Internal Medicine, vol. 174, no. 10, 1 Aug. 2014, p. 1668., doi:10.1001/jamainternmed.2014.4005.

[100] Livingston, Melvin D., et al. "Recreational Cannabis Legalization and Opioid-Related Deaths in Colorado, 2000–2015." American Journal of Public Health, vol. 107, no. 11, Nov. 2017, pp. 1827–1829., doi:10.2105/ajph.2017.304059.

with opponents' "gateway theory" and may actually be contributing to the decline.

Potency

Similar to beer, wine, and hard liquor, cannabis products can contain varying amounts of THC and other cannabinoids. There must be standardized testing and labeling requirements for cannabis related products so that consumers can safely know what they are purchasing and consuming. In fact, every state with a modern marijuana program on the books requires testing and accurate labeling to ensure consumers and patients know the potency of the product before consuming it – a safeguard that only exists in the legal and regulated market. Any federal cannabis policy reform should continue to allow states to decide how to best regulate product potency.

Conclusion

The cannabis industry has evolved into a national commercial enterprise generating significant tax revenue, generating hundreds of thousands of jobs, and providing people access to plant-based medicines that work to alleviate pain and treat symptoms of myriad diseases. State laws that have replaced the criminal markets with systems that provide for tightly regulated production and sale of cannabis to patients and adults over 21 are improving public safety. But, the unnecessary burdens caused by outdated federal policies must be resolved to benefit our communities' entrepreneurs while also safeguarding consumers and the general public. It is for these reasons that NCIA supports the de-scheduling and regulation of cannabis. Of all the proposals put forward this Congress, the clearest path toward the aforestated goals is the passage of the MORE Act, along with the addition of a robust regulatory structure. While imperfect, the MORE Act deschedules cannabis and provides social equity fixes that are long overdue.

I want to thank the Chair, Vice Chair, Ranking Member, and members of the Subcommittee for your time to discuss the future of cannabis policy in the new decade. As always, NCIA remains ready to work with Congress on public policy solutions that will benefit the burgeoning American cannabis industry, small and large businesses, lawmakers, and the American public.

* * *

Letter of August 1, 2020, From Over 100 Organizations in Support of H.R. 3884, to Ms. Nancy Pelosi, et al., Submitted by Ms. Eshoo

August 1, 2019
Speaker Nancy Pelosi
1236 Longworth H.O.B.
Washington, DC 20515

House Minority Leader Kevin McCarthy
2468 Rayburn H.O.B.
Washington, DC 20515

House Majority Leader Steny Hoyer
1236 Longworth H.O.B.
Washington, DC 20515

House Minority Whip Steve Scalise
2049 Rayburn H.O.B
Washington, DC 20515

House Judiciary Chairman Jerrold Nadler
2141 Rayburn H.O.B.
Washington, DC 20515

House Judiciary Ranking Member Doug Collins
1504 Longworth H.O.B.
Washington, DC 20515

RE: Support the Marijuana Opportunity Reinvestment and Expungement (MORE) Act

Dear Members of Congress,
On behalf of the more than 100 undersigned organizations, we write to express our support for the Marijuana Opportunity Reinvestment and Expungement

(MORE) Act (H.R. 3884). We request that this critical criminal and racial justice legislation be swiftly marked up and immediately scheduled for floor consideration. The MORE Act will de-schedule marijuana and fund social equity programs for individuals and communities most harmed by the war on drugs.

We are encouraged by the progress around marijuana reform at the state and federal level. Today 33 states and the District of Columbia provide legal access to medical marijuana and 11 states plus the District of Columbia provide legal access to recreational marijuana.[101] At the federal level, Congress has introduced a number of bills that would reform the nation's marijuana laws. This Congress has held a record-number of hearings on marijuana reform, including a historic hearing on July 10, 2019 on the need to reform marijuana laws and address racial justice.[102] Indeed, the tide has turned on marijuana reform. A 2018 Center for American Progress and GBA Strategies poll found that 68 percent of voters support marijuana legalization.[103] The poll also found that 73 percent of voters support the automatic sealing of marijuana offenses.[104] While this progress is promising, we insist that any marijuana reform or legalization bill considered by Congress include robust provisions addressing social justice and criminal justice reform.

The war on drugs, which includes the war on marijuana, devastated the lives of generations of African American and Latinx Americans from low-income communities.[105] These individuals were disproportionately targeted and brought into the criminal justice system for engaging in marijuana activity that is increasingly lawful. A 2013 ACLU study found that Black people are nearly four times more likely than white people to be arrested for marijuana

---

[101] Jeremy Berke and Skye Gould, "Illinois just became the first state to legalize marijuana sales through the legislature—here are all the states where marijuana is legal," Business Insider, June 25, 2019, available at https://www.businessinsider.com/legal-marijuana-states-2018-1.

[102] Angelica LaVito, "US lawmakers look to legalize pot in 'historic' marijuana reform hearing," CNBC, July 10, 2019, available at https://www.cnbc.com/2019/07/10/us-lawmakers-look-to-legalize-pot-in-historic-marijuana-reform-hearing.html.

[103] Center for American Progress, "New Polling From CAP and GBA Strategies Shows 68 percent of Voters Support Marijuana Legalization; 73 Percent Support Automatic Sealing of Marijuana Offenses," June 20, 2018, available at https://www.americanprogress.org/press/release/2018/06/20/452451/release-new-polling-cap-gba-strategies-shows-68-percent-voters-support-marijuana-legalization-73-percent-support-automatic-sealing-marijuana-offenses/.

[104] Ibid.

[105] Drug Policy Alliance, "Race and the Drug War," available at http://www.drugpolicy.org/issues/race-and-drug-war.

possession despite similar usage rates in both groups.[106] In 2018, *The New York Times* reported that black and Hispanic New Yorkers were arrested for low-level marijuana charges at eight times and five times the rate of white New Yorkers, respectively, notwithstanding similar marijuana usage rates across groups.[107] Criminal justice involvement deprives individuals from low-income communities of color equal access to economic opportunity.[108] Incarceration robs families and communities of breadwinners and workers. Thus, any marijuana reform bill that moves forward in Congress must first address criminal justice reform and repair the damage caused by the war on drugs in low-income communities of color.

The MORE Act is the most far-reaching marijuana reform bill introduced in Congress that would address historical and current racial inequities. The MORE Act will:

- De-schedule marijuana, removing it from the Controlled Substances Act.
- Instruct the Bureau of Labor Statistics (BLS) to collect demographic data on the marijuana industry.
- Provide a process for courts to expunge marijuana convictions and re-sentence people with marijuana convictions.
- Establish that no person will be denied federal benefits on the basis of use or possession of marijuana.
- Prohibit immigration penalties based on marijuana.
- Create a Cannabis Opportunity Trust Fund from federal marijuana tax revenue that will establish (1) the Community Reinvestment Grant Program to fund community organizations providing services in communities most harmed by the war on drugs; (2) the Cannabis Opportunity Program to fund Small Business Administration loans to support socially and economically disadvantaged individuals who own marijuana businesses; and (3) the Equitable Licensing Grant

---

106 ACLU, "Report: The War on Marijuana is Black and White," available at https://www.aclu.org/report/report-war-marijuana-black-and-white?redirect=criminal-law-reform/war-marijuana-black-and-white.

107 Benjamin Mueller, Robert Gebeloff, and Sahil Chinoy, "Surest Way to Face Marijuana Charges in New York: Be Black or Hispanic," *The New York Times*, May 13, 2018, available at https://www.nytimes.com/2018/05/13/nyregion/marijuana-arrests-nyc-race.html?module=inline.

108 Maritza Perez, Olugbenga Ajilore, and Ed Chung, "Using Marijuana Revenue to Create Jobs," Center for American Progress, May 20, 2019, available at https://www.americanprogress.org/issues/criminal-justice/reports/2019/05/20/470031/using-marijuana-revenue-create-jobs/.

Program to provide jurisdictions with funds to develop and implement equitable marijuana licensing programs targeting individuals most adversely impacted by the war on drugs.

The MORE Act's targeted programs will serve to empower historically underserved communities that bore this nation's drug war. It will also reduce racial disparities in the criminal justice system and protect people from unequal marijuana enforcement. Justice requires that marijuana reform policy in Congress first de-schedule and repair past harms.

We ask Members of Congress to support the MORE Act and take this critical step to bolster communities ravaged by the war on drugs. We urge Members of Congress to swiftly mark-up this bill and send it to the floor for consideration.

Thank you for the opportunity to submit this letter. Please contact Maritza Perez, Senior Policy Analyst for Criminal Justice Reform at the Center for American Progress, with any questions at mperez@americanprogress.org or 202.796.9719.

Sincerely,

4Front Ventures
A New PATH
African American Ministers In Action
American Civil Liberties Union AOUON
Blacks in Law Enforcement of America
Broken No More
Buds & Roses
California NORML
Cannabis Consumers Campaign
Center for American Progress (CAP)
Center for Law and Social Policy (CLASP)
Center for Living and Learning
Central Florida NORML
Clergy for a New Drug Policy
Coalition for Humane Immigrant Rights (CHIRLA)
Colorado NORML
Community Mediation DC
Contra Costa County NORML
Delaware NORML

Dignity & Power Now
Drug Policy Alliance
Due Process Institute
Empire State NORML
Families ACT
Family Law and Cannabis Alliance (FLCA)
FedCURE
Federal Public and Community Defenders
From Prison Cells To PhD
Generation Progress
Harm Reduction Coalition
Health Equity Alliance
Heartland Alliance
Human Rights Defense Center
Human Rights Watch
Immigrant Legal Resource Center
Institute of the Black World 21st Century
Interfaith Action for Human Rights
International CURE
Jewish Council for Public Affairs
Justice Roundtable
Justice Strategies
JustLeadershipUSA
LatinoJustice PRLDEF
Law Enforcement Action Partnership
Leadership Conference on Civil and Human Rights
Legal Aid Society
Lehigh Valley NORML
life for pot
Maryland Marijuana Justice
Maryland NORML
Michigan NORML
Minority Cannabis Business Association
MomsRising
NAACP
National Action Network
National Association of Criminal Defense Lawyers
National Association of Social Workers
National Center for Lesbian Rights

National Center for Transgender Equality
National Council on Independent Living (NCIL)
National Employment Law Project
National Immigrant Justice Center
National Immigration Law Center
National Juvenile Justice Network
National LGBTQ Task Force Action Fund
NETWORK Lobby for Catholic Social Justice
Nevada NORML
New York City NORML
NORML
NORML Long Island
NORML of Florida
Pittsburgh NORML
Point of Discovery
PolicyLink
Prevention Point Pittsburgh
Progressive Leadership Alliance of Nevada
Protect Families First
Public Justice Center
Quad Cities Harm Reduction
Rights Restoration Project
Roanoke Valley NORML
Roc NORML
Safe Street Arts Foundation
SENSIBLE FLORIDA
Southeast Asia Resource Action Center
Southern Arizona NORML
SPARC
St. Ann's Corner of Harm Reduction, Inc.
StoptheDrugWar.org
Students for Sensible Drug Policy
Takoma Wellness Center
Texas Criminal Justice Coalition
Texas NORML
Texas Organizing Project
The Brotherhood/Sister Sol
The Holy Trinity Community of Ethiopia Restoration House in D.C.
The Legal Aid Society

The Ordinary People Society
The Sentencing Project
United We Dream
United Food and Commercial Workers International Union
Urban Survivors Union and NC Survivors Union
VOCAL-NY
Washington NORML
Washington Office on Latin America (WOLA)
West Ga NORML Women's Alliance
Witness to Mass Incarceration
Women Who Never Give Up, Inc.
Women with a Vision, Inc.
Wyoming NORML
Youth Justice Coalition

* * *

Letter of January 15, 2020, from Aaron Smith, Executive Director, National Cannabis Industry Association

January 15, 2020

Chairwoman Anna Eshoo
Subcommittee on Health, Committee on Energy & Commerce
202 Cannon House Office Building
Washington, DC 20515

Ranking Member Michael Burgess
Subcommittee on Health, Committee on Energy & Commerce
2161 Rayburn House Office Building
Washington, DC 20515

Dear Chairwoman Eshoo & Ranking Member Burgess:
As organizations that collectively represent thousands of state-legal cannabis businesses around the country, ancillary industries, and our communities, we applaud your decision to hold a hearing on cannabis policy so early in the new legislative session. This is a wonderful opportunity to continue the robust and

groundbreaking discussion on this issue that took place in Congress last year and we commend your leadership in carrying it over into 2020.

While this is a complex and nuanced issue, the cannabis industry stands united in its support for policies under your jurisdiction that would help ensure access to safe legal cannabis products.

These policies include, but are not limited to:

- *Federal regulatory oversight:* Any discussion of cannabis policy for the new decade must have federal regulatory oversight as a key component. The states that have reformed their cannabis laws ahead of the federal government have established regulatory frameworks to govern their markets and protect public health. We support robust federal regulatory guidance and oversight that informs the development of additional safety protocols and produces greater regulatory consistency of product marketing, safety and oversight across state and national borders.
- *Descheduling vs. Rescheduling:* We ultimately support the full removal of cannabis from the federal list of controlled substances. While rescheduling on its own may provide some benefit in terms of facilitating research, it could complicate the federal-state relationship with respect to cannabis. If the sole goal of Congress is to facilitate research, it can take alternative steps, such as those described in the following paragraph.

  Research: We support removing current barriers to research on cannabis and its derivatives in order to provide policymakers, regulators, and consumers with the most accurate and updated information possible and to keep pace with innovation and technological developments in the market. This includes ending the NIDA monopoly on the cultivation of cannabis for research purposes, and allowing researchers to easily and legally study products that are currently available in regulated state cannabis markets. We also support policies and additional funding for research that address current healthcare disparities and the unique needs of women, veterans, and people of color.
- *Access by minors:* The National Minimum Drinking Age Act of 1984 required all states to prohibit the purchase and public possession of alcohol by individuals under the age of 21. Failure to impose this standard would result in a state losing federal highway funds. As part

of an overall scheme to end cannabis prohibition at the federal level, we support a similar federal incentive for states to establish 21 as the minimum age for the purchase of cannabis in the U.S. and enact non-criminal penalties for underage possession. Such a federal law, however, should be crafted so that it does not diminish the rights and well-being of state-legal medical cannabis patients. Currently, all states with legal adult cannabis markets have instituted age limits, including uniformly setting the legal, non-medical possession of cannabis age at 21, and industry compliance is outperforming that of other age-restricted products.

- *Labeling:* We support clear and accurate labeling of cannabis products that include cannabinoid content, potential health risks, and other applicable information such as allergen risks and dietary profile as appropriate for individual products.
- *Advertising:* We support limits on advertising to prevent targeting minors and ensure products and packaging are not designed to appeal to children.
- *Testing:* We support federal guidelines on best testing practices and the ability to conduct product recalls for anything found to be contaminated or deemed unsafe for human use.
- *Ending federal cannabis prohibition:* As an industry, we strongly support an immediate end to the blanket federal prohibition of cannabis.
- *Social equity and social justice:* As we consider cannabis policy for the new decade, we must acknowledge that the cannabis policies of the past have had a demonstrably severe and detrimental impact on health and well-being in low-income communities and communities of color. The end of cannabis prohibition at the federal level should be paired with policies at the federal, state, and local level that right past wrongs and ensure that the benefits of legalization flow to individuals and communities that have borne the brunt of prohibitionist policies. Furthermore, emerging policies must seek to address healthcare disparities including access to affordable medicine, representation in research, and additional funding for women, veterans, and people of color.

As an industry, we understand that many lawmakers have concerns about the impact of the changing legal status of cannabis. We do not take these concerns lightly. These concerns underscore the need to establish a legal federal cannabis framework, as current federal policies can cause and exacerbate these concerns.

We welcome the opportunity to work with lawmakers and regulators to determine the best paths forward as state and federal cannabis policy evolves. Thank you for continuing this conversation and providing a venue to further explore these issues.

Sincerely,
Aaron Smith
Executive Director
National Cannabis Industry Association

Saphira Galoob
Executive Director
National Cannabis Roundtable

Randal John Meyer
Executive Director
Global Alliance for Cannabis Commerce

Neal Levine
CEO
Cannabis Trade Federation

Jason Ortiz
President
Minority Cannabis Business Association

Statement of California Cannabis Industry Association

California Cannabis Industry Association ("CCIA") is pleased to submit this statement for the record and applauds Chairwoman Anna Eshoo, Ranking Member Michael Burgess, Chairman Frank Pallone and the members of the Subcommittee on Health for the Committee on Energy & Commerce for holding a hearing entitled "Cannabis Policies for the New Decade." We appreciate your commitment to modernizing our nation's cannabis laws and wish to offer our input and suggestions as policy continues to develop on the federal level.

CCIA is uniquely positioned to weigh in on cannabis policy. Representing over 600 businesses and 15,000 employees from all aspects of the cannabis supply chain, including plant touching and ancillary businesses, CCIA promotes the growth of a responsible and legitimate cannabis industry. The California cannabis industry is the largest, and most regulated, cannabis market in the world with legal sales topping $3 billion dollars for 2019 according to analysis by the sales-tracking firms Arcview Market Research and BDS Analytics.[109] Unfortunately, due to federal illegality, and at times burdensome regulation by the state of California, these legal sales account for only a fraction of cannabis sold in the state when including the illicit market (estimated to be $8.7 billion in 2019).[110]

For the past two and a half decades California has been a pioneer in developing and passing cannabis legislation and regulation. This has led to many positive developments that protect consumer safety, but also some growing pains that have proven to be overly burdensome to industry. As the federal conversations shifts from not if, but how, cannabis should be legalized, California can serve as model of both what regulations are effective – and perhaps more importantly pitfalls to avoid as a federal regulatory framework is considered.

While the regulation of cannabis at the federal level will certainly be a complex process, one thing is clear: the current federal-state conflict is untenable, and any contemplated federal regulation of cannabis must at minimum contemplate removing cannabis from its Schedule I classification.

Adverse Events and Product Recalls

Perhaps the best argument for federal regulation of cannabis is that regulated markets provide stronger protections for consumer safety. While some of the bills before the committee contemplate federal legalization, they do not fully

---

[109] Sean Williams, *California's Cannabis Black Market is Insanely Larger Than Its Legal Market,* MOTLEY FOOL, (Sept. 19, 2019), https://www.fool.com/investing/2019/09/14/californias-cannabis-black-market-is-insanely-larg.aspx, *See also*, Patrick McGreevy, *California Now Has the Biggest Legal Marijuana Market in the World. Its Black Market is Even Bigger,* LA Times, (Aug. 15, 2019), https://www.latimes.com/california/story/2019-08-14/californias-biggest-legal-marijuana-market.

[110] *Id.*

address the role of the federal government from a regulatory prospective. To be sure, numerous federal agencies will need to be involved in the event cannabis is legalized at the federal level, including but not limited to the FDA, Department of Treasury, IRS, NIDA, EPA, and NIST. The cooperation of these agencies must at minimum be able to ensure that cannabis and cannabis products are appropriately tested and marketed (i.e., not advertised towards minors), and that consumers will have options for recourse if a product is revealed to be injurious or detrimental to public health.

Illicit market sellers do not test products for contaminants, pesticides or dangerous additives such as Vitamin E Acetate, a chemical that has been linked to many cases of lung injury during the CDC's investigation of vaping products.[111] Reports have shown that Vitamin E Acetate was used by illicit operators to mimic the appearance and viscosity of cannabis concentrate oil, to increase production while minimizing costs.[112] Quality control is central component to a regulated market. While California has not been immune to the lung injury cases associated with vaping, not a single product from the state's regulated market has been identified as the sole cause for lung injury. In fact, in Utah, a state where the consumption of cannabis is not yet permitted, there were nearly ten times more cases of lung injury per capita than in California.[113] Many of the cases in California were clustered in counties that prevented cannabis sale through local regulations, so consumers had no choice but to turn to illicit sources because regulated cannabis was not easily accessible. California's regulated market has the most stringent standards for testing for solvents, pesticides and heavy metals and similar product safety guardrails should be implemented by the federal government.

Another area where the Federal Government can build from California policy is recall and adverse event reporting.[114] As federal legalization of cannabis is contemplated, there must be strong regulatory protocols in place that allow for recalls of potentially dangerous products and the effective reporting of adverse events. Current FDA recall protocols allow for medicines,

---

[111] Benjamin C. Blount, et al., *Vitamin E Acetate in Bronchoalveolar-Lavage Fluid Associated with EVALI*, N. J. MED., (Dec. 20, 2019), https://www.nejm.org/doi/full/10.1056/NEJMoa1916433.

[112] *See e.g.,* David Downs, *Amid Vape Pen Lung Disease Deaths: What exactly is Vitamin E Oil?*, LEAFLY, (Sept. 11, 2019), https://www.leafly.com/news/health/vape-pen-lung-disease-vitamin-e-oil-explained.

[113] David Downs, *Legal Vape Markets Literally 1000% Safer Than Street*, LEAFLY, (Dec. 19, 2019), https://www.leafly.com/news/strains-products/vapi-evali-states-analysis-leafly.

[114] *See e.g.,* Michelle Wiley, *State Regulators Order Recall of Hundreds of Marijuana Products,* The California Report, (Dec. 22, 2018), https://www.kqed.org/news/11714412/state-regulators-order-recall-of-hundreds-of-marijuana-products.

foods, and devices to be pulled off the market for contamination, defects, and undeclared additives. On the state level, California cannabis producers should be able to afford themselves to the same public health safeguards as other products regulated by the FDA. Allowing cannabis producers to take advantage of the FDA recall procedures would be beneficial to public health in the event of undisclosed ingredients or harmful additives.

Packaging and Labeling

To promote consumer safety, California requires clear and accurate packaging and labeling. Cannabis products must be labeled accurately with cannabinoid content, a unique identification and tracking number, allergens, weight, a universal symbol, nutrition info, and other disclosures.[115] While it may be challenging for the subcommittee to develop a uniform federal label without the assistance of executive agencies, federal legalization should consider the massive existing market and the labels that exist on it presently. The current labeling processes that exist for alcohol may have to be modified for cannabis products. Currently, when a new alcoholic product enters the marketplace, the label must be approved by the Alcohol and Tobacco Tax and Trade Bureau ("TTB") prior to sales of the beverage. However, as many cannabis companies and brands have existing pockets of consumers, label approval may need to take place while products are still on the market rather than requiring producers to pull their products before receiving label approval from TTB or another agency.

Taxation and Illicit Market

Tax revenue is oft cited as a primary reason why states move forward with legalization, however, over taxation can result in unintended consequences, and further growth of the illicit market. At least one of the bills considered by the subcommittee, the MORE Act (H.R. 3884), proposes leveraging a federal excise tax on the cannabis industry. CCIA applauds many of the principles contained in the MORE Act but cautions against any excessive federal

[115] *See generally, Labeling Requirements,* Cal. Dept. Pub. Health, (last visited Jan. 14, 2020), https://www.cdph.ca.gov/Programs/CEH/DFDCS/MCSB/CDPH%20Document%20Library/LabelingChecklist-Products.pdf.

taxation of cannabis. While CCIA appreciates that tax revenue from cannabis can be used for a variety of programs, it is critical that prices in the regulated market are not so high as to drive consumers to the illicit market. At the state level in California, taxation of cannabis and cannabis products can reach effective rates of 80%[116] making it incredibly difficult for licensed producers to compete with the lower prices of the illicit market.

Recently, Governor Gavin Newsom proposed streamlining cannabis taxation, but this may not be sufficient enough to keep prices at a rate competitive with the illicit market. As federal regulators look to strike the balance between fairness to businesses and revenue generation, we urge them to exempt state legal cannabis businesses from Internal Revenue Code § 280E so these businesses can take standard business deductions like any other non-cannabis company.

Expansion of Research and Centers of Excellence

CCIA is pleased that the committee is considering a variety of research proposals. Currently, the requirements to conduct a clinical trial or other study with cannabis are incredibly burdensome due to the plant's Schedule I status. Researchers are fearful of losing federal funding if they engage in cannabis research, and are frustrated by the the lack of genetic and cannabinoid diversity available through the NIDA Cannabis Farm at the University of Mississippi.[117] As Congress considers research proposals, a central tenet should be the availability for researchers to source cannabis from private sources.

The cannabis commercially available in California is markedly different from the cannabis grown at the Mississippi NIDA facility. California cannabis differs in THC and cannabinoid content, formulation, and undergoes far more rigorous testing than cannabis grown under NIDA's supervision. For example, there is no readily available testing protocols for cannabis grown at the NIDA facility, while California requires testing in over a dozen different categories including cannabinoid content, impurities, pesticides, heavy metals and

---

[116] Cal. Dep't. of Tax and Fee Admin, *Cannabis Special Notice – L270*, (last visited Jan. 14, 2020), https://www.cdtfa.ca.gov/formspubs/L720.pdf.

[117] Owen Daugherty, *Risk of Losing Federal Funding Reason Why Medical Marijuana Research Won't Happen,* (Aug. 23, 2017), https://www.thelantern.com/2017/08/risk-of-losing-federal-funding-reason-why-medical-marijuana-research-wont-happen/.

mycotoxins.[118] Allowing cannabis to be sourced from private industry would provide researchers the opportunity to more appropriately align their research studies with what is going on in the marketplace.

As the committee considers research proposals, they should also consider establishing centers of excellence for cannabis research. Top California universities including UCLA, and Berkley have developed substantial research programs. UC San Diego is home to the Center for Medicinal Cannabis Research. By allowing for California universities to become Centers of Excellence, Congress could facilitate grants to universities who have made substantial progress in research. Centers of excellence have been established in agriculture, marine & maritime issues, and other policy areas.[119]

Conclusion

CCIA deeply appreciates the subcommittee holding this hearing and for its willingness to reexamine the current framework surround cannabis. As the subcommittee and the committee at large continue to contemplate how to effectively regulate cannabis, we are happy to serve as a resource and provide guidance and feedback to the committee as appropriate. Please contact Executive Director Lindsay Robinson at lindsay@cacannabisindustry.org with any questions or if additional information is needed.

Statement of Congressman Hakeem Jeffries, Testimony on H.R. 2843 the "Marijuana Freedom and Opportunity Act of 2019,"

Good Morning,

Thank you to Chairwoman Eshoo and Ranking Member Burgess for considering H.R. 2843, the "Marijuana Freedom and Opportunity Act" as a part of this hearing on "Cannabis Policies for the New Decade."

---

[118] Bureau of Cannabis Control, *Required Testing Chart,* (last visited Jan. 14, 2020), https://bcc.ca.gov/about_us/documents/17-261_required_testing_chart.pdf.

[119] *See e.g.,* U.S. Dep't Treasury, *Centers of Excellence Research Grants Program,* (last updated Oct. 15, 2019), https://www.thelantern.com/2017/08/risk-of-losing-federal-funding-reason-why-medical-marijuana-research-wont-happen/.

While states have led the charge in legislating on cannabis over the past decade, it is important that Congress crafts federal policies and addresses the matters that are within our jurisdiction. In doing so, Congress must take a broad approach, considering a number of potential fixes to our current laws.

That is what the Marijuana Freedom and Opportunity Act strives to do. It enables states to act as labs of democracy and decide how to regulate marijuana in a way that makes the most sense for their residents, while taking federal action to allow for better information and enhanced safety. In addition to decriminalizing marijuana at the federal level, the Marijuana Freedom and Opportunity Act takes significant steps to address the harms our current marijuana laws have caused through the creation of grant programs and increased opportunities.

It makes targeted investments that are necessary to protect public health and safety, including research to better understand health impacts of marijuana, the effects of THC on the human brain and the efficacy of marijuana as a treatment for specific ailments. In order to ensure that marijuana businesses are not allowed to target children, this legislation also requires the promulgation of regulations that restrict advertising and promotion of products as is currently done with tobacco products.

As federal legislators, we must be thoughtful in our approach to updates in this space, and this hearing is significant in moving us forward. Thank you again for taking the time to discuss these issues and for considering this important legislation.

Written Statement of Kris Krane, President of 4Front Ventures

Thank you to Chair Eshoo and the Energy and Commerce Subcommittee on Health for holding this hearing on cannabis policies, its schedule status in the Controlled Substance Act ("CSA"), and the related barriers to research that are impeding public health knowledge. With 33 states with regulated medical cannabis programs and 11 with regulated adult-use systems, millions of Americans are purchasing cannabis that is packaged and sold in accordance with state law. Support for these programs is substantial with 91% of Americans supporting medical cannabis 67% supporting adult use, including majority support across nearly every age group and political ideology.[120] But in the two-and-a-half decades since states began to permit legal access to cannabis, federal law has not kept up with the states or the American public.

Despite the lack of evolution in federal law, this session of Congress has seen substantial movement on the issue, with the SAFE Banking Act (H.R. 1595) passing on the House floor with strong bipartisan support and the MORE Act (H.R.3884) which would remove ("deschedule") cannabis from the CSA, receiving a favorable markup in House Judiciary. We appreciate the Health Subcommittee holding this hearing to examine impacts of changing the CSA status of cannabis and barriers to research.

Schedule Status of "Marijuana"

Cannabis has been a Schedule I drug since the CSA was signed into law in 1971; however, lawmakers only placed it in the most restrictive schedule as a placeholder. It ended up there permanently for political reasons. President Nixon convened the National Commission on Marijuana and Drug Abuse (more commonly known as the Shafer Commission) to examine the potential harms of cannabis legalization and make a recommendation on schedule placement within the CSA. The Shafer Commission recommended that personal possession of cannabis be decriminalized and even recommended fines over prison for amounts greater than personal possession.[121] Nixon ignored the commission's recommendation. In a lawsuit challenging the president's decision, the DEA's own administrative law judge ruled: "Marijuana, in its natural form, is one of the safest therapeutically active substances known to man," while recommending that it's placement in Schedule I was inappropriate.[122]

---

[120] "Nearly eight-in-ten Democrats and Democratic-leaning independents (78%) say marijuana use should be legal. Republicans and Republican leaners are less supportive, with 55% in favor of legalization and 44% opposed."https://www.pewresearch.org/fact-tank/2019/11/14/americans-support-marijuana-legalization/.

[121] The Shafer Commission report is available at: https://www.ncbi.nlm.nih.gov/pmc/articles/PMC1749335/pdf/bullnyacadmed00168-0058.pdf.

[122] United States Department of Justice, Drug Enforcement Administration, in the Matter Of Marijuana Rescheduling Petition," Opinion and Recommended Ruling, Findings of Fact, Conclusions of Law and Decision of Administrative Law Judge Francis L. Young, Administrative Law Judge, Sept. 6, 1988, http://www.druglibrary.org/schaffer/library/studies/young/young4.html.

To date, neither Congress nor any administration has implemented these recommendations. However, states have taken it upon themselves to remove criminal penalties for cannabis. In 1996, California became the first of 33 states to enact medical cannabis laws. By 2018, 2.3 million Americans were registered as patients in state-legal medical cannabis programs.[123] Under these programs, physicians recommend cannabis to treat conditions ranging from cancer to seizure disorders. Among the 33 state programs, there are well over 100 conditions that physicians can legally recommend cannabis to their patients as a therapeutic treatment option.[124] And yet, the CSA claims Schedule I drugs have no currently accepted medical use.

The fact that millions of patients are using cannabis to treat a medical condition based on a physician's recommendation means that its Schedule I status does not meet the laugh test, let alone scientific rigor. Therefore, the placement of cannabis in Schedule I undermines the integrity of the CSA itself. As a result, the conversation then turns to whether cannabis should be rescheduled elsewhere in the CSA or whether it should be descheduled and removed from the CSA.

Rescheduling vs. Descheduling

It may seem like a reasonable initial step to move cannabis to a less restrictive schedule status; however, that could have disastrous unintended consequences. If Congress were to move cannabis to Schedule II, as would be done under the LUMMA Act (H.R. 171), the state medical and adult-use laws could be preempted and nullified. This could lead to federal agencies aggressively shutting down the regulated cannabis programs, which could have adverse health consequences for patients and adult-use customers, alike.

For medical cannabis patients, shutting off state-regulated access to their physician-recommended treatment option would leave them with two options: either they would stop using medical cannabis and would likely replace it with pharmaceutical options that may be more harmful or expensive, or two, they could turn to unregulated sources of cannabis. In other words, rescheduling means that Congress would be getting in the way of decisions between doctors and patients, while simultaneously driving patients towards unregulated and untested products.

---

[123] Number of Legal Medical Marijuana Patients (as of May 17, 2018), Pro-Con.org, https://medicalmarijuana.procon.org/number-of-legal-medical-marijuana-patients/.

[124] A current list of each of the approved conditions under the various state medical cannabis laws is compiled by Americans for Safe Access, available here: https://www.safeaccessnow.org/condition.

There is evidence to suggest that shutting off access to regulated medical cannabis would create substantial burdens on Medicare Part D expenditures. Research has shown that in 2013, when there were just 17 medical cannabis programs operating, there was a savings of $165.2 million and that if expanded to all 50 states, the savings would be closer to $468.1 million.[125] As the nation's Baby Boomer population ages, there will be increased strain on Medicare Part D expenditures. Rescheduling cannabis to Schedule II or even Schedule V (the least restrictive schedule) could impose even greater stress on the prescription drug program.

Additionally, evidence suggests that cutting off access to medical cannabis would worsen opioid abuse issues. States that have created medical cannabis access have seen significant decreases in the total number of opioid doses prescribed in the state.[126] Moreover, states with regulated cannabis programs have been demonstrated to have significantly fewer fatal opioid overdoses.[127] This shows that preemption of state cannabis laws could have fatal implications for concerns around opioid use.

For both medical cannabis patients and adult-use consumers, shutting down the state-regulated systems would mean they will no longer have access to tested products from programs featuring recall mechanisms and chain-of-custody traceability. The recent news around illnesses caused by vaping illustrates the public health differences between criminalization and regulation. The overwhelming majority of the cases were from unregulated cannabis sources. States were able to pull potentially dangerous products off the shelves of stores and were able to investigate the likely source of the problem and have begun to ban Vitamin E acetate and other contaminants from vaping products.

Under the unregulated market, consumers do not have the advantages of lab testing and product safety recalls. Preemption of state cannabis programs by rescheduling the plant elsewhere within the CSA could lead to a situation where untested products that have a greater likelihood of being dangerous are the only ones available. Given the hundreds of thousands of cannabis arrests

---

125 "Medical Marijuana Laws Reduce Prescription Medication Use In Medicare Part D," HEALTH AFFAIRS 35, NO. 7 (2016): 1230–1236, https://www.healthaffairs.org/doi/pdf/10.1377/hlthaff.2015.1661.

126 "Association Between US State Medical Cannabis Laws and Opioid Prescribing in the Medicare Part D Population" JAMA Intern Med. 2018;178(5):667-672, https://jamanetwork.com/journals/jamainternalmedicine/fullarticle/2676999.

127 "The Effects of Recreational Marijuana Legalization and Dispensing on Opioid Mortality," Economic Inquiry, August 2019. https://onlinelibrary.wiley.com/doi/abs/10.1111/ecin.12819.

each year, we know that millions of Americans would continue to use cannabis if the state programs were to be preempted. Instead, Congress should deschedule and look at ways to empower Alcohol and Tobacco Tax and Trade Bureau to regulate cannabis in manner similar to alcohol.

Barriers to Research

There is a bit of a paradox when it comes to the volume of peer-reviewed cannabis research that has been conducted. There are over 700 peer-reviewed studies examining the medical efficacy of cannabis, making it one of the most studied substances on the planet.[1289] The majority of the studies show evidence of medicinal benefits from cannabis to treat certain conditions or symptoms.

The paradox is that there is hardly any federally approved clinical research. This is almost exclusively due to the Schedule I status of cannabis under the CSA. Schedule I status presents significant red tape for researchers to get projects approved. Once approved, researchers can only obtain cannabis from one federally approved source. Researchers have reported that the cannabis available from this source is of low quality and does not mirror the types of cannabis millions of Americans are purchasing from tested and regulated state-licensed sources.

Scientific research on cannabis should more accurately reflect the types of cannabis that are being used every day by Americans. If cannabis remains in Schedule I, clinical research will continue to be compromised. But given that rescheduling cannabis to somewhere between Schedule II and V could risk the aforementioned public health problems that would likely arise if the state programs are preempted by rescheduling, the prudent step to take would be to remove cannabis from the CSA.

Public Health and Criminalization

The conversation around cannabis and public health is often framed by examining the possible negative health consequences that could come with ending criminalization. This is a prudent thing to examine but it should not exclusively dominate the public health narrative around ending cannabis criminalization. In addition, we should also be examining the adverse public consequences of maintaining criminalization. We know that cannabis criminalization leads to incarceration and we know that incarceration raises

---

[128] Compiled list of peer reviewed studies available here: https://www.cannabis-med.org /studies/study.php.

the risk of contracting infectious diseases.[129] This demonstrates a clear link between criminalization causing negative public health consequences.

Additionally, a cannabis conviction can make it more difficult to obtain employment, leading to both unemployment and underemployment.[130] There is evidence that shows a link between unemployment and negative public health consequences.[131] This factor is exasperated by Aid Elimination Penalty in the Higher Education Act, which strips away federal student loan money if a currently enrolled student is convicted for a crime involving a controlled substance. If cannabis were to be rescheduled, this penalty will still apply.

Federal resources should be directed toward studying the public health consequences of cannabis criminalization and the full array of ancillary consequences. Thankfully, none of the barriers to clinical research of cannabis would stand in the way of these types of studies.

For these reasons, 4Front strongly urges Congress to take action to pass legislation that would remove cannabis from the Controlled Substances Act. We urge the members of the Subcommittee on Health to support the MORE Act to remove cannabis from the CSA, which would serve the dual benefit of enabling greater research while not endangering cannabis consumers by shutting off their tested and regulated sources.

Statement of January 15, 2020, from Americans for SafeAccess, submitted by Ms. Eshoo

Americans for Safe Access (ASA) would like to thank Chairman Pallone, Ranking Member Walden, Chairwoman Eshoo, Ranking Member Burgess, and members of the Subcommittee for holding this hearing. As the nation's largest member-based organization of patients, medical professionals, scientists, and concerned citizens working to promote safe and legal access to cannabis for therapeutic use and research, ASA is grateful for the opportunity to submit testimony regarding cannabis policy in the United States. As we

[129] "...prison places inmates at a disproportionate risk of acquiring infectious diseases such as tuberculosis, hepatitis, HIV, sexually transmitted infections, and methicillin-resistant Staphylococcus aureus." https://www.ncbi.nlm.nih.gov/pmc/articles/PMC6124689/pdf/nihms981983.pdf.

[130] Study observed a call-back rate for job seekers without a drug conviction was 13.6%, while those with a drug conviction only had an 8.5% call back rate. https://repository.law.umich.edu/cgi/viewcontent.cgi?article=2892&context=articles.

[131] https://www.hindawi.com/journals/isrn/2012/483432/.

enter a new decade and examine the impact of past and current policies, hearings such as this play a vital role in determining the appropriate approach to cannabis policy moving forward. While the ravages of the War on Drugs extend far beyond its effects on members of the medical cannabis community, this testimony will focus on the impact of federal law on medical cannabis patients.

California enacted the nation's first medical cannabis law in 1996. Currently, 47 states, the District of Columbia, Puerto Rico, the U.S. Virgin Islands, the Commonwealth of the Northern Mariana Islands, and Guam have passed laws that allow residents with a recommendation from a healthcare provider to obtain medical benefit from cannabis, and it is estimated that more than three million people now use cannabis for medical purposes.[132] At their most basic, these laws merely provide compliant patients with an affirmative defense should they be arrested for possessing cannabis oil. At their best, these laws approach the subject in a holistic and comprehensive manner to provide important civil protections, safeguard patient rights, and create robust medical cannabis programs with regulated sales channels through which patients can obtain a diverse set of products that are subject to stringent safety and quality standards and laboratory testing. Even in those states that do best at providing patients with access to medical cannabis, the conflict between state and federal law makes the status quo untenable. A comprehensive medical cannabis program with strong patient protections, such as provisions against housing and employment discrimination, is urgently needed at the federal level.

Cannabis has been used medicinally for millennia, and it was listed in the *United States Pharmacopoeia* from the mid-1850s through the early 1940s.[133] Nevertheless, for the past 50 years, cannabis has been classified as a Schedule I substance under the Controlled Substances Act (CSA), which is predicated in part on a determination by the federal government that cannabis does not have accepted medical value. In spite of the fact that there exists conclusive or substantial evidence that cannabis and constituents thereof are effective means by which to treat chronic pain, nausea and vomiting, and persistent

---

132 Americans for Safe Access. *2019 State of the States Report: An Analysis of Medical Cannabis Access in the United States*. (2019). Available from http://www.safeaccessnow.org/sos.

133 The National Academies of Sciences, Engineering, and Medicine. *The Health Effects of Cannabis and Cannabinoids: The Current State of Evidence and Recommendations for Research.* (2017).

muscle spasms,[134] the federal government has spent five decades criminalizing those who rely on cannabis to treat debilitating conditions.

The harm resulting from this approach is staggering. Being perpetually criminalized and stigmatized by the federal government takes a physical, mental, and economic toll on the 3,000,000+ people who participate in medical cannabis programs. Those who live in federally subsidized housing risk losing their homes. Those who travel must decide whether to risk their freedom or their health. Health insurance can't be used to pay for medical cannabis or the costs of program participation (e.g., registration fees), meaning only those in medical cannabis jurisdictions who can afford to pay these expenses out of pocket on an ongoing basis are able to obtain relief. Every day, the government robs medical cannabis patients of their peace of mind. Additionally, millions of people who could improve their health and quality of life through the medicinal use of cannabis – including our nation's veterans – are denied access and are suffering needlessly.

Last year, the World Health Organization's Expert Committee on Drug Dependence recommended to the United Nations that international drug control conventions be amended to remove cannabis and cannabis resin from the category of strictest control (Schedule IV).[135] More than 30 countries have already legalized medical cannabis at the federal/national level, including both of the countries with which we share national borders.[136] In addition to complicating or frustrating seriously ill people's efforts to effectively treat their conditions, the government's practice of ignoring the reality that cannabis is effective in treating an array of chronic and debilitating conditions erodes people's trust in the federal government.

Descheduling cannabis would reduce stigma around a relatively safe and effective treatment option and set the stage for the nationwide availability of medical cannabis and preparations therefrom. Patients suffering from multiple sclerosis, epilepsy, chronic pain, and other severe, chronic, or debilitating conditions would be able to try medical cannabis originating from a licit source under an authorized healthcare provider's supervision. This would be vastly preferable to the current situation, which forces many patients to resort

---

[134] Ibid.

[135] Adhanom Ghebreyesus, Tedros. Letter to António Guterres. 24 January 2019. TS. Available from https://www.who.int/medicines/access/controlled-substances/UNSG_letter_ECDD41_recommendations_cannabis_24Jan19.pdf?ua=1. Accessed on 14 January 2020.

[136] Hawryluk, Markian. "America's marijuana growers are the best in the world, but federal laws are keeping them out of global markets." *The Washington Post*, 27 December 2019. Accessed on 14 January 2020.

to using cannabis of unknown composition and quality that is sourced from illegal channels. Such cannabis is not subject to laboratory testing to determine its chemical profile and to ensure that it is not contaminated or adulterated, meaning that a lack of access to licit medical cannabis puts patients' well-being at greater risk.

Furthermore, descheduling cannabis would immediately make it easier for researchers to conduct important experiments with the same cannabis and cannabis products that patients and consumers currently obtain from dispensaries. Instead of having to rely on the University of Mississippi to provide plant material that bears very little resemblance to what is found in dispensaries, scientists would be able to work with a much wider range of products with varying chemical profiles, which could aid in the development of targeted therapies. Given that studies conducted using cannabis supplied by the University of Mississippi may not reveal the plant's full therapeutic potential, millions of people throughout the United States stand to gain from such research.

Medical cannabis patients must be able to travel between states without fear of arrest or anguish and must not otherwise be deprived of their rights. Veterans must be able to seek medical cannabis recommendations/ prescriptions from VA healthcare providers. All authorized healthcare providers must be free to recommend/prescribe cannabis for any illness for which it may provide relief. Insurance companies must be able to cover medical cannabis without violating federal law. Researchers must be able to obtain the same products patients and consumers currently use in order to produce useful data.

The needless suffering inflicted on the millions of people who cannot access cannabis and those who have gone to or fear ending up in jail because of it is immeasurable. It is time to abandon this cruel, misguided experiment in prohibition and deschedule cannabis.

Americans for Safe Access is grateful to have been able to submit testimony on this important topic and would like to thank the members of the subcommittee again for giving us the opportunity to do so.

National Cannabis Industry Association (NCIA), Adapting a Proven Regulatory Framewor, for the Emerging Cannabis Industry

Executive Summary

For almost a century, the United States government has criminalized the production, distribution, and sale of cannabis. However, this era of prohibition has been crumbling in the face of voter and, increasingly, legislative revolt. Even as these federal laws remain unchanged, most states have legalized some form of medical cannabis, and eleven states and the District of Columbia have changed their laws to regulate adult-use cannabis in a manner similar to alcohol. Moreover, Congress recently removed hemp (and any cannabinoids derived therefrom) from the Controlled Substances Act (CSA), legalizing a subset of cannabis plants and derivatives that contain less than 0.3% THC. With momentum building and public support ever-increasing, the critical question has shifted from "Should cannabis be legalized?" to "How will we regulate the commercial cannabis market at the federal level?"

As the leading policy voice for the state-regulated cannabis industry, the National Cannabis Industry Association (NCIA) herein offers reasoned and responsible approaches that the federal government could adopt to regulate cannabis products after the last vestiges of federal prohibition are removed.

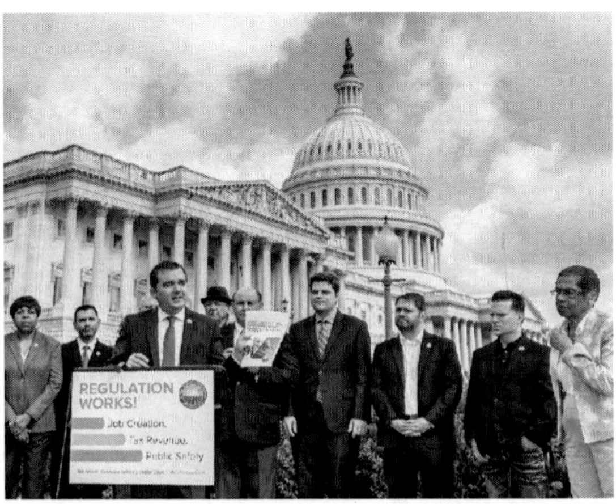

The diversity of products that contain cannabis means that a "one-size-fits-all" regulatory framework would be ineffective. Under such a framework, some products would be overregulated, while others might be underregulated. Instead, different regulatory structures, or "lanes," could be utilized based on the characteristics and intended uses of the products to leverage existing federal regulatory expertise. This will lead to an effective and efficient review process for existing government agencies that avoids unnecessary bureaucracy, costs, and delays for cannabis companies. Indeed, because human consumables are already regulated by the federal government through a variety of regulatory lanes designed for these purposes, most cannabis products could simply follow analogous products already being sold legally through these lanes. By building off existing systems and making modifications where necessary, all cannabis products could be properly regulated by existing federal agencies without reinventing the wheel.

Currently, because of marijuana's status as a Schedule I drug under the CSA, the Drug Enforcement Administration (DEA) is the primary federal regulator of cannabis, with criminal enforcement serving as the sole regulatory tool for the law enforcement agency. The first and most important step of a comprehensive regulatory system for cannabis would be for Congress to remove marijuana and its derivatives, including delta-9 tetrahydrocannabinol (THC), from the CSA, otherwise known as "descheduling."[137] Descheduling is the only way for cannabis to be regulated in the manner proposed herein, and it is the only way to truly reform federal cannabis policy in a sensible manner. Our proposal calls for cannabis products, like other highly regulated consumables, to be regulated by the government agencies that currently regulate most food and drugs, primarily the Food and Drug Administration (FDA) and the Alcohol and Tobacco Tax and Trade Bureau (TTB) within the U.S. Department of the Treasury.

Under our plan, cannabis products would be divided into four categories, based on chemical components, safety, intended use, and consumption method. Each of these groups would be regulated through a separate regulatory "lane" tailored to the public policy issues raised by that particular classification. The four lanes are: (1) Pharmaceutical drugs; (2) Ingested, inhaled, or topically applied products with more than de minimis amounts of THC; (3) Ingested and inhaled products with de minimis amounts of THC; and (4) Topically applied products with de minimis amounts of THC.

---

[137] Some politicians advocate moving marijuana to a different/lower schedule (rescheduling within the CSA). However, rescheduling would limit most cannabis products to sales only through the current pharmaceutical drug system (Lane #1).

Lane #1 — Pharmaceutical drugs (e.g., Epidiolex; Marinol) (Regulated Like Prescription/OTC Drugs; Lead Federal Regulator: FDA)

Lane #1 includes all products approved as pharmaceutical drugs, over which FDA currently exercises jurisdiction under the authority of the Federal Food, Drug, and Cosmetic Act. This category currently includes approved drugs such as Epidiolex and Marinol and would include any cannabis derivative (whether extracted or synthetic) that is approved as a new drug or authorized for use as an active pharmaceutical ingredient under a tentative or final over-the-counter (OTC) monograph. Products in Lane #1 are subject to FDA's existing rigorous drug approval process. Once the products have been approved by FDA, substantiated disease claims could be made about them, consistent with the terms of the FDA's approval and existing limitations governing off-label uses. These products would be sold alongside prescription or OTC drugs, depending on whether they are approved for use by prescription or OTC.

Necessary Legislation: Lane #1 requires no legislative modifications, other than "descheduling" cannabis to facilitate further drug research and vest FDA with sole regulatory authority.

Lane #2 — Ingested, inhaled, or topically applied products with more than de minimis amounts of THC (+0.3%) (Regulated Like; Lead Federal Regulator: TTB)

Lane #2 includes edible, inhalable, and topically applied cannabis products that are not approved as pharmaceutical drugs by FDA under Lane #1 but that contain more than a de minimis amount of THC (greater than 0.3% by dry weight). The intoxicating properties of these cannabis products raise public policy and safety concerns that are not present for the low-THC products in Lanes #3 and #4. Accordingly, these products would be sold through a network of state-licensed retail stores to individuals meeting state age requirements and/or qualifying medical condition requirements, as appropriate. Here, the states would assume the primary regulatory responsibility for these products, with TTB playing a significant oversight role at the federal level. Of course, thirty-three states already have regulations in place for the sale of medical marijuana through state-licensed dispensaries, and eleven states have legalized recreational sales through state-licensed retail facilities.

Necessary Legislation: Congressional action would be needed to deschedule marijuana and THC (above 0.3%). Legislation would also be needed to grant authority to TTB to regulate these substances (similar to the regulation of alcohol) and to facilitate interstate shipment of the products, as the 2018 Farm Bill did for hemp. Consistent with the model for alcohol, FDA and the states would retain important regulatory roles. Congressional action would be needed to authorize FDA to establish manufacturing requirements for inhalable products. Most cannabis products currently being sold through state adult-use or medical cannabis programs would be regulated through this lane.

Lane #3 — Ingested and inhaled products with de minimis amounts of THC (<0.3% THC) (e.g., CBD, CBN, and CBG) (Regulated Like Food/Dietary Supplements; Lead Regulator: FDA)

Lanes #3 and #4 are the least restrictive lanes and cover products containing no more than de minimis amounts of THC. Currently, federal law provides for the inclusion only of hemp and hemp derivatives with a THC concentration below 0.3%.

Numerous non-intoxicating cannabinoids such as CBD, CBN, THC-A, and THC-V may be derived from either the marijuana plant or the hemp plant. The 2018 Farm Bill created an arbitrary dividing line between marijuana and hemp plants, based entirely on their THC concentration. This has resulted in an overregulation of popular non-intoxicating products based on the THC level of the plant source material instead of the THC level of the finished product (e.g., CBD derived from the marijuana plant). We propose remedying this problem by classifying any final product containing less than 0.3% THC within Lane #3, rather than focusing on the THC content of the plant source material or of any intermediate product.

Based on existing research, these low-THC products carry relatively attenuated public safety risks (see below). Products in Lane #3 would be regulated by FDA to protect the public health and ensure accurate labeling, with regulatory oversight varying based on the products' intended use and any health-related claims made. Sales would be allowed anywhere food or dietary supplements are currently available, without a special retail license requirement. Products with more than the statutorily allowable THC level (currently 0.3%) would be considered adulterated and prohibited from being sold through this lane.

Necessary Legislation: Congressional action is necessary to clarify that non-intoxicating products derived from the marijuana plant should be treated the same as non-intoxicating products derived from the hemp plant, so long as the final product contains no more than 0.3% THC. To expedite the ongoing FDA review process and to meet the significant public demand for these products, congressional action would also make explicit that low-THC products are allowed in food and dietary supplements. Congressional action would also be needed to: (1) authorize FDA to regulate inhalable products, and (2) establish parameters for permissible claims for such products. Congress should also make clear that FDA is the primary regulatory body for this lane.

Lane #4 — Topically applied products with de minimis amounts of THC (<0.3% THC) (e.g., CBD, CBN, and CBG topicals) (Regulated Like Cosmetics; Lead Federal Regulator: FDA)

Lane #4 includes products with low levels of THC that are not consumed orally or inhaled (e.g., topical lotions, creams, balms, etc.). Like products in Lane #3, these products would be regulated by FDA to protect the public health and ensure accurate labeling. Sales would be allowed where other cosmetics are sold without any special retail license. Products with more than the statutorily allowable THC level (currently 0.3%) would be considered adulterated and prohibited from being sold through this lane.

Necessary Legislation: To expedite the ongoing FDA review process related to CBD and to meet the significant public demand for these products, congressional action is needed to make explicit that low-THC products are permitted in topically applied products. This legislation would also set maximum allowable THC levels for products sold through this lane.

Next Steps

It is clear that the era of prohibition is coming to a close. It is now incumbent on the federal government to devise an efficient and effective regulatory system for cannabis products. By leveraging the existing infrastructure and expertise of federal regulators already engaged in analogous tasks, Congress can act to create a system for ensuring a safe product supply chain (as demanded by voter-consumers) without reinventing the wheel or adding layers of unnecessary bureaucratic red tape. This approach is tailored by product category to avoid underregulation and overregulation, both of which advance only the interests of the cartels supplying the illicit market with untested, unregulated, and potentially unsafe products. After a failed century of prohibition, the public deserves and demands safe access to appropriately regulated cannabis products.

Acknowledgments

NCIA's Policy Council would like to thank the professionals who donated their time, energy, and ideas as members of our Regulating Cannabis Working Group. We could not have produced the thoughtful recommendations in this document without their collective insight and expertise.

NCIA's Policy Council Contributors

- Andrew Kline, National Cannabis Industry Association
- Michael Cooper, MadisonJay Solutions
- Khurshid Khoja, Greenbridge Corporate Counsel
- Kris Krane, 4Front Ventures
- Eduardo Provencio, Mary's Medicinals
- Nick Etten, Acreage Holdings
- Douglas Fischer, Greenlane
- Sabrina Fendrick, Berkeley Patients Group
- Alena Rodriguez, Rm3 Labs
- Ian Stewart, Wilson Elser
- Arun Kurichety, KushCo
- Tyler Williams, ASI Food Safety
- Chelsey McKrill, Kikoko
- Chaney Turner, The People's Dispensary
- Steven Hawkins, Marijuana Policy Project
- Trevor Morones, Control Point
- Jason Horst, Horst Legal Counsel
- Jeanine Moss, AnnaBis

- Barton Morris, Cannabis Legal Group
- Patrick Maloy, Cansortium
- Tyler Beuerlein, Hypur
- Jeff Kang, RabbitSwag Inc.
- Kirk Fredrickson, 2Accept
- Sylvan Gerish, Cova
- Hanna Shanes, 365 Cannabis
- Phillip Neiman, JAMS
- Gary Seelhorst, Flora
- Tim Shu, VETCBD
- Brittany Cohen, Global Cannabis Alliance

NCIA Board Members

- AC Braddock, NCIA Board Chair and CEO, Eden Labs
- Manndie Tingler, COO, Khemia Manufacturing
- Mark Passerini, Co-Founder, Om of Medicine
- Sean McAllister, Founding Partner, McAllister & Garfield

Other Significant Contributors

- Ricardo Carvajal, Hyman, Phelps & McNamara
- Bryant Godfrey, Arnold and Porter
- Dan Smith, VS Strategies
- Jordan Wellington, VS Strategies
- Andrew Livingston, VS Strategies
- Rebecca Stamey-White, Hinman & Carmichael LLP
- Erin Kelleher, Hinman & Carmichael LLP

Introduction

For much of the last century, with few exceptions, the U.S. government misguidedly deemed the cannabis plant too dangerous to possess. During this time, millions of people were arrested and billions of dollars were spent on enforcement. Nonetheless, cannabis consumption continued unabated.

However, over the past few decades, a grassroots coalition of Americans across the nation and political spectrum has started chipping away at this near-total prohibition. States, often through ballot initiatives responding to the will of the electorate, have begun to liberalize their cannabis laws. To date, thirty-three states and the District of Columbia have legalized medical cannabis, and eleven states and the District of Columbia have legalized cannabis for adult use.[138] The Agriculture Improvement Act of 2018 (2018 Farm Bill) removed hemp, defined as cannabis and its derivatives, extracts, and cannabinoids with no more than 0.3% THC, from the CSA.[139]

Demand for products containing the cannabinoid cannabidiol (CBD) has exploded recently, with the global CBD product market potentially reaching $22 billion by 2022.[140] Polls consistently show that a clear majority of the public now supports cannabis legalization. For example, 65% of respondents in an April 2019 CBS News poll supported marijuana legalization, with clear majorities of Republicans, Democrats, and Independents favoring the end of prohibition.[141]

A great deal of work nevertheless remains before we see the end of prohibition. While NCIA continues to endorse incremental legislation that achieves piecemeal progress, only descheduling and a new robust federal regulatory framework will ultimately suffice. Part of our ongoing work is envisioning how the cannabis plant should be regulated after it is descheduled. We need to start focusing on the regulatory structure now so that we are not caught flat-footed once descheduling legislation passes both chambers of Congress and is signed by the President.

Non-cannabis consumables for humans and animals are regulated differently depending on ingredients, safety concerns, intended use, and consumption method. Below, we propose appropriate regulatory schemes for each different lane, based on the characteristics of the products, using the regulatory model of similar products as a guide for cannabis regulation.

The first and most important step of this new regulatory process involves removing marijuana and THC from the CSA (descheduling). Proposals to reschedule (as opposed to deschedule) marijuana and THC have been made in the past, but rescheduling would actually create more problems than it would solve. Specifically, moving marijuana and THC to another schedule (below

---

[138] Jeremy Berke and Skye Gould, *Illinois just became the first state to legalize marijuana sales through the legislature — here are all the states where marijuana is legal*, Business Insider (June 25, 2019), https://www.businessinsider.com/legal-marijuana-states-2018-1.

[139] 2018 Farm Bill, Pub. L. No.115-334, 132 Stat. 5018.

[140] *CBD Market Insights,* Brightfield Group, https://www.brightfieldgroup.com/products/cbd-market-research (last visited Sept. 5, 2019).

[141] Jennifer De Pinto, *Support for Marijuana Legalization Hits New High,* CBS News (April 19, 2019), https://www.cbsnews.com/news/support-for-marijuana-legalization-hits-new-high-cbs-news-poll-finds/.

Schedule 1) would still require companies to go through the FDA drug approval process. Merely rescheduling would cause an irreconcilable conflict with the adult-use and medical cannabis systems that have been broadly supported by the public. It would also keep the DEA as a regulator and delay sales while pharmaceutical companies performed the expensive and lengthy clinical drug studies required for FDA drug approval. In short, rescheduling is not just suboptimal—it is simply incompatible with state cannabis laws and runs counter to the will of the voters. Rescheduling is plainly bad public policy.

Removing marijuana and THC from the CSA entirely ("descheduling") is also by itself an inadequate solution without a comprehensive regulatory system in place at the federal level. In the absence of a consistent national regulatory structure, cannabis products will struggle to enter the legal marketplace, and either such products will continue to be sold in the illicit market or legitimate sales will be hampered by ongoing legal uncertainty.[142]

One (suboptimal) option would be to create a new federal agency to regulate the large variety of cannabis products that have market demand. However, creating a new agency is time-consuming, expensive, and unnecessary. The best path forward is to design a regulatory scheme that leverages existing government agencies' expertise and the lessons learned from the many states that have legalized cannabis, while making the necessary legal adjustments to smooth the transition into a post-prohibition world where cannabis products are treated similarly to non-cannabis products. This involves tailoring the regulatory framework of each group of products to address relevant public policy concerns.

The regulatory system proposed here begins by embracing the current methods through which human consumables are regulated, leveraging existing systems and agencies with relevant institutional knowledge to group cannabis products into different regulatory lanes. This approach allows these products to have tailored regulatory structures that address product-specific concerns without applying unnecessary regulatory burdens. By leveraging existing agencies, our proposal can increase efficiency and reduce cost and regulatory uncertainty. For example, both FDA and TTB have significant experience regulating similar products and have previously implemented successful

---

[142] For example, without further guidance from Congress, FDA could consider cannabis extracts "adulterants" and keep them out of consumable products. Similarly, a comprehensive regulatory system would facilitate interstate commerce in these products.

regulatory schemes. Given this available expertise, reinventing the regulatory wheel makes little sense.

> *"The first and most important step of this new* regulatory process involves removing marijuana and THC from the CSA (descheduling)."

Indeed, almost all cannabis product types have comparable offerings currently available through existing regulatory schemes. The proposals outlined below would allow for all cannabis products to be safely produced, sold, and consumed in any state that chooses to permit their sale, ending a lost century where millions of lives were ruined in a misguided attempt to prevent reasonable access to the cannabis plant.

Legal Status of Cannabis in the United States

For much of modern history, cannabis existed with very little regulatory oversight and was widely grown as a cash crop. The plant was used for many industrial products like rope, textiles, and building materials. The effects of consuming cannabis were widely known, and cannabis was used for both medical and recreational purposes. It was not until the end of the nineteenth century and the beginning of the twentieth century that the push to restrict and regulate cannabis gained momentum. This movement to regulate was part of a larger push to improve public health and regulate human consumables. Alcohol prohibition and the first food and drug safety statutes were implemented at around the same time. It should be noted that scholars of this effort to regulate cannabis have identified race as an important impetus, given that government officials and the public portrayed "marijuana" as a dangerous drug brought to the United States by Mexican immigrants.[143] The restriction and criminalization of cannabis continued to accelerate over the next few decades until the passage of the CSA, which essentially created the criminal cannabis regulatory system we have today.

Under the CSA, cannabis (other than hemp and pharmaceutical drugs approved by FDA) is classified as a Schedule I drug, meaning that the substance is considered to have a high potential for abuse, it has no accepted

---

[143] Olivia B. Waxman, *The Surprising Link Between U.S. Marijuana Law and the History of Immigration*, Time (Apr. 20, 2019), https://time.com/5572691/420-marijuana-mexican-immigration/.

medical use, and there is a lack of accepted safety for the use of the substance under medical supervision.[144] Of course, that classification is fundamentally irreconcilable with reality. There is no serious debate that numerous cannabinoids have accepted medical use. One blatant example of this dichotomy is the patent in the hands of the federal government. In 2003, the United States Department of Health and Human Services was awarded a patent entitled "Cannabinoids as Antioxidants and Neuroprotectants."[145] So the fact is that despite cannabis having been classified as having no medicinal use, the United States government itself has a patent on its medicinal use. Meanwhile, there is no consensus in the scientific community that cannabis has a high potential for abuse. Non-scheduled substances such as alcohol and tobacco are widely considered to have a much higher potential for abuse than cannabis.

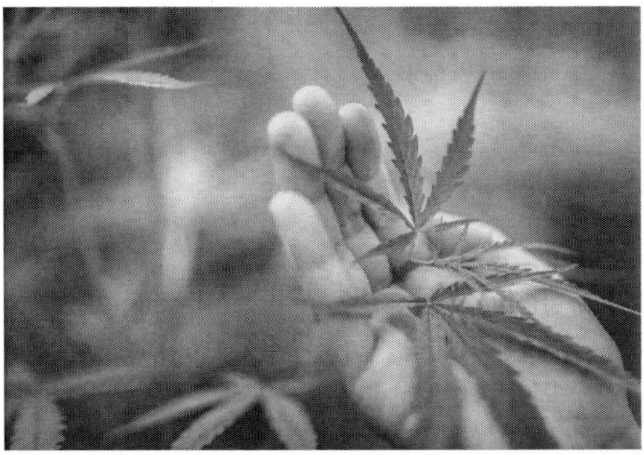

Commercial production and sale is currently prohibited at the federal level for all Schedule I substances, and this prohibition is enforced with severe federal criminal penalties. Not only are nearly all cannabis-related activities criminalized at the federal level, but an individual may be punished as a principal for aiding, abetting, counseling, commanding, inducing, or procuring another person to engage in a cannabis-related transaction that violates the CSA.[146] Further, monetary transactions involving a violation of the CSA are separately criminalized under federal money-laundering statutes.[147] In short, the federal scheduling of cannabis results in possible federal criminal liability

[144] *Drug Scheduling*, DEA, https://www.dea.gov/drug-scheduling.
[145] U.S. Patent No. 6,630,507 (filed Apr. 21, 1999).
[146] 18 U.S.C. § 2.
[147] 18 U.S.C. § 1956.

for all those who work to produce or sell cannabis products, who provide services related to cannabis products, or who handle funds from the production or sale of cannabis products, regardless of state law. This has created an unsustainable federalism clash, with the states operating in direct contravention of federal criminal law.

There has been significant movement cutting against this full federal prohibition. First, numerous states (thirty-three at the time of this writing), in direct conflict with federal law, have licensed cannabis sales and consumption. Second, the federal government began to protect some of these state regimes through guidance memos and language included in appropriation bills.[148] Third, Congress, first as a pilot program in the 2014 Farm Bill, and then permanently in the 2018 Farm Bill, bifurcated the legal status of cannabis, allowing for legal production and sale of products containing less than 0.3% THC (hemp) while keeping products with THC levels above 0.3% (marijuana) federally criminalized and classified as a Schedule I drug.[149]

These efforts have left cannabis in a unique and unsustainable legal status. Products containing THC are sold both for adult use and medical purposes by state-licensed facilities, but they remain criminalized at the federal level. The federal government (through FDA) has approved the use of some drugs that contain cannabis derivatives or their synthetic equivalents (e.g., Marinol, Epidiolex), while regulatory restrictions on wide-scale cannabis research prevents many other potentially beneficial drugs from being developed. The 2018 Farm Bill descheduled a vast number of hemp-derived products, but regulations have not yet been completed by the U.S. Department of Agriculture (USDA) to govern hemp cultivation or by FDA to permit the production and sale of CBD products as foods or dietary supplements. And CBD derived from the marijuana plant (as opposed to the hemp plant) remains federally illegal, regardless of THC content, and notwithstanding the identical chemical composition derived from either source. FDA has been internally evaluating how to allow popular, widely consumed CBD products to be lawfully marketed, particularly for use in ingestible form. Comprehensive reform is needed to address all these issues and the many more that will arise during the transition from prohibition. The piecemeal approach that some in Congress are supporting will not solve the federalism problems and will not

---

148 Memorandum from James M. Cole, Deputy Attorney General, Guidance Regarding Marijuana Enforcement, (Aug. 29, 2013), https://www.justice.gov/iso/opa/resources/3052013829132756857467.pdf.

149 2018 Farm Bill, Pub. L. No. 115-334.

serve to support this burgeoning industry that has proven to be an essential revenue driver for the states that have allowed it to flourish.

Current Legislative Efforts

There have been scores of legislative efforts in Congress to change the current regulatory system for cannabis. Although none of them are as comprehensive as the plan we present here, they all continue the piecemeal process of liberalizing the cannabis laws of the country. Legislative proposals include highly publicized efforts like the Strengthening the Tenth Amendment Through Entrusting States Act (STATES Act), which would allow each state to determine how it wants to regulate adult-use and medical cannabis within its borders, and the Secure and Fair Enforcement Banking Act of 2019 (SAFE Banking Act), which would clarify that banks and financial institutions can provide services to the cannabis industry. There are also efforts to fully deschedule cannabis, such as the Marijuana Opportunity Reinvestment and Expungement Act (MORE Act) or the Marijuana Justice Act. State governments also continue to push efforts to legalize cannabis forward, with Illinois recently becoming the first state to allow for adult-use cannabis sales through legislative action, as opposed to ballot initiative.

NCIA supports all of these efforts as an intermediate step. However, merely rescheduling, providing access to banking, providing for state autonomy, or even removing criminal penalties at the federal level will continue to leave the industry in a precarious gray area. We need a plan to actively regulate production and sales of cannabis. NCIA therefore calls upon Congress, and the federal agencies referenced herein, to work to implement a comprehensive federal regulatory system that begins with descheduling cannabis.

Cannabis Products

Few plants have as many possible applications as cannabis. It is consumed and used for industrial purposes. It can be intoxicating. It can be medicinally therapeutic. It can be inhaled, ingested, and applied topically. But there are a few distinctions between these products that are important to note. Most importantly, we must differentiate between products consumed or otherwise ingested (hereinafter "consumable" products) and those that are not. These consumable products will be the focus of our proposal, given that our aim is to design a regulatory scheme for such products. While there are innumerable uses for industrial hemp fibers and other cannabis products, those uses fall beyond the scope of this regulatory plan.

Within the segment of consumable products, there are still important distinctions that should form the basis for different product regulatory frameworks. Cannabis products can be classified based on whether or not they are intoxicating, whether they are intended for a medical or therapeutic purpose, their cannabinoid concentration levels, consumption method, and myriad other ways. These distinctions are important in determining how each product should be regulated. Inhaling an intoxicating product raises much different policy concerns and requires a different regulatory system than applying a non-intoxicating infused lotion. In general, however, the level of regulation should be proportionate to the potential harm the product can cause and be adequately tailored to that product's intended use.

Below, we present a proposed regulatory structure that encompasses consumable and non-consumable products, including:

- combustible/vaporizable products, like flower, trim, concentrates, and "vape pens"
- orally consumed products, like food or drinks infused with cannabis, pills and capsules, and concentrates intended for oral consumption
- skin and body products, like topicals and patches

Removing the Outdated Regulatory Structure

Cannabis is currently regulated under the CSA, which classifies drugs into five schedules depending on factors such as medical usage, potential for abuse, safety, and potential for forming dependence. Schedule I drugs are those with a high potential for abuse, no currently accepted medical use, and no accepted safe usage under medical supervision. Schedule II drugs are those that have a high potential for abuse and whose abuse may lead to severe psychological or physical dependence but that have a currently accepted medical use. Schedule III drugs are those that have less abuse potential than Schedule I or II drugs, whose abuse may lead to moderate or low physical dependence or high psychological dependence, and that have a currently accepted medical use. Schedule IV drugs have a lower abuse potential, have more limited dependence issues than Schedule III drugs, and have a currently accepted medical use. Schedule V drugs are those that have low abuse potential, have more limited dependence issues than Schedule IV drugs, and have a currently accepted medical use.[150]

Remarkably, marijuana and THC, except in low concentrations in hemp, are currently both classified as Schedule I drugs. This classification is plainly contrary to the facts. For instance, FDA has approved multiple cannabis-related therapeutic drugs, there is a lack of evidence linking cannabis to dependence, and there are no documented cases of overdose. The most direct path to resolve this misclassification is for Congress to act by descheduling cannabis and establishing a comprehensive regulatory framework.

While some politicians have called for rescheduling, that will create far-reaching problems and is unworkable as a solution. Removing all products derived from the cannabis plant from the CSA will lead to fairer outcomes and mirrors how similar products are currently being regulated. There are clear precedents as well: Most recently, the 2018 Farm Bill used this method when creating a regulatory structure for hemp. Similarly, alcohol and tobacco have long been exempted from the CSA. This is because these products are not well-suited to regulation through the CSA model, notwithstanding their addictive properties and potential for harm.

Keeping marijuana and THC scheduled (even at a lower schedule) would only allow for the sale of any non-hemp-derived cannabis product through the current FDA-approved drug model. It would have dramatic negative consequences for the popular legal medical cannabis systems in thirty-three states. The practical result would be the destruction of the current medicinal and recreational cannabis industry and the resurgence of the illicit marijuana market.

> *"Remarkably, marijuana and THC, except in* low concentrations in hemp, are currently both classified as Schedule I drugs. This classification *is plainly contrary to the facts."*

Accordingly, the most efficient blueprint for cannabis regulation begins with descheduling, followed by the implementation of a series of product category-specific regulatory frameworks to deal with the unique policy concerns raised by each product category. In short, cannabis products have too many practical and medicinal uses to be regulated within the limited structure

150 *See supra* note 8.

of the CSA and to face the continued specter of criminal enforcement by the DEA.

Removing marijuana from the CSA also solves many of the related issues plaguing the industry. It would remove restrictions under section 280E of the Internal Revenue Code, facilitate badly needed research into the medical benefits of cannabis, permit full access to banking and payment processing, end criminal sanctions to cannabis-related activities, and facilitate interstate commerce. Descheduling is therefore the most important first step and is a necessary precondition to any effective federal regulatory system.

Establishing a New Regulatory Framework

Americans enjoy the benefits of a broad federal regulatory system designed to promote public health and safety. Consumers benefit every time they take a new prescription drug that FDA has approved or safely consume food that has passed through the USDA inspection process. To date, Americans who purchase cannabis products from state-regulated markets have not been able to enjoy those same benefits. Fortunately, however, this existing federal regulatory system encompasses enough diversity to sufficiently and adequately regulate all cannabis products, provided that certain regulatory and statutory adjustments are made.

Our proposed regulatory system involves existing agencies that will regulate different aspects of the process, ranging from cultivation to retail sales. Under this approach, cannabis products would be grouped into different regulatory lanes, each subject to targeted regulation to address the specific public policy issues raised by that particular group. The four proposed lanes are as follows:

- Lane #1 — Pharmaceutical drugs
- Lane #2 — Ingested, inhaled, and topically applied THC products (+0.3%)
- Lane #3 — Ingested and inhaled cannabinoid products with low/no THC
- Lane #4 — Topically applied cannabinoid products with low/no THC

Further, the proposed system would strive to maximize regulatory certainty and protect orderly markets. This includes creating baseline regulations to facilitate interstate commerce. Recognizing that the well-entrenched (and untaxed) illicit market is unlikely to disappear overnight with the creation of a legal market, regulators must be mindful of overregulation that undermines the efforts of participants in these regulated (and taxed) markets to produce safe products while competing against their unlicensed rivals. Efficiently regulating cannabis products, like similarly situated products, in a safe and consistent manner promises to hasten the demise of the illicit market supplying Americans with unregulated, untested products.

Lane #1 would include all products approved as pharmaceutical drugs by FDA. Products in Lane #1 would be regulated by FDA, and sales would take place through the existing pharmaceutical model, both by prescription and over the counter.

Lane #2 would include all products that are not regulated through Lane #1 and contain more than a de minimis amount of THC. These products would be regulated in a manner similar to alcohol, with TTB, FDA, and the states all having regulatory roles to play. Most products currently being sold through state adult-use or medical cannabis programs would be regulated through this lane.

Lane #3 would include orally consumed and inhaled cannabinoid products with minimal THC concentration. These products would be regulated by FDA in a manner similar to food and dietary supplements. Sales would be allowed anywhere food or dietary supplements are currently available without a special retail license requirement but subject to specific label requirements.

Lane #4 would include topically applied cannabinoid products with minimal THC concentration (e.g., topical lotions, creams, and balms). Like the products in Lane #3, these products would be regulated by FDA, and sales would be allowed where other cosmetics are sold without any special retail license.

This four-lane structure would allow for adequate controls and retail restrictions over products that have intoxicating effects, while allowing greater consumer access to non-intoxicating cannabinoid products. The two primary agencies recommended to regulate cannabis are FDA, which is part of the U.S. Department of Health and Human Services, and TTB, which is part of the U.S. Department of the Treasury. These agencies have extensive experience creating safe and predictable markets for regulated consumer products and are best suited for regulating cannabis.

FDA is the primary federal regulatory agency that oversees food (including food additives and dietary supplements) and drugs (both prescription and OTC). TTB regulates alcohol and tobacco, although FDA retains certain regulatory responsibilities for both products. While most consumable products fall under these agencies' jurisdiction, the agencies have different regulatory mandates. FDA ensures that food products are safe to consume and are properly labeled, and it verifies that drugs are adequately tested to ensure that they are safe and effective for their intended use. To that end, FDA works to prevent or stop the marketing of adulterated or misbranded foods and drugs. By contrast, TTB collects taxes on alcohol, protects consumers, combats the illicit alcohol market, and enforces liquor laws. It is worth noting that these regulators are highly trusted by the public, which generally has high confidence in the quality of the American food and drug supply, and has little concern with bootleggers that sell illicit alcohol. Cannabis deserves the same level of effective regulation. And again, there is no reason to reinvent the wheel.

An illustrative example of the unique charges of the two agencies is the differences in their labeling requirements. FDA requires a declaration of ingredients on food products as well as a nutritional facts panel that consumers can use to understand the relevant nutritional value of the products, with information on such aspects as serving size, calories, fat content, and percentage of daily vitamins. TTB requires different label information on alcoholic beverages, including specific mandated warning language. Both labeling regimes inform the public about important attributes of a product based on the product's contents and intended use, but the form and content are tailored to the product category.

Social Equity

There are other regulatory goals that policymakers should incorporate into any new regulatory framework. Most notably, the federal government must prioritize opportunities for people of color in this developing industry. NCIA's Policy Council recently published a white paper entitled "Increasing Equity in the Cannabis Industry: Six Achievable Goals for Policy Makers."[151] All of the goals from that paper are compatible with the regulatory framework presented here. We urge policymakers to heed the message of our paper and incorporate social equity priorities into any new regulatory framework.

---

[151] *Increasing Equity in the Cannabis Industry: Six Achievable Goals for Policy Makers,* NCIA (Mar. 2019), https://thecannabisindustry.org/reports/ increasing-equity-in-the-cannabis-industry-six-achievable-goals-for-policy-makers/.

LANE #1: Pharmaceutical Drugs
• Products: Products approved as pharmaceutical drugs by FDA • Regulator: FDA • Model: Pharmaceutical drugs • Policy goal priorities: Public health; consumer protection • Retail locations: Drugstores—by prescription or over the counter • Health-related claims: Detailed disease claims allowed

Lane #1 would require no modification to existing law other than descheduling marijuana and THC to allow for robust research and development and to decriminalize possession of the plant. The sole federal regulator for this lane would be FDA.

In fact, there is already a regulatory path that enables cannabis products to legally make it to market in this lane. But at present, that regulatory path is hindered by restrictions on research due to the current scheduling of cannabis. Though FDA has approved a handful of cannabis-derived products or their synthetic equivalents as drugs, including Epidiolex, Marinol, and Cesamet, the research to secure approval was unnecessarily challenging because of cannabis's current CSA schedule. That said, this cannot be the sole lane for cannabis products to reach the market, particularly given that the drug approval process is expensive and complex. In 2016, the Journal of Health Economics estimated the average cost per approved drug at well over $1 billion.

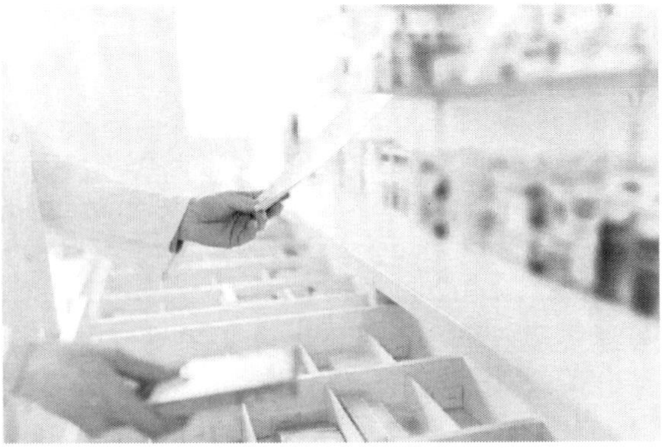

Products in Lane #1

If a cannabis product is approved by FDA as a drug, it would be sold through this lane in a manner that is consistent with any other FDA-approved drug.

Lane #1, like the regulatory lanes governing other pharmacologically active compounds and concentrations that have received FDA approval, would supersede all other regulatory lanes for cannabis-derived products that are intended to treat, cure, prevent, mitigate, or diagnose a disease. Because product approval through this lane is a function of well-established medical and scientific principles, there are no additional content or concentration restrictions in Lane #1 beyond those specified as a condition of approval.

Policy Areas Implicated in Lane #1

FDA is best situated to promote the primary policy goals of this lane: promoting public health by unleashing the potential of the cannabis plant through research and protecting the health and safety of consumers.

This lane provides an opportunity to market cannabis products that, having been approved through a rigorous scientific process, can make disease claims. Once approved, cannabis products can be marketed, sold, and consumed to address specific diseases or ailments consistent with the terms of FDA's approval and current restrictions governing off-label use. Because of the rigorous approval process, this system protects public health by preventing businesses from making false or unsubstantiated disease claims. As a result of the need to achieve these important policy goals and protect consumers, this lane is heavily regulated and requires significant cost outlays for companies trying to bring a product to market that wish to make disease claims. We nevertheless recommend adopting this process for Lane #1 because the FDA approval process facilitates public trust that a cannabis product marketed as a drug has been approved as safe and effective for its intended use.

> "*Regulation of cannabis products under Lane #1* would be no different than the current FDA drug approval process for non-cannabis products."

An important benefit of proceeding entirely within the current regulatory structure is that these products would go to market under an orderly system that operators and consumers understand. The market is stable, companies understand how to operate within the system, and customers are familiar with purchasing FDA-approved drugs. Moreover, this lane offers access to consumers for these cannabis drug products. Consumers will be able to access these drugs through their existing local pharmacy network and can obtain coverage for them alongside other comparable FDA-approved drugs through their health insurance plan.

What Regulation Would Look Like Under Lane #1

Regulation of cannabis products under Lane #1 would be no different than the current FDA drug approval process for non-cannabis products. FDA regulates the safety and efficacy of drugs. This includes premarket review and approval and postmarket monitoring to ensure that a drug is safe. FDA exercises ongoing jurisdiction while the drug is sold.

The FDA approval process normally begins with testing in the laboratory setting. A prototype is developed and the pharmaceutical or biotechnology company submits an Investigational New Drug (IND) application. If this is authorized, the company can then begin testing the product on humans through a series of clinical trials. Three phases of clinical trials are required, with increasing numbers of patients in each subsequent phase. Information collected through the trials is submitted to FDA as a New Drug Application (NDA).

The NDA is reviewed by FDA with a focus on (1) the safety and efficacy of the drug's proposed use; (2) the appropriateness of the proposed labeling; and (3) the adequacy of manufacturing methods to assure the drug's identity, strength, quality, and purity. There are certain limited pathways for some drugs to be approved faster, but generally the process from initial research through final approval is difficult, time-consuming, and expensive.

After approval, the drug may be sold in the United States, but it remains subject to heavy oversight by FDA. The sale of many FDA-approved drugs requires a prescription from a doctor, but some drugs are approved for OTC sales. Whether prescription drugs or OTC drugs are at issue, FDA retains and exercises its authority to oversee product integrity, labeling, adverse event reporting, and advertising through product and facility registrations, inspections, chain-of-custody documentation, mandatory reporting requirements for adverse events, updates to labels and product inserts, and other post-approval monitoring and enforcement efforts.

As noted above, some cannabis-derived products and their synthetic analogues have received approval under this system. We expect that many more pharmaceutical products will be developed after cannabis is descheduled. The main barrier to cannabis products through the pharmaceutical lane so far has been cannabis's Schedule I status. The Schedule I classification has prevented the research and development necessary at the early stages to lead to IND applications, which in turn lead to NDAs. Removing these restrictions will allow research and development that will directly lead to new approved drugs containing THC, CBD, and other compounds found in the cannabis plant.

OTC monographs offer an alternate path for the marketing of cannabis drug products. An OTC monograph sets out standards for the marketing of an OTC drug that is not covered by a new drug application and specifies the permissible active ingredients and labeling (including indications for use). Through the submission of a petition, FDA can be asked to amend a monograph to add ingredients and new indications for use.

LANE #2: Ingested, Inhaled, or Topically Applied THC Products

- Products: All ingested, inhaled, or topically applied products with THC levels above the federally allowable hemp limit that are not otherwise approved as drugs by FDA through Lane #1
- Regulators: TTB, FDA, and state regulatory authorities
- Model: Alcohol
- Policy goal priorities: Public health; public safety; eliminating the illicit market; regulatory certainty and efficiency; and revenue and tax generation
- Retail locations: Allowed only in state-licensed locations
- Health-related claims: State lists of qualifying conditions remain in place; structure/function claims and general wellness claims are allowed under state law for medical cannabis products sold through state-licensed dispensaries

Cannabis products containing more than de minimis levels of THC have stood at the center of debate around reform. It is clear that access to safe and regulated products containing THC has served as an important driver of the cannabis reform movement sweeping the nation. Given the potential for intoxication from use of products that contain THC, the regulatory structure for these products would largely follow the alcohol model. That system also was designed to transition a widely consumed intoxicating product from a robust illicit market to a legal marketplace while protecting public health. And that system succeeded by any measure: today, bootlegging and concerns over the source of alcohol products have largely been consigned to the dustbin of history.

Of course, ending cannabis prohibition is not identical to ending alcohol prohibition, and certain necessary modifications are addressed below. However, many of the larger regulatory concepts would remain the same. Producers, processors, and wholesalers would be regulated at the federal level by TTB. FDA would have a secondary role in Lane #2 regulation (as it does with alcohol), exclusively focused on public health. Age restrictions and retail sales location restrictions would be imposed and enforced by state and local governments.

Products in Lane #2

Lane#2 wouldencompassalloftheproductsthatcontain THCataconcentration above that of "hemp" (as defined in the 2018 Farm Bill) and that are not otherwise approved as drugs by FDA through Lane #1. These would include inhalables (flowers, concentrates, etc.), edibles, other ingestible products, and topically applied products with elevated concentrations of THC. Congress has already defined a THC concentration dividing line in the 2018 Farm Bill between hemp and cannabis: hemp is defined as the cannabis plant or any parts or extracts thereof with a THC concentration of "not more than 0.3 percent on a dry weight basis."[152] This lane would contain all products with more than a de minimis level of THC.

As a result, this lane would contain most of the products sold under the state adult-use and medical cannabis systems. Under this regulatory structure, what today exists as adult-use and medical products would be treated the same through the cultivation, processing, and wholesale phases. These products would be produced, tested, and labeled in a manner similar to that currently allowed under state regulations, and medical cannabis could be prescribed consistent with existing lists of qualifying conditions maintained by the states. Where distinctions remain between these state adult-use and medical cannabis systems, namely tax rates and permissible claims, they are addressed below.

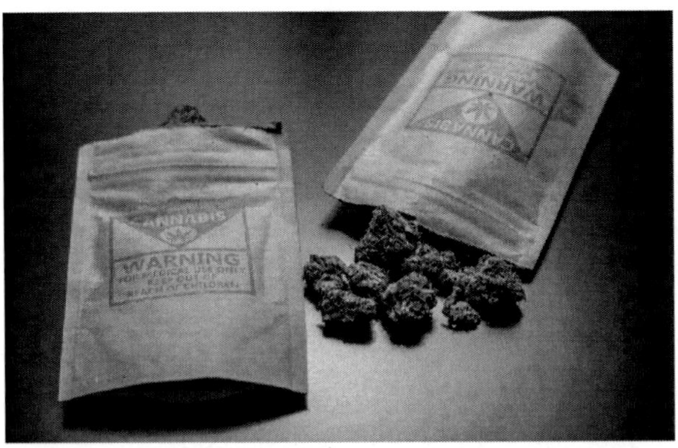

[152] 2018 Farm Bill, Pub. L. No. 115-334, 132 Stat. 4908.

Policy Areas Implicated in Lane #2

The century-long prohibition on cannabis has created a major competitor: the illicit market. The illicit market will not evaporate merely because the government deschedules cannabis. The legal market needs to compete with this market on price and access. A legal cannabis market that is properly regulated with sufficient product quality, access, and price will keep cannabis consumers out of the criminal justice system and put illicit cannabis sellers out of business. The regulatory structure should be set up to continue to protect public safety by emphasizing policies that will reduce ancillary criminal activity. Likewise, by reducing consumption of untested, unregulated products from the illicit market, public health is simultaneously promoted.

Successful development of a regulatory lane for these products is essential to achieving key policy goals: promoting public health, improving public safety, eliminating the illicit market, creating regulatory certainty and efficiency in the legal market, and generating public revenues, both direct and indirect.

To promote public health, the system should be designed to keep adulterants and harmful substances out of consumable products. Notably, unlike in Lanes #3 and #4, THC above 0.3% would not be a prohibited adulterant in Lane #2. As with other products with potentially intoxicating properties, appropriate warning labels should be developed and retail locations should be licensed by the state.

This well-regulated, efficient regulatory lane will also promote interstate commerce by developing certain universal standards applicable to the production and sale of cannabis. Through Lane #2, policymakers can impose labeling restrictions, age restrictions, and other reasonable limits on consumption. Consumers will soon familiarize themselves with standard warnings, symbols, and instructions so they can properly identify products and understand the effects and the potential dangers of consumption. To be explicit, state control over the retail tier will permit each state to restrict sales in ways that reflect the wishes of the local community. National standards nevertheless play an important role in facilitating interstate commerce.

Finally, this lane should allow for revenue collection to fund this regulatory system and other important public policy goals, including social equity. We recognize that the other non-cannabis products regulated in this manner are subject to an excise tax. While we do not attempt to determine an appropriate level of taxation, the amount set should account for the following realities. First, the level of taxation should be sufficient to cover the costs of a new federal regulatory system. Second, unlike many other industries, legal cannabis sales are competing directly with an entrenched illicit market in which participants do not pay any taxes—they avoid paying not merely excise taxes but also taxes on corporate profits and taxes on employee wages. Taxes imposed therefore should be calibrated so that legal cannabis is cost-competitive with the illicit market, including existing state-specific cannabis taxes. None of these public policy goals can be accomplished if the illicit market is not displaced, and that will not happen if consumers do not transition to the legal market because prices are too high. One important caveat to this revenue-generating system is that we recommend that products intended for state-medical cannabis systems should be excluded from this excise tax at the federal level.

Importantly, this model has a clear precedent for success. As with alcohol regulation, which successfully transitioned most illicit alcohol commerce to the legal market, this model will help consumers, operators, and law enforcement agencies better navigate the new regulatory landscape.

What Lane #2 Regulation Would Look Like

Lane #2 would use alcohol as a regulatory model and leverage the state regulatory systems that already exist.[153] State officials would still have an important role in regulating cannabis. Here, Congress would provide TTB with the authority to regulate products containing more than de minimis levels of THC that are not included in the Lane #1 approval process. TTB has the expertise to hit the ground running here. TTB already enforces the Federal Alcohol Administration Act (FAA Act), which involves permitting certain

[153] While we recognize that FDA has the authority under the Family Smoking Prevention and Tobacco Control Act ("Tobacco Control Act") (Pub. L. 111-31) to regulate products made or derived from tobacco and intended for human consumption, we do not believe that cannabis-derived products in any of the categories outlined in this paper should be regulated akin to tobacco-derived products for numerous reasons. By way of example, the findings made by Congress in Section 2 of the Tobacco Control Act (which provides the rationale for granting FDA the authority to regulate tobacco products and serves as the basis for the Act's ensuing requirements) are specific to tobacco use (and the tobacco industry generally) and are inapplicable to the cannabis-derived product space. Moreover, tobacco-derived products are highly addictive because of the drug substance nicotine naturally found in the tobacco plant. Cannabis and cannabis-derived products, on the other hand, do not contain nicotine and are generally non-addictive. Third, cannabis and cannabis-derived products have the potential to produce intoxicating effects, depending on the presence and level of THC found within the product. Whereas, these intoxicating effects are generally not associated with tobacco-derived products. For these reasons, we believe that cannabis-derived products warrant different regulatory treatment than products made or derived from tobacco, and that any additional authority granted to FDA to regulate cannabis-derived products acknowledges these distinctions.

businesses in the alcohol industry, collecting taxes, approving truthful labels, performing inspections and audits, regulating imports, and ensuring that only "qualified persons" work in the industry. As with cannabis, this system was designed to regulate a product emerging from prohibition, with a particular emphasis on shifting sales from a robust illicit market to a legal but regulated market. Many of the methods used by TTB to regulate alcohol would be applicable to the regulation of intoxicating cannabis products and should be adopted.

In this proposal, TTB would be supported by FDA in a manner similar to the alcohol model. The two agencies have previously entered into memoranda of understanding delineating their relationship for regulating alcohol, and we recommend that Congress direct them to enter into a similar agreement for cannabis regulation. For cannabis products in Lane #2, FDA would play the same role that it performs in alcohol regulation: protecting public health by registering production facilities, performing inspections in accord with standards most directly applicable to the product, evaluating the safety of non-cannabis-derived ingredients, and monitoring for adulterants. States would continue to regulate the composition and potency of cannabis-derived ingredients.

Licensing

All producers, manufacturers, and wholesalers of products regulated under this lane would have to receive a permit from TTB. Producers and manufacturers would also have to register with FDA. Retail facilities would not have to register with the federal government and would be regulated solely at the state and local level.

The permitting systems for cannabis products and for alcohol products under TTB would be very similar. In both cases, the state would set minimum conditions for persons eligible to hold these permits. There would be no limit on how many permits could be issued. Facilities would then be subject to safety inspections.

All facilities producing or manufacturing cannabis products would also be required to register with FDA. This allows FDA to know where human consumables are being produced. FDA would have the authority to inspect these facilities for compliance with the most directly applicable manufacturing requirements and to monitor products for harmful adulterants. The law would clarify that no substance derived from the cannabis plant could be considered an adulterant for products sold through Lane #2.

Retail Sales

Intentionally absent from the proposed federal permitting system are retail locations. In this system, the federal government would not issue permits for retail locations. Instead, each state that chooses to permit product sales through Lane #2 would develop a permitting structure for retail sales. This is consistent with how alcohol is regulated and allows each state flexibility and autonomy. States would have the ability to develop regulations to limit sales, make decisions about the location of sales establishments, impose purchase limits, etc. This split system, with the states regulating retail and the federal government and the states regulating all of the upstream commerce, strikes an important balance between providing clarity for businesses while respecting state laws and local political conditions.

Labeling

Label regulation for alcohol is one of the primary functions of TTB, and it would fulfill that role for cannabis as well. Here, TTB would ensure that labels are accurate, do not mislead the public, provide adequate information about the contents and quality of the product, and are regulated for other qualities determined by policymakers (e.g., prohibiting obscenity).

In addition to the standardized labels, TTB would have authority to create a standardized warning label and universal THC symbol to affix to all products. This standardization is of great importance for interstate commerce because it enables companies to move products from state to state without having to comply with fifty distinct labeling requirements.

We propose one major change from the alcohol labeling system, however. The current alcohol labeling system requires preapproval of all labels before a product can be sent to market. This system was designed for a different technological era and a different industry. With today's rapid communication networks and the diversity of cannabis products that will be entering the market, a preapproval process would unnecessarily overburden regulators without providing any additional benefit to consumers. Rather, we propose a system in which the agency issues detailed guidance on labeling as well as a standardized warning label, a universal symbol, and a standard template for information on ingredients and potency. Then the producer or manufacturer can release the products to market without preapproval but must submit a copy of the label to TTB. Businesses can then begin selling the product into the market, but if TTB finds that the label violates agency guidance, it may require the company to revise the label and, for egregious violations or potentially harmful misrepresentations, may order an immediate recall of all products bearing that label. TTB may also conduct periodic audits to ensure accuracy.

Taxation

Under this proposal, a federal excise tax could be imposed at the retail level on all nonmedical products. While we remain silent on the level of taxation, we again emphasize that the legal cannabis market is directly competing with an unregulated and untaxed illicit market. While taxes should be sufficient to cover the necessary regulatory structure, the rate should be kept reasonable to allow legal cannabis to compete against the illicit market. We further propose that products sold through this lane's state-regulated medical retail outlets be exempt from federal tax.

Product Safety

Under our proposal, TTB and FDA would work in tandem to protect public health. FDA currently oversees a wide range of ingested and inhaled products that could be infused with cannabis. While TTB would have authority over the "cannabis" side of these products, FDA would have shared regulatory authority over product safety. TTB would consult with FDA regarding the safety of non-cannabis ingredients. FDA would be responsible for inspecting production facilities to ensure that they follow the most directly applicable standards, including but not limited to Good Agricultural Practices (GAPs), Good Manufacturing Practices (GMPs), and/or preventive controls.[154] Further, FDA would supervise recalls of products that pose a health risk; however, any recall would be made in concert with TTB given TTB's primary enforcement powers.

Health-Related Statements

Most products regulated by TTB are not permitted to make health-related claims. However, the unique status of cannabis makes this default position untenable, and certain health-related claims should be allowed for a limited subset of Lane #2 products as permitted under state law. These claims would also be strictly limited to avoid consumer confusion with products sold through Lane #1 and would mirror the health-related claims that makers of dietary supplements can make regarding their products.

---

[154] Federal legislation would be needed to authorize FDA to establish GMPs for inhalable products. As an alternative, industry could develop and implement model GMPs, ideally in consultation with FDA and its state counterparts.

We recommend this regulatory carve-out because, as mentioned earlier, thirty-three states and the District of Columbia have adopted medical cannabis programs. Countless patient testimonials and doctor recommendations credit cannabis with health benefits. Today, millions of patients rely on cannabis for health purposes, but because of federal prohibition, this medical cannabis system grew independently from the traditional FDA-regulated drug system. When dismantling the prohibition-era policies, care should be taken to avoid destroying the systems that have flourished in the majority of the states.

Cannabis products regulated in Lane #2 would continue to be prescribed in accord with lists of qualifying conditions maintained by the states. In addition, manufacturers could make certain limited health-related claims if permitted under state law, provided those products are sold through a state-licensed medical cannabis dispensary. The claims allowed, like those for dietary supplements, would be structure/function claims and general wellness claims. As with dietary supplements, these products would include a disclaimer on their labels stating that FDA has not evaluated the accuracy of the claim. To be clear, no products could claim that they could diagnose, cure, mitigate, treat, or prevent a specific disease, and products would be misbranded if they made any such claims. Such claims could only be made for products approved through Lane #1.

"Today, millions of patients rely on cannabis for health purposes, but because of federal prohibition, this medical cannabis system grew independently from the traditional FDA-regulated drug system."

Inapplicable Alcohol Regulations

There are provisions of TTB's alcohol regulations designed to target particular issues facing the alcohol industry. Those should not be applied reflexively to the cannabis industry. One such regulation is the mandatory "three-tiered system." The federal government requires, in most cases, that alcohol producers sell their products to wholesale distributors, who then sell to retailers. This requirement emerged from circumstances unique to alcohol prohibition, and imposing it upon cannabis businesses would not further the public policy goals summarized here. Today, states have engaged in a broad federalist experiment to determine the optimal tiered structure for cannabis regulation. Many states have adopted a distribution tier, and many have not. Accordingly, wholesale distributors should be allowed and permitted, but they should not be required.

Another issue that TTB addresses in the alcohol context (that should not be imposed on the cannabis industry) is the "tied house" prohibition. Tied house rules prohibit breweries from having exclusivity contracts with drinking establishments, effectively prohibiting vertical integration. These rules were imposed in an effort to stop aggressive practices of certain large breweries that are not applicable to the cannabis context. In fact, many states have required cannabis companies to be vertically integrated. With a recognition that Congress and TTB could revisit these issues in the future if necessary, we recommend that tied house rules not be adopted at present.

LANE #3: Ingested and Inhaled Cannabinoid Products with Low/No THC

- Products: Cannabis products with de minimis THC sold as food and food ingredients (including dietary supplements and dietary ingredients) in various forms (including tinctures and capsules), as well as non-intoxicating (e.g., CBD) inhaled products
- Regulator: FDA
- Model: Food and dietary supplements
- Policy goal priorities: Public health; regulatory certainty and efficiency; consumer protection
- Retail locations: Wherever food and dietary supplements are sold; no further restrictions
- Health-related claims: Health claims and structure/function claims for dietary supplements and foods, consistent with existing requirements

Lane #3 would govern the large number of ingested and inhaled products that are hitting shelves around the country containing CBD, hemp extract, and other low-THC cannabis compounds. Since the passage of the 2018 Farm Bill, FDA has begun working to identify how to properly regulate these products. Due to various restrictions (discussed below), many of these products are not currently able to flow smoothly through this lane and to market. Statutory changes should be made to help allow these products, which are non-intoxicating and provide myriad nutritional and health benefits, to safely reach the public.

Numerous non-intoxicating cannabinoids such as CBD, CBN, THC-A, and THC-V may be derived from either the marijuana plant or the hemp plant.

The 2018 Farm Bill created an arbitrary dividing line between marijuana and hemp based entirely on THC concentration. This has resulted in an overregulation of popular non-intoxicating products based on the THC level of the plant source material instead of the THC level of the finished product. We propose remedying this problem by classifying any final product containing less than 0.3% THC within Lane #3, rather than focusing on the THC content of the plant source material or any intermediate product.

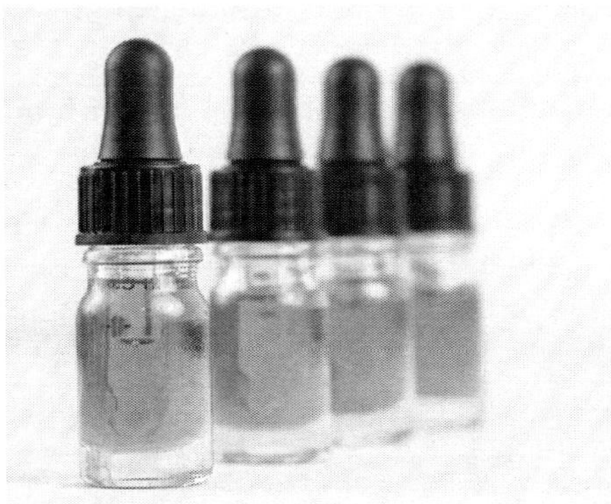

This lane encompasses products that would be regulated as food for humans (including dietary supplements), food for animals, and products that are inhaled. The regulatory scheme should reflect the low risk associated with these products. The exact regulatory requirements would depend on the intended use and whether any health-related claims are made. FDA would serve as the federal regulator for this lane.

Products in Lane #3

Many of the products included in this lane are already governed by the current federal definitions of the terms "food" at 21 U.S.C. § 321(f), "food additive" at 21 U.S.C. § 321(s), and "dietary supplement" at 21 U.S.C. § 321(ff).[155] Though FDA does not currently regulate non-nicotine vaporized products as such, those products would also fall into this category of relatively benign products.

The federally mandated Current Good Manufacturing Practice (cGMP) rules for both foods and supplements already require goods in these categories to take measures to prevent hazards or contamination that may adulterate a

[155] Lane #3 includes food products for humans and animals. The definition of food, pursuant to 21 U.S.C. § 321(f), includes food for humans and "other animals."

product, through the implementation of preventive controls and good manufacturing practices, as applicable. Testing is an important means of ensuring that specifications are met and that hazards are controlled, and it will help ensure that these products are not intoxicating. All of the regulating responsibilities under this lane with respect to ingested products fall under the purview of FDA and existing state agencies that ensure food safety. Federal legislation would be needed to (1) grant FDA authority over inhalable products, and (2) establish parameters for permissible claims for such products.

Under certain circumstances, existing law prohibits the use in foods and supplements of approved drugs or investigational drugs that are undergoing clinical trials. FDA's interpretation of this law has created a regulatory barrier for products in Lane #3 that contain CBD because CBD is the active pharmaceutical ingredient in an approved drug (Epidiolex). Although FDA has recognized that certain hemp-derived ingredients can be added to food, none of those ingredients contain more than trace levels of CBD. FDA has expressed its intention to consider creating a regulatory "pathway" for the use of CBD in foods and supplements but has also recognized that congressional action could resolve this issue. Similar regulatory or statutory pathways should also be facilitated for other non-intoxicating cannabinoids such as CBN and CBG. Once these issues are addressed, this lane will require the fewest modifications to the existing structure for regulation of ingested products.

In the interim, responsible marketers of non-intoxicating products that contain hemp and hemp-derived ingredients, including CBD, should operate as if the existing regulatory structure governed their operations. For example, each such company should be registered with FDA as a food facility; its manufacturing operations must comply with the relevant cGMP rule(s); product labels must refrain from making any disease claims, conform to the relevant nutrition labeling regulation (i.e., with Nutrition Facts for foods and Supplement Facts for supplements), and disclose major food allergens, if present; safety obligations must be met for any substance in a food (through food additive or "generally recognized as safe" (GRAS) provisions) or for any new dietary ingredient in a supplement (through the "new dietary ingredient" (NDI) notification process, if applicable); and supplement marketers must submit to FDA required information about any serious adverse event report they receive in association with their products.

Under this proposal, any product in this lane would be considered adulterated if it contains a THC concentration greater than 0.3%. There are already cannabis products regulated through this lane, including hemp seed and hemp seed oil.

Policy Areas Implicated in Lane #3

Public health is the primary policy concern for products in Lane #3, as it is for all the other lanes. This lane includes products ingested for nutritional purposes, to supplement a person's diet, and to promote general wellness.

The regulations adopted by FDA should facilitate these products entering the market without bureaucratic hurdles, and an emphasis should be placed on allowing members of the public to make informed decisions about the products that they consume. Thus, a well-functioning regulatory system that provides clear guidance for appropriate claims provides an important benefit for producers and consumers alike.

There is no justifiable public health policy reason to continue restricting access to these products beyond the standard restrictions for food and dietary supplements. Moreover, foods and dietary supplements have a long-standing regulatory system built upon best practices that consumers know and trust to keep them safe. Given the limited public safety concerns regarding these products and the absence of an entrenched illicit market, it is critical to narrowly tailor regulations to legitimate public health concerns and avoid overly burdensome regulations that would prevent the United States from being competitive in the emerging global market for these popular products.

With respect to inhalable products, standards would have to be developed to make sure that such products do not contain toxic substances at levels that could pose a health hazard and that they are manufactured in such a way as to help ensure product safety and quality.

> "There is no justifiable public health policy reason to continue restricting access to these products beyond the standard restrictions for food and dietary supplements."

What Lane #3 Regulation Would Look Like

Ingested Products

FDA ensures the safety of food through enforcement of the Federal Food, Drug, and Cosmetic Act (FFDCA). This enforcement is designed to protect public health and involves regulating the products and ingredients that enter the food supply, including dietary supplements, which are subject to some additional requirements.

Before substances can enter the food supply, the FFDCA requires that they be demonstrably safe. In general, there are two ways in which a substance can be lawfully used in conventional food (as opposed to dietary supplements): (1) its use is determined to be GRAS by virtue of common use in food prior to 1958 or through scientific procedures, or (2) its use is approved as a food additive by FDA before it goes to market.[156]

Dietary supplements have a related but slightly different regulatory system. A dietary supplement is a product that contains one or more dietary ingredients such as a vitamin, mineral, or botanical and that is used to supplement the diet. If a dietary supplement includes a "new dietary ingredient" (NDI), which is defined as a dietary ingredient not marketed in the United States before October 15, 1994, that NDI must be present in the food supply as an article used for food in a form in which the food was not chemically altered, or it must be the subject of a notification submitted to FDA at least 75 days prior to marketing a dietary supplement containing the NDI. The notification must provide the basis for the manufacturer's conclusion that the NDI will reasonably be expected to be safe when used under the conditions recommended or suggested in the labeling of the dietary supplement.

The current FDA position is that many cannabis products cannot be sold as food or dietary supplements due to statutory restrictions. A substance cannot be added to food or marketed as a dietary supplement if the substance is already an active ingredient in an approved drug or if it has been authorized for investigation as a new drug, substantial clinical investigations have been instituted, and the existence of those investigations has been made public (the "drug exclusion rule").[157] Because cannabis products are already being sold through Lane #1, FDA has interpreted the drug exclusion rule to prohibit CBD products from being marketed as food or dietary supplements.[158] There is an exception to this rule for products with a prior history of marketing as food or supplements (the "prior use exception"), but FDA has stated that CBD does not currently meet that exception without additional substantiation.

FDA does have the authority, upon notice and public comment, to promulgate a regulation allowing CBD products to be marketed as food or dietary supplements. Indeed, FDA Principal Deputy Commissioner Amy Abernethy, M.D., Ph.D., clarified in a July 2019 letter that the agency is

---

[156] Overview of Food Ingredients, Additives & Colors, IFIC and FDA (Apr. 2010), https://www.fda.gov/food/food-ingredients-packaging/overview-food-ingredients-additives-colors.

[157] 21 U.S. Code § 331.

[158] *Id.*

committed to evaluating the regulatory framework for non-drug uses of CBD, including products marketed as foods and dietary supplements. Dr. Abernethy acknowledged that the statutory provisions behind the drug exclusion rule "allow the FDA to issue a regulation creating an exception, and some stakeholders have asked that the FDA consider issuing such a regulation to allow for the marketing of CBD in conventional foods or as a dietary supplement, or both."[159] She further acknowledged that this process would likely involve determination of a threshold CBD level that could appropriately be considered safe for foods and dietary supplements.

"In the absence of prompt action by FDA, we recommend that Congress act to clarify the status of these products."

Former FDA Commissioner Scott Gottlieb, M.D., previously expressed similar opinions. He testified in February 2019 before the U.S. House Appropriations Committee that CBD could potentially exist "in a high concentration, pure formulation as a pharmaceutical product" while also existing at lower concentrations in products that could be sold as foods and dietary supplements.[160] More recently, in an article published in The Washington Post on July 30, 2019, former Commissioner Gottlieb also acknowledged the ability of FDA to "approve the sale of some CBD products immediately, while effecting a framework for their safe and proper regulation and a pathway for an enforceable market for these goods."[161] This would involve a combination of manufacturers providing new ingredient submissions and FDA exercising enforcement discretion to allow CBD to be marketed in food and supplements so long as the products meet certain conditions. Former Commissioner Gottlieb further acknowledged that "Congress can help by passing language saying that the FDA doesn't need to

[159] 23 Amy Abernethy & Lowell Schiller, *FDA is Committed to Sound, Science-based Policy on CBD*, FDA (July 17, 2019), https://www.fda.gov/news-events/fda-voices-perspectives-fda-leadership-and-experts/fda-committed-sound-science-based-policy-cbd.

[160] Kyle Jaeger, *FDA Head Reveals New Details About Agency's CBD Regulation Plans*, Marijuana Moment (Feb. 27, 2019), https://www.marijuanamoment. net/fda-head-reveals-new-details-about-agencys-cbd-regulation-plans/.

[161] Scott Gottlieb, *The CBD craze is getting out of hand. The FDA needs to act.*, Washington Post (July 30 2019), https://www.washingtonpost.com/ opinions/the-cbd-craze-is-getting-out-of-hand-the-fda-needs-to-act/2019/07/30/94c8024c-b211-11e9-8f6c-7828e68cb15f_story.html?noredirect=on.

issue a broad regulation on CBD and can instead rely on petitions filed by individual, prospective producers."[162]

In the absence of prompt action by FDA, we recommend that Congress act to clarify the status of these products. There is immense public desire for these products, and numerous clinical studies have shown that CBD is safe and well-tolerated in humans, even at very high (> 30 mg/kg/day) doses. This dose is approximately equivalent to 2,800 mg per day for the average adult male, 2,000 mg per day for the average adult female, and 550 mg per day for the average child. In humans, CBD exhibits no effects indicative of any abuse or dependence potential.[163,164,165,166]

It is important to recognize that, but for federal prohibition, many of these products would very likely have proceeded to market many years ago and thereby qualified for the prior use exception. Accordingly, congressional action should be taken to accomplish the following:

- Clarify that non-intoxicating products derived from the marijuana plant should be treated the same way as non-intoxicating products derived from the hemp plant, so long as the final product contains no more than 0.3% THC;
- Clarify that CBD and other non-intoxicating cannabinoids are not prohibited from being marketed in or as dietary supplements solely because they are the subject of clinical trials conducted under an IND or have been approved for use as new drugs;
- Clarify that CBD and other non-intoxicating cannabinoids are not prohibited from being added to food solely because they are drugs that have been the subject of clinical trials or have been approved for use as new drugs; and
- Require periodic audits of cannabis products sold through this lane for label accuracy.

---

[162] *Id.*

[163] Orrin Devinsky, et al., *Randomized, dose-ranging safety trial of cannabidiol in Dravet syndrome*, 90 Neurology e1204 (Apr. 3, 2018).

[164] Kerstin Iffland & Franjo Grotenhermen, *An Update on Safety and Side Effects of Cannabidiol: A Review of Clinical Data and Relevant Animal Studies*, 2.1 Cannabis Cannabinoid Research 139 (2017).

[165] Mateus Machado Bergamaschi, et al., *Safety and Side Effects of Cannabidiol, A Cannabis sativa Constituent*, 6 Current Drug Safety 237 (2011).

[166] Linda C. Laux, et al., *Long-term safety and efficacy of cannabidiol in children and adults with treatment resistant Lennox-Gastaut syndrome or Dravet syndrome: Expanded access program results*, Epilepsy Research, Aug. 2019, at 13.

After Congress takes this action, these cannabis products would be regulated like any other food or dietary ingredient, which would require the following:

Registration and Inspection

All food facilities must register with FDA. This would include all facilities that manufacture, process, pack, or hold Lane #3 products products destined to enter the food supply. These facilities would then be subject to inspection by FDA and all of the current food quality and safety regulations.

Product Approval

For a substance to enter the food supply, its use must be (1) determined to be GRAS; or (2) allowed pursuant to a food additive regulation promulgated by FDA. Most substances that enter the food supply go through a GRAS determination. Some cannabis products like hemp seed, hemp seed oil, and hulled hemp seed have already been determined to be GRAS with no objection from FDA. That pathway should be available for these products as well.[167]

A GRAS determination is typically made by a company, sometimes with the help of outside consultants or organizations. That determination can then be voluntarily communicated to FDA. In response, the agency can issue a "letter of no objection" or a letter that raises questions about the determination. The congressional action recommended above would enable such notifications to be voluntarily submitted to and considered by FDA, because they would not be rejected solely because of the ingredient's presence in an investigational or approved drug. This approach will allow research to continue without foreclosing the possibility that these hemp derivatives could be used in or as

---

[167] Currently, most GRAS determinations are based on scientific procedures (as opposed to experience based on common use in food prior to 1958). Scientific procedures include the application of scientific data (including, as appropriate, data from human, animal, analytical, or other scientific studies), information, and methods, whether published or unpublished, as well as the application of scientific principles, appropriate to establish the safety of a substance under the conditions of its intended use. Note that general recognition of safety may be based only on the views of experts qualified by scientific training and experience to evaluate the safety of substances directly or indirectly added to food. General recognition of safety requires common knowledge throughout the scientific community knowledgeable about the safety of substances directly or indirectly added to food that there is reasonable certainty that the substance is not harmful under the conditions of its intended use. General recognition of safety based upon scientific procedures requires the same quantity and quality of scientific evidence as is required to obtain approval of a food additive. Further, it must be based upon the application of generally available and accepted scientific data, information, or methods, which ordinarily are published, as well as the application of scientific principles. See 21 C.F.R. §§ 170.3(h),170.30(a-b).

food. Similar congressional action could also enable NDI notifications to be submitted to and considered by FDA, notwithstanding an ingredient's presence in an investigational or approved drug.

Product Safety

FDA requires all facilities to follow certain manufacturing standards intended to ensure safety and quality. These standards would apply to all Lane #3 products. There are different GMP standards for food and dietary supplements. Applicable standards would depend on the nature, type, components, marketing, and intended use of the product. These GMP standards ensure that final products do not include the wrong ingredients or contaminants, bear improper labeling, etc.

Labeling

Food and dietary supplements are both subject to detailed labeling requirements. Product labels must include a statement of identity, state the net quantity of contents, provide nutrition information (i.e., with Nutrition Facts for foods and Supplement Facts for supplements), declare ingredients, and disclose major food allergens. A cannabinoid or other cannabis-derived substance included in a product would be listed as an ingredient. Products marketed as dietary supplements are subject to additional requirements. These include the provision of a standard disclaimer coupled to structure/ function claims.

Health Claims

There are similarities and differences between food products and dietary supplements with regard to the distinct types of health-related claims that can be made about each product. Neither type of product can bear a claim to diagnose, cure, mitigate, treat, or prevent a specific disease. However, both products can bear a health claim (meaning a claim that characterizes the relationship between a nutrient and a disease or health-related condition), provided that the claim has been approved by FDA or FDA has been notified of it. More specifically, health claims are allowed if FDA "determines, based on the totality of publicly available scientific evidence (including evidence from well-designed studies conducted in a manner which is consistent with generally recognized scientific procedures and principles), that there is significant scientific agreement, among experts qualified by scientific training and experience to evaluate such claims, that the claim is supported by such evidence."[168] Health claims are also allowed based on statements from federal scientific bodies. Qualified health claims may be allowed based on lesser scientific evidence if authorized by FDA.

In addition, both types of products can bear a structure/function claim (meaning a claim of an effect on a structure or function of the body). In the case of dietary supplements, such a claim must be submitted to FDA within thirty days of the product being marketed and must be coupled to a disclaimer stating that the claim has not been evaluated by FDA and that the product is not intended to diagnose, treat, cure, or prevent any disease. In the case of conventional foods, there is no requirement for notification or the use of a disclaimer; however, FDA's position is that any claimed effect on a structure or function of the body must derive from nutritive value.

Retail Sales

Assuming no contrary state regulations, these hemp and cannabinoid products would be permitted for sale in all retail outlets that are able to sell food or dietary supplements now, with no age restrictions or additional regulatory barriers.

Inhalable Products

Currently FDA does not regulate inhalable products, unless such a product makes a claim that renders the product a drug (i.e., a disease claim or a structure/function claim) or the product qualifies as a tobacco product. Therefore, congressional action would be needed to grant FDA authority to regulate cannabis-derived inhalable products and to secure a pathway for marketing of inhalable products that make structure/function claims or other appropriate non-disease claims. Enabling legislation could specify the safety standard applicable to such products, designate substances that are prohibited for use, and establish GMPs, mandatory labeling elements, parameters for permissible claims, and restrictions on retail sales. Pending enactment and implementation, the cannabis industry could voluntarily develop and implement guidelines to address these issues so as to help ensure the safety and quality of these products.

---

[168] 21 U.S.C. § 343 (r)(3)(B)(i).

LANE #4: Topically Applied Low THC Products

- Products: Low-THC cannabis products that are topically applied
- Regulator: FDA
- Model: Cosmetics
- Policy goal priorities: Public health; regulatory certainty and efficiency; consumer protection
- Retail locations: No restrictions
- Health-related claims: Not allowed

Topically applied products, both those that contain cannabis and those that do not, are generally believed to pose more limited public health concerns than orally consumed products. FDA, which regulates cosmetics, recognizes this and applies a less comprehensive regulatory system to these products than it does to food or drugs.

The existing regulatory structure for cosmetics should be used for clarity and consistency, with hemp derivatives being just one of the many allowed ingredients in cosmetics. This system would provide appropriate oversight while ensuring that customers can access cannabis cosmetic products in all stores that sell cosmetics.

Products in Lane #4

Lane #4 will contain all cannabis products that do not contain more than a de minimis level of THC and are "intended to be rubbed, poured, sprinkled, or sprayed on, introduced into, or otherwise applied to the human body ... for cleansing, beautifying, promoting attractiveness, or altering the appearance," consistent with the current statutory definition of "cosmetic."[169] Such products can come in various forms, such as lotions, creams, and balms. This lane is very similar to Lane #3, again involving the introduction of non-intoxicating, safe cannabis products into an already existing regulatory framework. But because topical products generally pose more attenuated potential health risks than food products, they should follow the federal regulatory framework of other cosmetic products.

[169] *Cosmetics & U.S. Law*, FDA (Nov. 3, 2017), https://www.fda.gov/cosmetics/cosmetics-laws-regulations/cosmetics-us-law.

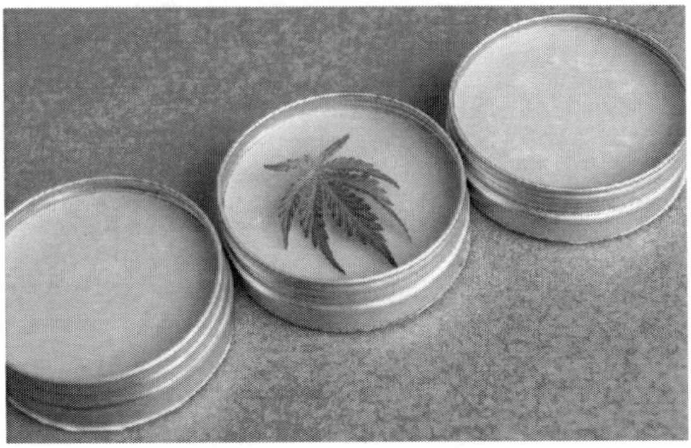

Policy Areas Implicated by Lane #4

Cosmetics are not orally consumed, reducing the public health risk. Moreover, cosmetics are not marketed with health-related claims or nutrition claims.[170] The goal of this regulatory system should be to protect the public from dangerous products and misleading claims, while not imposing unnecessary burdens on businesses or consumers.

The current cosmetic regulatory system does exactly that and should be applied to products that contain cannabis. Cosmetics crossing the THC threshold would be considered adulterated and subject to FDA enforcement actions. Cosmetics making disease or structure/function claims would be considered misbranded. This ensures that consumers have ready access to low-THC products that raise few policy concerns, while creating a path for products with higher levels of THC through Lane #1. Although the mere presence of a cannabis derivative is not sufficient to render a cosmetic a "drug," we recommend that this be made clear in any enabling legislation.

What Lane #4 Regulation Would Look Like

FDA has the authority to regulate cosmetics under the FFDCA. The FFDCA, the Fair Packaging and Labeling Act, the Color Additive Amendments Act of 1960, the Poison Prevention Packaging Act, and related regulations constitute the law governing cosmetics.

In many ways, FDA's regulation of cosmetics is a less burdensome version of Lane #3. Given that some of the public health concerns are inapplicable to cosmetics due to the nature of these products, the more onerous regulatory requirements have been deemed unnecessary. The focus remains

[170] Although a cosmetic product might have a structure/function effect, that effect cannot be the subject of a labeling claim, because such a claim would render a cosmetic a drug.

on adulterated and misbranded products. FDA may still seize products in violation of the FFDCA, may issue injunctions, and may enforce the law with criminal penalties in some instances. It also may conduct inspections. However, much of the rest of the regulatory environment for cosmetics takes the form of guidelines and self-regulation. Registration of manufacturers is voluntary. There is no requirement to use GMPs, although FDA has set out recommended GMPs in a draft guidance. There are no premarket notification requirements except those involving color additives.

Conclusion

With the prohibition era nearing its end, it is imperative to begin discussing how to shape an effective, comprehensive cannabis regulatory framework. The system proposed here would allow all cannabis products to flow to the market through a regulatory scheme designed to best advance the policy goals raised by these products. It builds off the existing expertise of federal agencies and the developing state-level industry. Potentially intoxicating products and those making medical claims will be sold through controlled systems that limit their availability, while non-intoxicating products will not be hampered by those same restrictions. The system proposed here would end prohibition in a thoughtful and comprehensive manner, ensuring that the mistakes of the previous era do not negatively affect the opportunities that are at our doorstep.

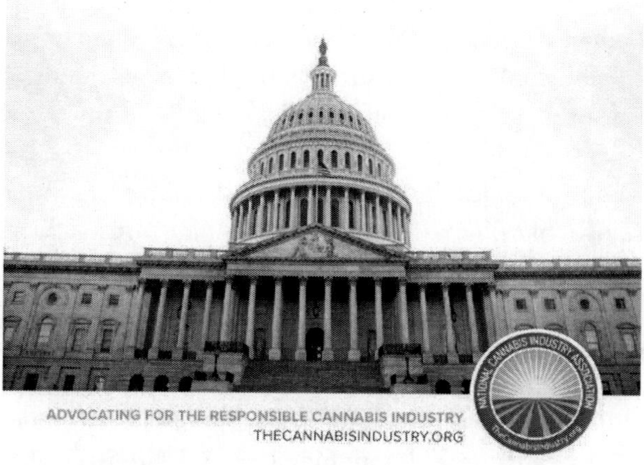

* * *

Letter of January 13, 2020, from Bruce A. Jarrell, M.D., Interim President, University of Maryland, to Mr. Sarbanes, submitted by Ms. Eshoo

January 13, 2020
The Honorable John A. Sarbanes
Congressman
2370 Rayburn House Office Building
Washington, DC 20515

Dear Congressman Sarbanes:

This week the US House Committee on Energy and Commerce will be holding a legislative hearing on *"Cannabis Policies for the New Decade."* As the interim president of the University of Maryland, Baltimore (UMB), Maryland's only public health, law, and human services university, I have significant interest in *H.R. 601, the Medical Cannabis Research Act of 2019* and *H.R. 3797, the Medical Marijuana Research Act of 2019* which are among the bills being discussed during this upcoming hearing.

Due to the federal prohibition on the possession and research on the strains of medical cannabis grown within the United States, there is an alarming gap on the science, policy and therapeutic benefits of medical cannabis. Specifically, health care professionals report significant gaps in cannabis-related knowledge, and the degree of this educational gap has been the focus of a number of studies. Published surveys of physicians, medical students and residents, nurse practitioners, pharmacists, and pharmacy students have described similar perceived knowledge gaps.

The University of Maryland, Baltimore (UMB) is essentially prevented from possessing marijuana and allowing our researchers to purify, characterize, synthesize and alter its derivatives so that it could be used for research. Federal law prohibits us from any action that aids or abets these activities as well as receiving funding from state-licensed marijuana companies. In effect, federal law not only prevents us from studying marijuana in the research lab, it also prevents us from clinical research on the effects of any chemical derived from the cannabis plant. Violations of these regulations could jeopardize UMB-ourlarge federally sponsored research grants are estimated at $250 million, and our US Department of Education student aid funding.

Throughout medical history, native plants have been the source for many important medical discoveries. Antibiotics to cure infections, digitalis to treat heart failure, drugs to stop cancers, narcotics to control pain, medications to induce anesthesia allowing surgeries to be performed-and many ot hers. Plants often have complex chemistry, which often produce miracle drugs to improve our health and well-being. The cannabis plant may also be one of these plants, and further and extensive research is crucial.

Cannabis is known to have over 400 unique chemicals in its composition. We know that one of these chemicals components produces the psychoactive effects known as a high, but we also know of another chemical in cannabis that can control nausea and loss of appetite seen during cancer chemotherapy treatment. The cancer drug has transformed care in certain instances. Another chemical entity prevents seizures in children. There are other compounds with active effect, although less proven. The remaining chemicals need research as well. In addition, we need to develop ways to measure levels of the drug in the body, a critical part of performing high quality clinical trials.

In 2017, the National Academies of Sciences, Engineering, and Medicine.[171] released a comprehensive report based on the review of more than 10,000 scientific abstracts from cannabis health research. This report made approximately 100 conclusions related to the therapeutic and health effects of cannabis and suggested approaches to stimulate and improve cannabis research. The report presents a national research agenda for cannabis, including a focus on research standards for medical cannabis, and for federal agencies to reduce the impact of regulatory barriers on cannabis research.

As a corollary, the University of Maryland School of Pharmacy (UMSOP) began offering a Master of Science in Medical Cannabis Science and Therapeutics beginning this past fall of 2019. As the number of states legalizing medical cannabis continues to grow, so does the need for an educated workforce to respond to the patient inquiries regarding the therapeutic effects of medical cannabis. In a 2015 survey[172] of health care providers (physicians, nurse practitioners, and pharmacists), a large knowledge gap was found related to medical cannabis dosing, the development of therapeutic treatment plans, knowledge on the similarities and differences between cannabis pro ducts, education related to safety, risks and

[171] The Health Effects of Cannabis and Cannabinoids: The Current State of Evidence and Recommendations for Research. Washington, D.C.: The National Academies Press; Online document at: www.nap.edu/read/24625/chapter/l, accessed February 15, 2019.

[172] Ziemianski D, Capler R, Tekanoff R, et al. Canna bis in medicine: A national educational needs assessment among Canadian physicians. BMC Med Educ 2015;15:52.

precautions for medical cannabis use, and the laws and regulations surrounding medical cannabis. For example, we do not even know simple things like safe dosing practices. A related survey[173] found lack of education regarding medical cannabis reported by 87% of respondents as a barrier to use in clinical practice, with 76% of respondents ranking the need for education to be strong or very strong. The UMSOP Master of Science in Medical Cannabis Science and Therapeutics will cover the principles of drug action and cannabinoid pharmacology; drug delivery and pharmaceutics; clinical use and effects of medical cannabis; current state and federal laws along with elective courses in research methodology, basic sciences, therapeutics, and policy.

I do hope that you and your colleagues take into consideration the need to allow research on marijuana and eliminate the barriers and onerous regulations to study this potentially useful plant to improve human health.

Sincerely,

Bruce A. Jarrell

Statement of the American Property Casualty Insurance Association

Introduction

Dear Chairwoman Eshoo, Ranking Member Burgess, and Members of the Subcommittee:

The American Property Casualty Insurance Association (APCIA) appreciates the House Energy and Commerce Subcommittee on Health's interest in the future of cannabis policy and welcomes the opportunity to submit comments for the Subcommittee's hearing titled "Cannabis Policies in the New Decade."

Representing nearly 60 percent of the U.S. property casualty insurance market, APCIA promotes and protects the viability of private competition for the benefit of consumers and insurers.

---

[173] Ziemianski D, Tekanoff R, Luconi F, Ware M. Cannabinoids in clinical practice: experiences and educational needs. In: Proceeds of the Canadian Pain Society 2012. Pain Research and Management 2012;17(3):229.

APCIA represents the broadest cross-section of home, auto, and business insurers of any national trade association. APCIA members represent all sizes, structures, and regions, which protect families, communities, and businesses in the U.S. and across the globe.

The following comments do not seek to promote views for or against the legalization of marijuana. However, to the extent that states decide to make marijuana "state legal," APCIA believes that Congress must play a role in providing legal certainty to businesses otherwise abiding state law as well as supporting expanded scientific research into the effects of marijuana on public health and safety.

APCIA supports full consideration of a broad range of necessary regulatory and enforcement standards and a resolution of the direct conflict between state and federal law on the legality of providing financial services, including insurance, to marijuana related business and activities. Specifically, APCIA supports S. 2201, CLAIM Act, and the house-passed version of H.R. 1595, SAFE Banking Act, providing a safe harbor allowing voluntary coverage of state legal marijuana related activities.

APCIA is also concerned about the growing risks of marijuana use and its effects on highway and workplace safety. Unfortunately, federal restrictions on scientific research into marijuana's effects has resulted in a lack of effort into the development of a meaningful impairment standard and related testing technology. Therefore, we would support legislation that would allow for expanded research of marijuana focusing on types of marijuana and products representative of those found in state-legal marketplaces.

Background

Thirty-three states and the District of Columbia have approved medicinal marijuana, twelve of which have also approved recreational use. These state laws conflict with federal law, which classifies marijuana as a Schedule I drug under the Controlled Substances Act (CSA), with no currently accepted medical use and a high potential for abuse.

As states continue to legalize marijuana, and its use increases, more people are getting behind the wheel and working under its influence. In states where marijuana is legal, studies have shown an increase in motor vehicle collision claim frequencies and an increase in traffic deaths involving drivers who tested positive for marijuana.

In the workplace, marijuana is the most commonly detected illicit substance in drug testing. The National Institute on Drug Abuse (NIDA) reported that employees who tested positive had 55 percent more industrial incidents and 85 percent more injuries. The National Safety Council has stated that no level of marijuana use is acceptable for those in safety sensitive positions.

Despite this, there has been very little high-quality scientific research on marijuana impairment. Unlike alcohol, the extent and effect of marijuana does not have a clear correlation with the amount of the psychoactive component, THC, in a user's blood. The amount of THC can peak before a user experiences impairment and remains in a user's system for weeks after use, which means a positive blood test is not a reliable indicator of impairment. *There is presently no objective standard for marijuana impairment and no reliable test to measure it.*

To ensure the safety of workplaces and roads, it is imperative that an objective impairment standard and a reliable test for impairment be developed. High-quality scientific study, using marijuana product comparable to what consumers can access in legal marketplaces, is key to that development.

Marijuana Impairment Research

Regardless of whether one supports or opposes legalizing marijuana, we can all agree on the importance of preventing marijuana impairment on our roads and in the workplace. There is no objective standard or reliable methodology to determine marijuana impairment. In comparison, when testing for alcohol impairment there is a clear correlation between the amount of alcohol in the blood and a level of impairment. Detecting marijuana impairment through a standardized test is more complicated.

Marijuana is metabolized by the body differently from alcohol. The level of THC (tetrahydrocannabinol), the psychoactive ingredient of marijuana, in the body can vary based on several factors, including how marijuana is ingested and the potency of the product. The level of THC can drop before a user experiences impairment, but traces of THC may still be found in the body weeks after using marijuana. This means that a positive test results for the present of marijuana in someone's system does not necessarily mean he or she is impaired.

APCIA Supports High Quality Scientific Research into the Health and Safety Impacts of Marijuana Use, Including Observational, Behavioral, and Physiological Studies Using Marijuana and Products Containing Marijuana

Few studies have evaluated the effect of marijuana use on driver and workers performance. Government agencies face difficulties in developing marijuana impairment standards and determining medical efficacy because of federal prohibitions and arduous requirements placed on scientists seeking to use marijuana in studies, due to its Schedule I classification. The federal application process, including clearance through the FDA, to study marijuana impairment can delay a research program by years.

- APCIA recommends allowing marijuana impairment research without application through the FDA Investigational New Drug program to expedite research to determine how marijuana impairs users and how impaired users impact public safety.

Additionally, marijuana's classification as a Schedule I drug under the CSA places it in the same category as heroin, LSD, and ecstasy (MDMA), and defines it as having high potential of abuse, and no currently accepted medical use. To study Schedule I drugs, researchers must complete an extensive application process through the Drug Enforcement Administration (DEA) that exceeds the already stringent requirements to study Schedule II and III drugs.

- APCIA recommends, allowing institutions and researchers already authorized to conduct research with controlled substances in Schedules II or III, to facilitate research while not reducing safety or diversion controls.

Once approved, marijuana for study can only be obtained through the National Institute on Drug Abuse (NIDA), which requires marijuana to be obtained from a single source. The marijuana available to researchers through NIDA's sole source contract is not representative of what is available in state-legal cannabis markets for either medical or recreational use. NIDA-sourced marijuana contains a much lower amount of THC than marijuana commercially available to consumers in states where marijuana is legal. The NIDA program produces cannabis containing 12 percent or less THC by weight. In comparison, states with legal marijuana offer flower containing 20-

30 percent THC, concentrates containing 60-90 percent THC, and edible products which may contain anywhere from five to hundreds of milligrams of THC.

A genetic analysis conducted by researchers at the University of Northern Colorado report the NIDA product is genetically related to hemp, which is unlike the plant material available to consumers. It is not representative of actual use of marijuana in the 33 states and the District of Columbia, where it is legal, and cannot produce scientifically meaningful and useful results when researchers test for medical efficacy or driving and workplace impairment.

- APCIA recommends, allowing authorized researchers and institutions in states where marijuana is legal to access marijuana and marijuana products that are representative of what adult consumers may legally obtain in those states.
- APCIA also recommends permitting the NIDA sole source program to provide marijuana products, that are representative of what adult consumers may legally obtain in states where marijuana-legal states, to authorized institutions and researchers located in states where marijuana is not legal.

Federal – State Conflict for Legal Businesses

In addition to the twelve states and the District of Columbia where is recreational marijuana is already legal, 23 states proposed legalization in 2019. Gallup polling reports continued increase in support for marijuana legalization, with 66 percent of Americans supporting in 2018, up from 51 percent in 2014. We expect this trend to continue and for the legal cannabis industry to continue to expand.

Like businesses in any other industry, a cannabis-related legal business (CRLB) requires commercial general liability, property, directors and officers, professional liability, and other insurance coverages. However, a CRLB may not have access to the same number of insurers, the same selection of policies, or the same limits as other non-cannabis-related businesses. This potential gap in insurance leaves consumers, employees, vendors, and businessowners without adequate financial protection in the event of a loss.

A key reason for this discrepancy is that cannabis remains illegal under U.S. federal law. Marijuana's Schedule I classification makes no exception for states that approved the legal use of marijuana. Possession, purchase, or sale of even small amounts is a violation of federal law. Title 18 of the federal criminal statutes expands the CSA to include the transportation or transmission of funds known to have been derived from the distribution of marijuana. The federal treatment of marijuana has varied and financial institutions, including insurers, fear federal prosecution should they provide coverage to a state legal CRLB. The house-passed H.R 1595, SAFE Banking Act is an important step toward legal certainty for consumers and the insurance industry and will encourage insurers to provide needed coverage for the financial exposures faced by these legal businesses.

Conclusion

APCIA appreciates the opportunity to provide feedback on this important issue. We strongly urge the passage of the SAFE Banking Act to resolve the legal predicament consumers, businesses, and insurers face under competing state and federal laws. Further, we support the committee addressing public safety by expediting the expansion and advancement of high-quality scientific research into marijuana impairment and the development of an objective impairment standard.

APCIA would be happy to answer any questions the Committee or its Members may have and look forward to engaging with Members, staff, and other stakeholders.

Written Testimony Submitted by Paul Armentano, Deputy Director, National Organization for the Reform of Marijuana Laws

Chairwoman Eshoo, Esteemed members of the Committee, and Interested Parties:

As is evident by the title of this hearing, our federal marijuana policies are stuck in the past. It is time for Congress to amend them in a manner that comports with our current political and cultural reality.

Congress initially classified the cannabis plant as a Schedule I controlled substance in 1970 – at a time when America knew far less about it than we now know today. Since that time, tens of millions of Americans have experimented with cannabis and according to the PubMed.gov database, over

30,000 peer-reviewed studies have been published about this plant. It is clear from both the scientific and empirical data that marijuana does not meet the specific definitions of a Schedule I controlled substance.

It does not possess a "high potential of abuse" as compared to substances placed in lower classifications, like cocaine and opioids. It does not lack "accepted medical use" in the United States. In fact, 33 states by statute now authorize medical cannabis use, and millions of Americans are using it under the supervision of their physician. And while cannabis is not altogether harmless, it certainly is not so dangerous as to assert that it lacks "accepted safety … under medical supervision."[174]

Voters and state governments are no longer wedded to these federal 'Flat Earth' policies and are pursuing alternative regulatory options. Over one in four Americans now reside in a jurisdiction where the adult use of cannabis is legal, and the majority of states regulate medical marijuana use and sales. Many of these latter statewide policies have been in place for the better part of two decades, while adult-use regulations in Colorado and Washington were initially approved in 2012.

To date, no state has ever repealed a marijuana legalization law after enactment, medical or otherwise. Further, two-thirds of adults — including majorities of self-identified Democrats, Republicans, and Independents — endorse making the plant legal, according to the latest nationwide Gallup poll.[175] As more states amend their cannabis laws, public support for legalization has continued to rise, increasing some 25 percent in just the past seven years.

This rising support is evidence that legalization laws are functioning largely as voters and lawmakers intended. This further illustrates the majority of the public is pleased with results. Contrary to the concerns of some, state-specific cannabis liberalization policies have not been independently associated with adverse effects on public safety, such as increased levels of crime[176], traffic safety[177], and youth access.[178]

This is why most Americans prefer a policy of cannabis legalization and regulation rather than continuing the failed strategy of marijuana

---

[174] Iverson. 2015. Long-term effects of exposure to cannabis. Current Opinion in Pharmacology 5: 69-76 – "Overall, by comparison with other drugs used mainly for 'recreational' purposes, cannabis could be rated to be a relatively safe drug."

[175] https://news.gallup.com/poll/267698/support-legal-marijuana-steady-past-year.aspx.

[176] https://norml.org/marijuana/fact-sheets/item/marijuana-regulation-and-crime-rates.

[177] https://norml.org/marijuana/fact-sheets/item/marijuana-regulation-impact-on-health-safety-economy.

[178] https://norml.org/marijuana/fact-sheets/item/marijuana-regulation-and-teen-use-rates.

criminalization. Congress would be wise to listen. The establishment of a pragmatic regulatory framework that allows for states to engage in the legal, licensed, commercial production and retail sale of marijuana to adults – but that continues to restrict and discourage its use among young people – best reduces the risks associated with the plant's use or abuse. By contrast, advocating for the marijuana's continued criminalization only compounds them.

By removing cannabis from its Schedule I status, as provided by The MORE Act[179], and descheduling it in a manner similar to alcohol, Congress would eliminate the growing and untenable conflict between state and federal law. Further, this policy change would permit those state governments that wish to continue to prohibit intrastate cannabis-related activities to do so. It will also allow those states that already have – or that in the future wish to – pursue regulatory schemes the authority to move forward. Of course, even in an environment where cannabis is descheduled, Congress and other federal agencies would still possess various regulatory authority over how marijuana products are produced, taxed, marketed, and sold – just as it possesses similar oversight authority over alcohol. The closest analogy would be federal limits on how certain alcoholic beverages may be advertised; mandated warning labels on alcohol products, minor federal excise taxes on alcoholic goods; and a prohibition on the sale of certain formulations of alcoholic products, such as those mixed with caffeine.

Further, descheduling cannabis will facilitate scientists' ability to conduct large-scale clinical trials evaluating cannabis' therapeutic efficacy in a manner that is simply not possible today.[180] Because federal regulations prohibit clinical testing on all forms of cannabis other than the limited varieties of flowers available from the US National Institute on Drug Abuse/University of Mississippi program, there exists no legal pathway for a commercial entity to clinically evaluate marijuana products in a way that would meet FDA requirements. In fact, the US Drug Enforcement Agency acknowledged this reality in 2016, when it stated, "[U]nder the historical system, there was no clear legal pathway for commercial enterprises to produce marijuana for

---

[179] HR 3884: The Marijuana Opportunity, Reinvestment, and Expungement Act.

[180] https://thehill.com/opinion/white-house/406693-The%20federal-government-must-stop-stifling-medical-marijuana-research.

product development."[181] Yet, despite promises to the contrary, neither the DEA nor NIDA has amended these undue regulatory hurdles.[182]

For these and other reasons, NORML encourages members of this committee to join your colleagues on the House Judiciary Committee and advance The MORE Act to the House floor. For some 50 years, the cannabis plant has been improperly categorized and criminalized by federal law. It is time to re-examine and amend this longstanding failed policy.

Thank you for your time and consideration.

Paul Armentano
NORML Deputy Director
Washington, DC
202-483-5500

* * *

Letter of August 27, 2019, from Norman E. Sharpless, M.D., Acting Commissioner, FDA and Francis S. Collins, M.D., Ph.D., Director, NIH to Mr. Schatz, submitted by Ms. Eshoo

August 27, 2019
The Honorable Brian Schatz
United States Senate
Washington, DC 205 I 0-1105

Dear Senator Schatz:

Thank you for your March 20 letter requesting information on research and regulatory issues related to the therapeutic use of cannabis and cannabinoid compounds. The National Institutes of Health (NIH) and the Food and Drug Administration (FDA) are committed to advancing research on the risks and potential benefits of cannabis for therapeutic uses, and we are pleased to share the following information about this important area of inquiry with you.

---

181 DEA 21 CFR Part 1301 [Docket No. DEA-447] https://s3.amazonaws.com/public-inspection.federalregister.gov/2016-17955.pdf.

182 https://thehill.com/opinion/civil-rights/458868-deas-latest-promise-to-facilitate-medical-cannabis-research-should-be.

NIH's research portfolio includes epidemiologic, basic, and applied research on cannabis, its constituent compounds, and the endocannabinoid system through which cannabinoids act. Much of the current evidence on cannabis and health was synthesized in a National Academy of Sciences report, "The Health Effects of Cannabis and Cannabinoids: The Current State of Evidence and Recommendations for Research,"[183] which was sponsored by the National Institute on Drug Abuse (NIDA), the National Cancer Institute (NCI), the Centers for Disease Control and Prevention, FDA, and other stakeholders. The report summarizes the evidence on the efficacy of cannabis or cannabinoids for chronic pain, as anti-emetics, and for improving patient-reported spasticity symptoms in multiple sclerosis, as well as evidence on the risks cannabis poses to respiratory health, brain development, and impaired driving.

Several NIH Institutes and Centers, including NIDA, the National Center for Complementary and Integrative Health (NCCIH), the National Institute of Neurological Disorders and Stroke, NCI, the National Institute on Alcohol Abuse and Alcoholism (NIAAA), the National Institute of Arthritis and Musculoskeletal and Skin Diseases, and the National Institute of Diabetes and Digestive and Kidney Diseases fund studies on the therapeutic potential of cannabis and cannabinoids as relevant to their respective missions. In fiscal year 2018, NIH estimates to have spent $148 million on cannabinoid research, broadly, and $38 million on therapeutics, specifically. NIH funds studies on delta-9-tetrahydrocannabinol (THC) and cannabidiol (CBD), two of the cannabinoid components of the cannabis plant, for the treatment of pain, including chronic pain, back pain, and neuropathic pain caused by HIV. Several studies are also examining the endogenous signaling system that cannabinoids influence as a potential target for new pain and addiction therapies, including difficult-to-treat issues such as pain cause d by sickle cell disease or diabetic neuropathy. As part of these efforts, NIH recently reissued a funding opportunity announcement (FOA) titled "Developing the Therapeutic Potential of the Endocannabinoid System for Pain Treatment," signaling its continued interest in this area. NIH supports research on the development of novel CBD therapies to further understanding of the therapeutic potential of CBD. NIH's research portfolio on cannabinoids has already helped to facilitate important therapeutic advances, providing some of

[183] National Academies of Sciences, Engineering, and Medicine. 2017. The health effects of cannabis and cannabinoids: Current state of evidence and recommendations for research. Washington, DC: The National Academies Press.

the early basic and preclinical work on CBD as an epilepsy therapy. FDA's June 2018 approval of Epidiolex (cannabidiol oral solution for the treatment of seizures associated with Lennox-Gastaut syndrome or Dravet syndrome) demonstrates the potential for CBD drug development.

FDA also has demonstrated extensive support for drug development with cannabis and plant-derived cannabinoids. The Epidiolex development program received a fast track designation in FDA's Center for Drug Evaluation and Research. The new drug application for Epidiolex had been given a priority review and was approved in its first review cycle under the shortened review period for priority review of a new molecular entity. In addition, FDA has granted fast track designation for other cannabis-derived investigational new drug programs. FDA will continue to support development of drugs from the cannabis plant, and will continue to leverage its expedited programs (e.g., fast track, breakthrough therapy designation, etc.) to facilitate this drug development whenever the relevant standards are met.[184] This support includes the development of guidance for formulating and developing botanical drugs, and engagement with companies in formal industry meetings to discuss their planned or ongoing drug development programs for drugs derived from cannabis or containing cannabinoids.

NIH is also interested in disentangling the distinct therapeutic benefits and potential health risks of different component compounds within cannabis. Several studies across NIH are examining whether THC, CBD, and other cannabis components might have distinct profiles of risk and benefit. To further facilitate such research, in early 2019, NCCIH released an FOA titled "Exploring the Mechanisms Underlying Analgesic Properties of Minor Cannabinoids and Terpenes," which focused on soliciting applications to study the therapeutic potential of non-THC/CBD components of cannabis as it relates to pain and nociception.

NIH also supports policy research on cannabis, including how it affects the use of other drugs. In 2017, NIAAA, NIDA, and NCI issued a program announcement for research on "Public Policy Effects on Alcohol-, Marijuana-, and Other Substance-Related Behaviors and Outcomes," which invites grant applications (through 2020) to study how changes in policy affect substance use. One project funded under this FOA is examining how local policies

[184] For example, a drug may be granted breakthrough therapy designation "if the drug is intended, alone or in combination with one or more other drugs, to treat a serious or life-threatening disease or condition and preliminary clinical evidence indicates that the drug may demonstrate substantial improvement over existing therapies on one or more clinically significant endpoints" (21 U.S.C. 356(a)(I)).

around both cannabis and opioids contribute to the use of both retail marijuana and prescription opioids within a particular jurisdiction. NIH is also supporting research to determine whether individuals in states with legalized medical marijuana transition to using cannabis as a replacement for prescribed controlled substances like opioids.

NIH and FDA strongly support the need for additional research on cannabis and its constituent compounds. A larger body of rigorous research, including on cannabis and cannabinoid product s that are already in use or that could be developed into FDA-approved medications, is key to furthering our understanding of their potential medical benefits and risks. Research on cannabis as an alternative or adjunctive to opioids for treating pain conditions is ongoing; however, the study of cannabis as a treatment for opioid use disorder (OUD) is a gap area, with the exception of some work using CBD. At present, there are no clinical data showing that cannabis is effective for treating OUD (though there are other FDA-approved medications with established safety and efficacy that are underutilized),[185] and the current evidence on the use of cannabis to replace or reduce opioid use for pain is inconclusive. These are important areas for further research.

There are a variety of barriers to conducting research on cannabis and cannabinoids. First, through a contract with the University of Mississippi, which is the only entity registered with the Drug Enforcement Administration (DEA) to cultivate marijuana for research purposes, NIDA is the only source of marijuana permitted for use in research, thereby limiting the diversity of products and formulations available to researchers and slowing the development of cannabis-based medications.[186] Although the University of Mississippi supplies cannabis for clinical trials, it does not have the capacity to manufacture a broad array of cannabis-derived formulations for research or to supply these cannabis products for commercial development. It is not clear how entities seeking to develop these products for commercial purposes would demonstrate equivalency between the University of Mississippi cannabis used

[185] National Academies of Sciences, Engineering, and Medicine. 2019. Medications for opioid use disorder save lives. Washington, DC: The National Academies Press. doi: https://doi.org/10.7226/25310.

[186] Marijuana is defined under the Controlled Substances Act as "all parts of the plant Cannabis sativa L., whether growing or not; the seeds thereof; the resin extracted from any part of such plant; and every compound, manufacture, salt, derivative, mixture, or preparation of such plant, its seeds or resin. Such term does not include hemp or the mature stalks of such plant, fiber produced from such stalks, oil or cake made from the seeds of such plant, any other compound, manufacture, salt, derivative, mixture, or preparation of such mature stalks (except the resin extracted therefrom), fiber, oil, or cake, or the sterilized seed of such plant which is incapable of germination." 21 U.S.C. § 802(16).

in clinical trials and the drug product that would ultimately be approved by the FDA for eventual marketing and sale. With this in mind, NIH and FDA support licensing additional entities to supply cannabis, including extracts and derivatives, to legitimate researcher s and drug product developers in the United States.

Second, another barrier to advancing cannabis research is that, under federal law, researchers are unable to purchase strains of marijuana or products containing marijuana from state dispensaries (even with non-federal funds), resulting in a significant gap in our understanding of these products and their imp act on health. Licensing additional entities to supply marijuana may improve the diversity of research products that more closely reflect what is currently consumed.

In addition, NIH and FDA support enabling researchers holding Schedule I licenses for marijuana to obtain products from state authorized dispensaries. Such products could be used for basic or clinical research, provided such materials to be used in clinical studies also comply with FDA chemistry, manufacturing, and control requirements for materials to be used in research conducted under an investigational new drug application.

The continued placement of marijuana in Schedule I of the Controlled Substances Act creates significant administrative and cost challenges that slow this research and may deter scientists from pursuing cannabis research altogether. For example, researchers have reported that the registration process can take more than a year to complete, that the process of adding different cannabinoids (e.g., THC, and individual *cannabimimetics)* to a researcher's Schedule I registration is time consuming, and that differing interpretations of the Schedule I registration process among local DEA field offices as well as dis tinct federal and state registration requirements greatly complicate the process. To address these challenges, NIH and FDA recommend streamlining the process for conducting research with cannabis and other Schedule I substances.

Thank you again for your inquiry on cannabis and cannabinoid research and for soliciting our input on the barrier s to conducting this research and how they could be addressed. Please do not hesitate to contact us if we can provide you with additional information on the role of NIH or FDA in advancing this important area of science.

Sincerely yours,

Norman E. Sharpless, M.D.
Acting Commissioner of
Food and Drugs

Francis S. Collins, M.D., Ph.D.
Director
National Institutes of Health

Letter of December 16, 2019, from Greg Walden, et al., to Hon. Pallone and Hon. Eshoo, submitted by Ms. Eshoo

December 16, 2019

The Honorable Frank Pallone, Jr.
Chairman
Committee on Energy and Commerce
2125 Rayburn House Office Building
Washington, DC 20515

The Honorable Anna G. Eshoo
Chairwoman
Subcommittee on Health
Committee on Energy and Commerce
202 Cannon House Office Building
Washington, DC 20515

Dear Chairman Pallone and Chairwoman Eshoo,

We write to request that the Committee on Energy and Commerce hold a hearing to review legislative initiatives aimed at improving federally-sanctioned research on cannabis, such as H.R. 171, Legitimate Use of Medicinal Marijuana Act (LUMMA); H.R. 601, Medical Cannabis Research Act of 2019; and H.R.3797, Medical Marijuana Research Act of 2019. It is critical that the Committee review the current state of cannabis research and hear from the U.S. Drug Enforcement Administration (DEA), the U.S. Food and Drug Administration (FDA), and the National Institute on Drug Abuse (NIDA).

Cannabis is a Schedule I controlled substance under the Controlled Substances Act (CSA).[187] Research on these substances must be conducted in accordance with the CSA and requires a DEA-approved protocol to conduct research. If a researcher desires to increase the quantity of a controlled substance used for an approved research project, the researcher must submit a request to do so, which is then reviewed and must be approved by the DEA and the FDA.[188] Any other changes to the research from what is outlined in the approved protocol must also be reviewed and approved by the DEA.[189]

The supply of research-grade cannabis is subject to the Single Convention on Narcotic Drugs,[190] which imposes certain obligations related to governmental oversight of its cultivation, NIDA has long acted as the agency responsible for overseeing the cultivation of cannabis for scientific research. For decades, the University of Mississippi's School of Pharmacy's National Center for Natural Products Research has had the sole contract with NIDA for the cultivation and procurement of research-grade cannabis.[191]

This single contract not only limits the supply, but also limits the diversity in quality, potency, chemical composition, and methods of consumption. Current research on the biological effects of cannabis might not replicate the experience of individuals using commercially available strains. Studies have found that cannabinoid levels in research-grade cannabis supplied by NIDA were not the same as those found in commercially available cannabis from state-legal dispensaries.[192] In fact, there is recent evidence that most of the commercially available cannabis was genetically distinct from the NIDA samples.[193] In 2016, the DEA announced it would allow additional growers to

---

[187] Comprehensive Drug Abuse Prevention and Control Act of 1970, P.L. 91-513 (Oct. 27, 1970).

[188] Research protocols, 21 C.F.R. 1301.18 (Mar. 9, 2010).

[189] *Id.*

[190] U.N. General Assembly, 1972 *Protocol Amending the Single Convention on Narcotic Drugs,* 1961 (Dec. 9, 1975), *available at* A/RES/3444, http://www.unodc.org/pdf/convention_1961_en.pdf.

[191] National Institute on Drug Abuse, NIDA's Role in Providing Marijuana for Research (Aug. 27, 2019), *available at* https://www.drugabusc.gov/drugs-abuse/marijuana/nidas-role-in-providing-marijuana-research.

[192] Vergara, Daniela, L. Cinnamon Bidwell, Reggie Gaudino, Anthony Torres, Gary Du, Travis C. Ruthenburg, Kymron Decesare, Donald P. Land, Kent E. Hutchison, and Nolan C Kane, *Compromised External Validity: Federally Produced Cannabis Does Not Reflect Legal Markets,* NATURE SCIENTIFIC REPORTS (Apr. 19, 2017), *available at* https://doi.org/10.1038/srep46528.

[193] Schwabe, Anna L., Connor J. Hansen, Richard M. Hyslop, and Mitchell E. Mcglaughlin. *Research Grade Marijuana Supplied by the National Institute on Drug Abuse Is Genetically Divergent from Commercially Available Cannabis,* B10Rx1v (Mar.'28, 2019), *available at* https://doi.org/10.1101/592725.

register in order to produce and distribute cannabis for research purposes.[194] Three years later, without any new approvals of additional manufacturers, the DEA announced in August that before making decisions on any pending applications, the agency would propose new regulations ·governing the growers program for scientific and medical research with a public comment period, which ended on October 28, 2019.[195]

Expanding the number of registered manufacturers is critical to understand fully the potential benefits and possible risks associated with cannabis use, as researchers must be able to study actual products that are currently used by consumers for both medical and·recreational use. However, because of the current restrictions on quality, quantity, and use of cannabis in scientific studies, high quality research on both potential risks and benefits associated with cannabis has been challenging.[196] Given that cannabis is still classified as a Schedule I drug with "no currently accepted medical use and a high potential for abuse,"[197] rescheduling the substance would necessitate robust data on potential medical uses. Recent evaluations conducted separately by the FDA and the National Academies of Sciences, Engineering, and Medicine illustrate the challenge of meeting the required standard of evidence for demonstrating effective medical use and have concluded that lack of research was a significant factor in denying the rescheduling petitions in 2016.[198]

While the detrimental effects of chronic, heavy, recreational use of cannabis among individuals is relatively well studied, a number of areas are still not fully understood. For example, more study is needed to clarify the impacts on the brain, short- and long-term consequences of high potency

---

[194] U.S. Department of Justice, Drug Enforcement Administration, *Applications To Become Registered Under the Controlled Substances To Manufacture Marijuana To Supply Researchers in the United States,* 81 F.R. 53846 (Aug. 12, 2016).

[195] U.S. Department of Justice, Drug Enforcement Administration, *Bulk Manufacturer of Controlled Substances Applications: Bulk Manufacturers of Marihuana,* 84 F.R. 44920 (Aug, 27, 2019).

[196] Taylor, Melissa, and Melissa Bailey, *Medical Marijuana's 'Catch-22': Limits On Research Hinder Patient Relief,* NPR (Apr. 7, 2018), *available at* https://www.npr.org/sections/health-shots/2018/04/07/600209754/medical-marijuanas-catch-22-limits-on-rcsearch-hinders-patient-relicf.

[197] Schedules of Controlled Substances, P.L, 91-513 (Oct. 27, 1970).

[198] U.S. Department of Justice, Drug Enforcement Administration, *Denial of Petition to Initiate Proceedings to Reschedule Marijuana,* 81 F.R 53687-53766 and 53767-53845 (Aug. 12, 2016); National Academies of Sciences, Engineering, and Medicine, *The health effects of cannabis and cannabinoids: Current slate of evidence and recommendations for research,* The NATIONAL ACADEMIES PRESS (Jan. 12, 2017), *available at* https://doi.org/lO.17226/24625.

products and novel modes of use, effects of cannabis use in older adults, and the safety and efficacy of existing products and those in development, ideally using clinical trial models.[199]

It is imperative that policy makers have scientific evidence to guide policy decisions.

Regarding cannabis, policy decisions have outpaced the science. For example:

> [S]tates that have legalized cannabis for adult use are doing so in an information-vacuum, with less understanding of what it is and what it does than virtua1ly any nutritional supplement currently on the market, and with far less information than they have on legal substances that are easily abused, such as alcohol or tobacco, Law enforcement officers don't even know at what point it is unsafe for marijuana users to drive.[200]

The urgency of addressing restrictions on cannabis research has been recently highlighted by recent legalization of one of its components, cannabidiol (CBD) derived from hemp. CBD is the second most prevalent of the active ingredients of cannabis and was removed from Schedule I if it is hemp-derived and produced in a manner consistent with the 2018 Farm Bill,[201] associated federa1 regulations, associated state regulations, and by a licensed grower. This substance is currently being marketed in a variety of products including drugs, food, dietary supplements, cosmetics, pet food, and other animal health products.[202] Although the FDA has approved one CBD-oral solution (Epidiolex) for the' treatment of seizures associated with two rare and severe forms of epilepsy, Lennox-Gastaut syndrome and Dravet syndrome,[203]

---

[199] Sagar, Kelly A., and Staci A. Gruber, *Marijuana Matters: Reviewing the Impact of Marijuana on Cognition, Brain Structure and Function, & Exploring Policy Implications and Barriers to Research,* INTERNATIONAL REVIEW OF PSYCHIATRY (July 3, 2018), *available at* https://doi.org/10.1080/0954026 1 :2018.1460334.

[200] Owermohle, Sarah, *Why We Don't Know Much about Pol,* POLITICO (Oct. 14, 2019), *available at* https://www.politico.com/agcnda/story/2019/10/14/cannabis-mcdical-marijuana-rescarch-000984.

[201] Agriculture Improvement Act of 2018, P.L. 115-33 (Dec. 20, 2018).

[202] U.S. Food and Drug Administration, What You Need to Know (And What We're Working to Find Out) About Products Containing Cannabis or Cannabis-derived Compounds, Including CBD (July 7, 20 19), *available at* https://www.fda.gov/Consumers/consumer-updates/what-you-need-know-and-what-were-working-find-out-about-products-containing-cannabis-or-cannabis.

[203] U.S. Food and Drug Administration, FDA approves first drug comprised of an active ingredient derived from marijuana to treat rare, severe forms of epilepsy (June 25, 2018), *available at* https://www.fda.gov/news-events/press-aimouncements/fda-approves-first-drug-comprised-active-ingredient-derived-marijuana-treat-rare- severe-forms.

it is illegal to market CBD as-a food additive or dietary supplement. There is no evidentiary base for the vast health claims being made around CBD and other non-FDA-approved cannabis-derived products that are currently on the shelves for consumers, and there are legitimate concerns that these claims may lead consumers to forego appropriate medical care. Many consumers who try CBD products believe there is no risk; however, the limited data available suggests CBD use may Pose serious health risks, including liver injury.[204]

Despite the accessibility of CBD on the market, research on this product remains challenging because of current law and cannabis's Schedule I status. Any cannabis-based research must use research-grade cannabis from the nation's sole provider of the product, The University of Mississippi's School of Pharmacy's National Center for Natural Products Research.[205] Uncertainty about the current legal landscape is further hindering research capabilities. Despite enactment of the Farm Bill and the legalization of CBD derived from hemp, regulato1y authorities have not made clear what, if any, restrictions remain in place for researchers seeking to study these substances.

The current public health crisis of e-cigarette, or vaping, product use associated lung injury (EVALI) further underscores the urgent need to review the current state of cannabis research. More than 2,000 people, most of them using vaping devices containing tetrahydrocannabinol (THC), the principal psychoactive constituent of cannabis, have been diagnosed withe-cigarette, or vaping, product use associated lung injury (EVALI), resulting in nearly fifty deaths.[206] The Centers for Disease Control and Prevention (CDC) identified vitamin E acetate as a chemical of concern among people with EVALI. Vitamin E acetate can be used as an additive, most notably as a thickening or diluting agent in e-cigarette, or vaping, products that contain THC.[207] Those in the state-legalized cannabis industry have stated that vaping products now

---

[204] U.S. Food and Drug Administration, FDA warns 15 companies for illegally selling various products containing cannabidiol as agency details safety concerns (November 25, 2019), *available at* https://www.fda.gov/news-events/press-announcemcnts/fda-warns-15-companics-illegally-selling-various-products-containing-cannabidiol-agency-details.

[205] Hudak, John, *The Farm Bill, Hemp Legalization and the Status of CBD: An explainer,* FIXGOV BLOG, Brookings Institution (Dec. 14, 2018), *available at* https://www.brookings.edu/blog/fixgov/2018/12/14/the-farm-bill-hemp-and-cbd-explainer/.

[206] Centers for Disease Control and Prevention, Outbreak of Lung Injury Associated with the Use of E-Cigarette, or Vaping, Products (Nov. 19, 2019), *available at* https://www.cdc.gov/tobacco/basic_infonnation/e-cigarettes/severe-lung-diseasc. html#latest-outbrcak-information.

[207] *Id.*

account for 30 percent or more of their business.[208] An analysis by The RAND Corporation found the fastest-growing segment of the state-legal cannabis market in Washington State was "extracts for inhalation," which includes vape pens and cartridges,[209] yet the scientific community's ability to research the use of THC in these products is limited.

We urge you to hold a legislative hearing regarding federally-sanctioned research on cannabis as soon as possible, with a panel of federal witnesses. This hearing would be an opportunity for members to learn about the aforementioned legislation that offers potential solutions to help improve the research landscape. Non-FDA-approved cannabis and cannabis-derived products are currently being used for the treatment of several medical conditions. In the absence of federally-sanctioned and scientifically-valid research on these products, all available evidence is generated in an uncontrolled study environment. The ability to study these products in clinical trial settings is necessary to assess the safety and effectiveness of these substances for the treatment of any disease or condition. Thank you for your consideration and we look forward to working with you to find solutions to cannabis research and all research on Schedule I substances.

Sincerely,

Greg Walden
Republican Leader

Michael C. Burgess, M.D.
Republican Leader
Subcommittee on Health

Cathy McMorris Rodgers
Member of Congress

H. Morgan Griffith
Member of Congress

* * *

---

[208] Richtel, Matt, *Marijuana and Vaping: Shadowy Past, Dangerous Present,* THE NEW YORK TIMES (Oct. 21, 2019), *available at* https://www.nytimcs.com/2019/10/21/health/marijuana-and-vaping-shadowy-past-dangerous-present.html.

[209] Kilmer, Beau, Steven Davenport, Rosanna Smart, Jonathan P. Caulkins, and Gregory Midgette, *After the Grand Opening: Assessing Cannabis Supply and Demand in Washington State,* RAND CORPORATION (2019), *available at* · https://www.rand.erg/pubs /research _reports/RR3I38.html.

Letter of January 22, 2019, from Ralph L. Sacco, President, the American Academy of Neurology, to Mr. Griffith, Submitted by Ms. Eshoo

January 22, 2019

The Honorable Morgan Griffith
United States House of Representatives
2202 Rayburn House Office Building
Washington, DC 20515

Dear Congressman Griffith,

The American Academy of Neurology (AAN), the world's largest association of neurologists representing more than 34,000 professionals, is strongly committed to improving the care and outcomes of persons with neurologic illness in a cost-effective manner. We would like to express our support for the Legitimate Use of Medicinal Marijuana Act.

Brain disorders such as Alzheimer's disease, Parkinson's disease, autism, epilepsy, schizophrenia, depression, and traumatic brain injury, are projected to be some of the most disabling and costly chronic diseases in the coming years. One in six Americans will be diagnosed with a brain or nervous system disorder this year and the annual cost of treating neurologic disorders is more than $500 billion.

The AAN supports all efforts to conduct rigorous research to evaluate the long-term safety and effectiveness of marijuana-based products. This includes requesting the reclassification of medical marijuana from their current Schedule 1 status to improve access for study of marijuana or cannabinoids under IRB-approved research protocols.

Regarding the use of medical marijuana, the AAN recognizes that there may be potential for the use of these agents in the treatment of neurologic disorders. However, there is not sufficient evidence at this time to make any definitive conclusions regarding the effectiveness of marijuana-based products for many neurologic conditions. Therefore, we are not advocating for legalization of prescriptions for medical marijuana-based products. Further research is urgently needed to determine the safety and medical benefit of various forms of marijuana in neurologic disorders.

Thank you for taking a leadership role on this critical issue. Please contact Derek Brandt at *dbrandt@aan.com* if you have questions or request additional information.

Sincerely,

Ralph L. Sacco, MD, MS, FAHA, FAAN
President, American Academy of Neurology

* * *

Letter of June 6, 2018, from Ralph L. Sacco, President, American Academy of Neurology, to Mr. Gaetz, Submitted by Ms. Eshoo

June 6, 2018

The Honorable Matt Gaetz
United States House of Representatives
507 Cannon House Office Building
Washington, DC 20515

Dear Congressman Gaetz:

The American Academy of Neurology (AAN), the world's largest association of neurologists representing more than 34,000 professionals, is strongly committed to improving the care and outcomes of persons with neurologic illness in a cost-effective manner. We would like to express our support for *H.R. 5634, the Medical Cannabis Research Act*.

One in six people live with a brain or nervous system condition, including Alzheimer's disease, Parkinson's disease, stroke, epilepsy, traumatic brain injury, ALS, multiple sclerosis, and headache. State legislatures and regulatory agencies have taken the first steps to making medical cannabis products available to patients. Nearly all conditions approved for state medical cannabis prescriptions are neurologic in nature, and patients visit their neurologist with requests for these products. However, neurologists are left with little scientific research to make appropriate prescribing decisions for their patients. Furthermore, many physicians are reluctant to approve their patients for medical cannabis due to the discrepancies between state and federal law. We applaud your legislation, which will make it easier for physicians to participate in legitimate medical research and for patients within the Department of Veterans Affairs to access high quality clinical trials for medical cannabis. Patients and physicians need this research to determine whether medical cannabis is an appropriate treatment option for neurologic disease. Physicians also need clarity on the divergent legal landscape so that they may appropriately prescribe any safe, effective, and approved cannabis-derived therapies supported by medical research.

The AAN applauds your efforts to support research on medical cannabis and its potential impact on patients living with devastating neurologic disease. Many of these sentiments are included in a recent update to our Medical Marijuana Position Statement, which was driven by member concerns on the lack of research available on medical marijuana products and the impact of the ambiguous environment on patients and physicians.

Thank you for taking a leadership role on this critical issue. Please contact Derek Brandt at *dbrandt@aan.com* if you have questions or request additional information.

Sincerely,

Ralph L. Sacco, MD, MS, FAHA, FAAN
President, American Academy of Neurology

Pot Imports Grow as U.S. Stalls on Medical Research

By Kristine Owram
January 12, 2020, 7:00 AM PST
Updated on January 13, 2020, 2:00 AM PST

Biopharmaceutical Research Co. acquired batch from Netherlands
'It saddens me that Americans aren't the ones producing'

One of the top advocates for allowing U.S. companies to grow cannabis for research purposes has imported a batch from the Netherlands, saying he had no choice because of the lack of progress at home.

California-based Biopharmaceutical Research Co., founded by former Navy SEAL George Hodgin, legally imported a small quantity of marijuana from Bedrocan International last month to use for scientific analysis with the goal of better understanding the plant.

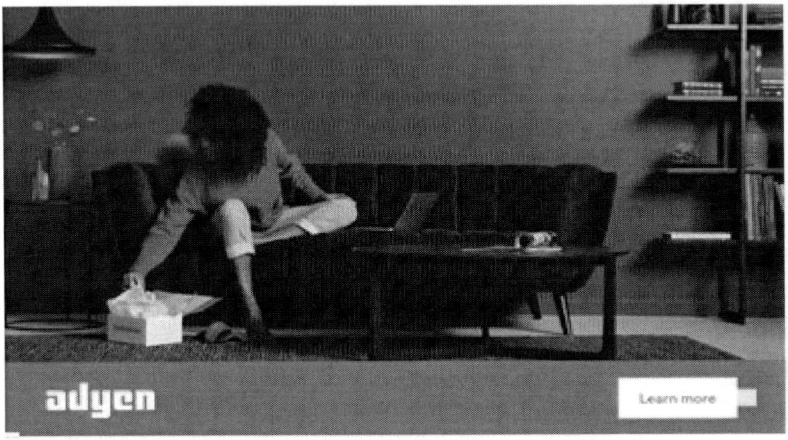

"As someone who fought for this country it saddens me that Americans aren't the ones producing the cannabis materials that we are researching," Hodgin said in an interview.

Canadian-grown cannabis has also been imported into the U.S. for research purposes. Tilray Inc., for example, has brought in pot for clinical trials at the University of California San Diego, New York University and Columbia University.

The restrictions on researching cannabis in the U.S. stem from a longstanding federal prohibition on the drug, despite it now being legal in 33 states for medical use and 11 for recreational use. Currently, there's only one government-approved farm at the University of Mississippi that grows pot for research purposes.

The Drug Enforcement Administration said in August that it would propose new regulations for growing marijuana for scientific and medical research, and would then make decisions on pending applications from growers. It first invited those applications in 2016.

Attorney General William Barr pledged in April to act on those pending applications, and said he was "pleased" the DEA was moving forward in August.

Then things stalled, said Senator Brian Schatz, a Democrat from Hawaii who sent a bipartisan letter to Barr last month urging the DEA to allow researchers to obtain products from state-legal dispensaries.

"The deadline for response was Dec. 20 and they did not get back to us," Schatz said in a phone interview. "This is another ominous sign that this administration opposes not just rescheduling or descheduling or decriminalization, but anything that has to do with cannabis, they're fighting it."

Schatz said he believes Congress can pass marijuana research legislation in 2020.

If it can't, Hodgin said his company is prepared to import more cannabis.

"I would much rather all of those tax dollars and intellectual property and job creation stay here in America, but if the federal government continues to be defined by inertia, then I suppose we'll have to look outside the United States for our research materials," he said.

Events This Week

TUESDAY 1/14

Aphria Inc. reports earnings pre-market

Organigram Holdings Inc. reports post-market

Several publicly traded cannabis companies present at the ICR Conference in Orlando, Florida

AltaCorp Capital and ATB Financial focus on cannabis stocks at the life sciences day of their institutional investor conference

Last Week's Top Stories

N.Y. Governor to Address Gig Worker Status, Legalize Pot

Aurora Cannabis Unlikely to Meet Debt Covenants, Analysts Warn

Hold My Beer: Legal Pot Hits Brew Consumption in Canada

Cannabis Vape Sales Slid 26% in 2 Months Following Health Crisis

Pot Frenzy Sweeps Thailand as Government Touts Medical Marijuana

Article, ''Support for the Medical Marijuana Research Act of 2019,'' by Mr. Blumenauer, et al., Submitted by Ms. Eshoo

U.S. Representatives Earl Blumenauer (D-OR), Andy Harris, M.D. (R-MD), Zoe Lofgren (D-CA), H. Morgan Griffith (R-VA), Debbie Dingell (D-MI), and Rob Bishop (R-UT)

Smart Colorado

Attributable to Diane Carlson, Co-Founder & National Policy Director, Smart Colorado:

> "We applaud the leadership of the congressional sponsors of The Medical Marijuana Research Act of 2019. They are from states that, like Colorado, have experienced the realities of marijuana legalization and know just how critical the need for more marijuana research is. For years Smart Colorado and its community partners and supporters have advocated for much-needed research to address information gaps. We believe this research is particularly important when it comes to today's new and very different marijuana products and unprecedentedly high THC potencies. This research could help protect kids and inform adults. In Colorado there is no age restriction when it comes to medical marijuana; that makes the need for sound science on its potential risks and benefits even more imperative. Just this past legislative session, Colorado state legislators overwhelmingly voted for marijuana potency to be studied, a goal that is supported by this congressional legislation. Again, we are grateful for the leadership provided by the sponsors and urge others to support The Medical Marijuana Research Act of 2019, which has important and far-reaching nationwide implications."

Smart Approaches for Marijuana (SAM Action)

"Dr. Harris is a leader in responsible research into medicines that could be derived from the marijuana plant, and we are glad to see him reintroducing this important bill. We hope that Congress will move swiftly to pass it and reduce barriers to researching marijuana to produce new FDA-approved medicines," said Kevin Sabet, PhD, President of Smart Approaches to Marijuana Action (SAM Action).

American Psychological Association (APA)

Attributed to Arthur C. Evans Jr. PhD, CEO of the American Psychological Association:

> "Scientists who have been discouraged from studying cannabis because of the hurdles associated with the registration process, redundant protocol reviews and security requirements will be encouraged by this bill, which greatly simplifies the whole process. Psychologists are interested in studying a wide range of scientific questions related to the use of real-world cannabis products, including cannabis use disorder, cognitive impairments, risk for psychosis and motor vehicle impairment, and the potential therapeutic uses for cannabis derivatives. Without access to an expanded range of cannabis products, scientific research cannot hope to keep pace with the expanding recreational and medicinal cannabis marketplace. This bill will facilitate the rapid approval of applications to manufacture cannabis products from non-government sources, resulting in a supply that can meet the needs of cannabis researchers."

Biopharmaceutical Research Company (BRC)

Attributed to George Hodgin, former Navy SEAL and founder and CEO of Biopharmaceutical Research Company (BRC):

> "For three years, I have waited for approval from the Drug Enforcement Administration to grow cannabis strictly for government-sanctioned research purposes. I have built a facility in compliance with federal regulations and hired a team ready to work, but we are stalled by federal bureaucracy.
>
> With thorough research and testing, patients across America could potentially benefit from medicinal cannabis, including many of my fellow veterans who struggle with chronic pain and post-traumatic stress. Lawmakers will also benefit as they consider policy to address the possible negative health consequences that can only be adequately understood through advanced research. The Medical Marijuana Research Act is an important step toward removing federal barriers to cannabis research, and I urge the Judiciary and Energy & Commerce Committees to promptly advance this bill."

Marijuana Policy Project (MPP)

"There isn't much that the Marijuana Policy Project and Congressman Harris agree on when it comes to the federal government's position on cannabis, but we applaud his sponsorship of the Medical Marijuana Research Act of 2019 which would reduce the barriers to cannabis research. The fact that such a bill is even necessary points out how out of touch the feds actually are," said Don Murphy, director of federal policies. "We stand with patients in calling for the best science available to determine marijuana's true medicinal value. We would add however that while this research is being conducted, patients should be given the care and compassion they deserve, not hand cuffs and convictions."

American Academy of Neurology (AAN)

"Many conditions that are the focus of potential medical cannabis treatments are neurologic in nature. However, neurologists are left with little scientific research to make appropriate prescribing decisions for their patients. The Medical Marijuana Research Act will help facilitate rigorous research that is needed to determine whether medical cannabis is an appropriate treatment option for neurologic disease," said James C. Stevens, MD, FAAN, President of the American Academy of Neurology.

* * *

July 16, 2019
The Honorable Andy Harris, MD
2334 Rayburn House Office Building
Washington, DC 20515

I write on behalf Smart Approaches to Marijuana Action (SAM Action). SAM Action is the affiliated 501(c)(4) of SAM, the leading, non-partisan national organization offering a science-based approach to marijuana policy. SAM was founded by former Congressman Patrick Kennedy, senior editor of *The Atlantic* David Frum, and myself, a White House advisor to the three U.S. administrations.

SAM Action supports the Medical Marijuana Research Act, legislation you have sponsored to facilitate legitimate research into the medicinal components of the marijuana plant. We have supported legitimate research as recommended by the National Academy of Sciences and National Institutes of Health into FDA-approved medications derived from marijuana since our inception, and SAM has published guides such as "Researching Marijuana's Medical Potential Responsibly: a Six Point Plan" promoting this approach. The Medical Marijuana Research Act (MMRA) would further these goals, and we urge Congress to take up and pass this legislation.

In working with stakeholders who conduct research into the hundreds of cannabinoids present in the marijuana plant, including medical researchers on SAM's science advisory board, we have been made aware of difficulties in the research process that can interfere with researching medicines that may be extracted from raw, plant-based marijuana. The MMRA takes a measured and thoughtful approach to reducing these barriers, without rescheduling or descheduling marijuana.

SAM Action looks forward to working with your office and other stakeholders, including medical researchers and the Drug Enforcement Administration (DEA), to ensure marijuana is not illegally diverted and is used only for legitimate research purposes. Thank you again for your diligence and care as you work to foster responsible, legitimate research for the benefit of all.

Sincerely,

Kevin A. Sabet, Ph.D.
President
SAM Action

* * *

July 15, 2019
The Honorable Andy Harris (MD)
U.S. House of Representatives
Washington, DC 20515

Dear Congressman Harris:

On behalf of the National Sheriffs' Association (NSA) and the more than 3,000 elected sheriffs nationwide, I write in support of the Medical Marijuana

Research Act. We believe that this bill is the necessary first step in the conversation of legalizing marijuana.

While the National Sheriffs' Association oppose efforts to legalize medicinal and recreational marijuana, we urge Congress to take the action necessary to ensure greater research on cannabis in order to make an informed decision. This bill will remove regulatory research barriers in a safe and effective manner. These barriers have undermined the ability to obtain clear, well-researched scientific evidence relevant to the use of cannabis for medical purposes and have prevented research that will lead to the ability to accurately quantify impairment levels of those who consume cannabis

The National Sheriffs' Association applauds your effort to push for further medicinal cannabis research before hastily legalizing marijuana on the national level. We believe this common-sense approach will allow trained professionals access to funding and resources required to ensure that law enforcement has the safeguards they need to protect their communities.

Sincerely,
Jonathan F. Thompson
Executive Director and CEO

CC: Representative Earl Blumenauer
Representative Morgan Griffith
Representative Mike Bishop
Representative Zoe Lofgren
Representative Debby Dingell

* * *

July 17, 2019

The Honorable Earl Blumenauer
United States House of Representatives
1111 Longworth House Office Building
Washington, DC 20515

The Honorable Andy Harris
United States House of Representatives
1533 Longworth House Office Building
Washington, DC 20515

Dear Representatives Blumenauer and Harris:

The undersigned national organizations are writing to strongly endorse the Medical Marijuana Research Act of 2019.

We applaud your initiative and that of your House co-sponsors to amend the Controlled Substances Act to lessen the regulatory burden and facilitate research on marijuana and its constituent compounds by qualified scientists. By creating an exception for marijuana from the current obstacles of Schedule I registration and review procedures, the bill provides a sensible streamlined approach for the review of applications and granting of registrations to conduct research with marijuana.

In addition, the bill amends the process for the Department of Justice (DoJ) approval of applications from individuals seeking to manufacture or dispense marijuana exclusively for legitimate medical research and requires DoJ to approve an application unless it is demonstrated that the issuance of such registration is not in the public interest.

Understanding the characteristics of a broader range of marijuana strains/varieties, including the potency (i.e., amount of tetrahydrocannabinol in the plant) and concentration of other components (e.g., cannabidiol), will be critical for studying the health effects of marijuana use. Rigorous research into the potential therapeutic benefits and public health consequences of marijuana use will lead to more refined cannabinoid medication development through identification of target chemical constituents associated with unique behavioral or physiological effects.

Further, the bill calls for the Department of Health and Human Services to review existing medical and other research on marijuana and to report to Congress on the results of the review. The National Institutes of Health provided funding of nearly $139 million for marijuana/cannabinoid research in 2018, and it recently convened a Neuroscience Research Summit on Marijuana and Cannabinoids to address the growing need to understand the basic pharmacology and potential therapeutic benefits of cannabinoids as well as their deleterious effects. Information from that Summit complemented the findings of a report published in 2017 by the National Academy of Medicine entitled "Health Effects of Marijuana: An Evidence Review and Research Agenda." Your bill will serve one of the principal recommendations of that report by proposing strategies for addressing the current barriers to the advancement of the cannabis research agenda.

Thank you again for introducing this bill. Our organizations represent a range of scientific, professional, and patient provider and advocacy groups which may differ on policies related to the legal status of marijuana but are united in their support of scientific research.

We are eager to assist in any way we can as this bill receives further consideration. If you have any questions or need additional information, please contact Geoff Mumford, PhD, directly at gmumford@apa.org.

Sincerely,

American Academy of Addiction Psychiatry
American Academy of Neurology
American Brain Coalition
American College of Neuropsychopharmacology
American Psychological Association
American Society of Addiction Medicine
American Society of Anesthesiologists
Child Neurology Society
Entertainment Industries Council EIC
Friends of the National Institute on Alcohol Abuse and Alcoholism
Friends of the National Institute on Drug Abuse
National Ataxia Foundation
Research Society on Alcoholism
Treatment Communities of America

* * *

July 2, 2019

The Honorable Earl Blumenauer
United States House of Representatives
1111 Longworth House Office Building
Washington, DC 20515

The Honorable Andy Harris
United States House of Representatives
1533 Longworth House Office Building
Washington, DC 20515

Dear Representatives Blumenauer and Harris:

We applaud your leadership and that of your co-sponsors to amend the Controlled Substances Act to lessen the regulatory burden and facilitate research on marijuana and its constituent compounds by qualified scientists. By creating an exception for marijuana from the current obstacles of Schedule I registration and review procedures, the bill provides a sensible streamlined approach for the review of applications and granting of registrations to conduct research with marijuana.

In addition, the bill amends the process for the Department of Justice (DoJ) approval of applications from individuals seeking to manufacture or dispense marijuana exclusively for legitimate medical research and requires DoJ to approve an application unless it is demonstrated that the issuance of such registration is not in the public interest. Understanding the characteristics of a broader range of marijuana strains/varieties, including the potency (i.e., amount of tetrahydrocannabinol in the plant) and concentration of other components (e.g., cannabidiol), will be critical for studying the health effects of marijuana use. Rigorous research into the potential therapeutic benefits and public health consequences of marijuana use will lead to more refined cannabinoid medication development through identification of target chemical constituents associated with unique behavioral or physiological effects.

Further, the bill calls for the Department of Health and Human Services to review existing medical and other research on marijuana and to report to Congress on the results of the review. The National Institutes of Health provided funding of nearly $139 million for marijuana/cannabinoid research in 2018, and it recently convened a Neuroscience Research Summit on Marijuana and Cannabinoids to address the growing need to understand the basic pharmacology and potential therapeutic benefits of cannabinoids as well as their deleterious effects. Information from that Summit complemented the findings of a report published in 2017 by the National Academy of Medicine entitled "Health Effects of Marijuana: An Evidence Review and Research Agenda." Your bill advances one of the principal recommendations of that report by proposing strategies for addressing the current barriers to the advancement of the cannabis research agenda.

Thank you again for introducing this bill. We are eager to assist in any way we can as this bill receives further consideration. If you have any questions or need additional information, please contact Dr. Geoff Mumford, APA's Associate Executive Director for Science Government Relations, at gmumford@apa.org or 202.336.6167.

Sincerely,

Russell Shilling, Ph.D.
Chief Scientific Officer

Katherine B. McGuire
Chief Advocacy Officer

* * *

July 15, 2019

The Honorable Andy Harris
United States House of Representatives
2334 Rayburn House Office Building
Washington, DC 20515

The Honorable Earl Blumenauer
United States House of Representatives
1111 Longworth House Office Building
Washington, DC 20515

Dear Representatives Harris and Blumenauer,

The American Academy of Neurology (AAN), the world's largest association of neurologists representing more than 36,000 professionals, is strongly committed to improving the care and outcomes of persons with neurologic illness in a cost-effective manner. We would like to express our support for the Medical Marijuana Research Act of 2019.

One in six people live with a brain or nervous system condition, including Alzheimer's disease, Parkinson's disease, stroke, epilepsy, traumatic brain injury, ALS, multiple sclerosis, and headache. State legislatures and regulatory agencies have taken the first steps to making medical cannabis products available to patients. Nearly all conditions approved for medical cannabis prescriptions are neurologic in nature, and many patients visit their neurologist with requests for these products. However, neurologists are left with little scientific research to make appropriate prescribing decisions for their patients. Furthermore, many physicians are reluctant to approve their patients for medical cannabis due to the discrepancies between state and federal law.

Patients and physicians need medical cannabis research to determine whether it is an appropriate treatment option for neurologic disease. Without this critical research, patients with neurologic disease will not be able to access potentially life-changing treatment. Physicians also need clarity on the divergent legal landscape so that they may appropriately prescribe any safe, effective, and approved cannabis-derived therapies supported by medical research.

The AAN applauds your efforts to support research on medical cannabis and its potential impact on patients living with devastating neurologic disease. Many of these sentiments are included in our Medical Marijuana Position Statement, which was driven by member concerns on the lack of research available on marijuana products and the impact of the ambiguous environment on patients and physicians.

Thank you for taking a leadership role on this critical issue. If you have any questions or requests for additional information, please contact Derek Brandt, Director, Congressional Affairs, at *dbrandt@aan.com.*

Sincerely,

James C. Stevens MD.

James C. Stevens, MD, FAAN
President, American Academy of Neurology

* * *

July 11, 2019
The Honorable Earl Blumenauer
United States House of Representatives
1111 Longworth House Office Building
Washington, DC 20515

The Honorable Andy Harris
United States House of Representatives
1533 Longworth House Office Building
Washington, DC 20515

Dear Representatives Blumenauer and Harris:

The American College of Neuropsychopharmacology (ACNP) endorses and supports the Medical Marijuana Research Act of 2019 which amends the Controlled Substances Act that aims to lessen the regulatory burden and facilitate research on marijuana and its constituent compounds by qualified scientists. By creating an exception for marijuana from the current obstacles of Schedule I registration and review procedures, the bill provides a streamlined approach for the review of applications and granting of registrations to conduct research with marijuana.

In addition, the bill amends the process of application approval from individuals seeking to manufacture or dispense marijuana exclusively for legitimate medical research from the U.S. Department of Justice unless it is demonstrated that the issuance of such registration is not in the public interest. This legislation will provide an annual assessment whether there is an adequate and uninterrupted supply of research-grade cannabis and be sure that there are at minimum four federally approved manufacturers at any given time. Currently, institutions that want to research cannabis, cannot as cannabis research poses a threat to their federal funding. This legislation provides refuge for researchers and institutions studying cannabis as well as the patients in medical cannabis clinical trials. This legislation will not interfere with the federal laws, state laws or local law enforcement and does not change the legal status of cannabis, but solely unlocks the potential for brain and behavioral research that could be beneficial to chronically ill persons.

Furthermore, the bill calls for the Department of Health and Human Services to review existing medical and other research on marijuana and to report to Congress on the results of the review. The National Institutes of Health provided funding of nearly $139 million for marijuana/cannabinoid research in 2018, and it recently convened a Neuroscience Research Summit on Marijuana and Cannabinoids to address the growing need to understand the basic pharmacology and potential therapeutic benefits of cannabinoids as well as their deleterious effects. Information from that Summit complemented the findings of a report published in 2017 by the National Academy of Medicine entitled "Health Effects of Marijuana: An Evidence Review and Research Agenda.". This bill will serve one of the principal recommendations of that report by proposing strategies for addressing the current barriers to the advancement of the cannabis research agenda.

As background, the ACNP is a professional organization of leading brain and behavior scientists. The principal functions of the College are research and education. Our goals in research are to offer investigators an opportunity for cross-disciplinary communication and to promote the application of various scientific disciplines to the study of the brain's effect on behavior, with a focus on mental illness of all forms. The College is an honorific society of just over 1200 members. Members are selected primarily on the basis of their original research contributions to the broad field of neuroscience. Founded in 1961, the membership of the College is drawn from scientists in multiple fields including behavioral pharmacology, brain imaging, chronobiology, clinical psychopharmacology, epidemiology, genetics, molecular biology, neurochemistry, neuroendocrinology, neuroimmunology, neurology, neurophysiology, pharmacology, psychiatry, and psychology.

Thank you again for introducing this bill. We are eager to assist in any way we can as this bill receives further consideration. If you have any questions or need additional information, please contact Sarah Timm at stimm@acnp.org.

Sincerely,

Sarah Timm

Sarah S. Timm, CAE, CMP-HC
Executive Director
American College of Neuropsychopharmacology

* * *

Letter of January 15, 2020, by George B. Hodgin, Biopharmaceutical Research Company

Re: Statement for the Record regarding United States House of Representatives Committee on Energy and Commerce, Health Subcommittee, Cannabis Policies for the New Decade

Chairman Pallone, Subcommittee Chairwoman Eshoo, Ranking Member Walden and Subcommittee Ranking Member Burgess, Biopharmaceutical Research Company ("BRC") appreciates the opportunity to submit a letter for the record regarding our experience attempting to produce federally compliant cannabis for federally approved research.

BRC is a Monterey, California based pharmaceutical company that maintains and operates an active DEA Registration for the handling of all schedules of Controlled Substances. BRC does not violate federal law or the Controlled Substances Act (CSA). I'm the CEO and Founder of BRC. I started BRC after serving as a Navy SEAL Officer for seven years, several of which were in combat in Afghanistan and SE Asia. After watching my teammates and fellow Veterans turn to cannabis after struggling with traditional therapeutics to treat their wartime wounds, I decided to start a business dedicated to answering the important questions of cannabis usage in a completely legal manner. My story should be one of the American dream. A Navy SEAL Veteran serves in combat, uses the G.I. Bill to get a graduate education at Stanford and then starts a business to answer nationally important questions around cannabis. Instead, my company sits and waits idly by for permission to grow cannabis for research while consumers, Veterans and policy-makers are being forced to make critical health decisions about cannabis blindly because the DOJ and DEA are preventing cannabis' production for research purposes. In the meantime, Veterans are killing themselves at a rate of 22 per day[210] and are twice as likely to die of an opioid overdose than a civilian.[211] Could cannabis help them? We don't know and we won't know until the DOJ and DEA make good on their promise to open the production of cannabis for research like they promised in 2016.

My premise has always been, if cannabis is indeed useful let's figure it out so we can help the most people possible. If it's harmful, we need to figure that out too so that consumers can make informed decisions. But to this day, despite the fact that 200 million Americans live in a state where they can access cannabis, scientists and doctors rely on a sole source of the drug for research. That source has been widely reported to be unsatisfactory in timely access and quality of material. Consumers have access to cannabis, scientists and doctors don't.[212]

The purpose of your hearing is to gain insights in order to better make smart cannabis policy for this new decade. The key to any meaningful cannabis policy in the United States is encouraging the DEA and DOJ to allow expanded production of cannabis for research. Until that happens, scientists, doctors, consumers and policy-makers will be making critically important decisions without appropriate health data.

---

210 https://www.stripes.com/news/us/va-reveals-its-veteran-suicide-statistic-included-active-duty-troops-1.533992.

211 https://www.whitehouse.gov/articles/fighting-pain-addiction-veterans/.

212 https://www.politico.com/agenda/story/2019/10/14/cannabis-medical-marijuana-research-000984.

I started my business in response to a 2016 US Drug Enforcement Administration (DEA) policy allowing for the licensure of companies to produce federally legal cannabis for exclusively scientific research purposes. This policy change was to be the first meaningful cannabis policy improvement in nearly 60 years and would indeed give scientists, policy-makers and consumers the answers to the questions around the safety and efficacy of cannabis. I started a business, hired a team, raised investment capital and built a pharmaceutical manufacturing facility because I trusted the federal government to follow through. Finally- the US government intended to allow cannabis to be produced for government-approved research purposes. Alas- to this day, nearly 3.5 years later, the US DEA and DOJ have refused to even examine my application. There have been nearly 20 bicameral and bipartisan letters to DOJ and DEA encouraging them to process these applications- but they have refused. In fact, they continue to move the permit applications through regulatory purgatory by asserting that they need to review the process of reviewing the applications first, to ensure conformity with the 1961 Single Convention on Narcotic Drugs.

The US produces every other federally controlled substance for research purposes. Why do they treat cannabis differently? While the DOJ and DEA hide behind a few sentences in a 1961 treaty in order to slow walk meaningful cannabis research reform, the rest of the world is lapping the United States in job creation, intellectual property generation and treating their patients. The following countries, all signatories to the same treaty as the USA, all have expansive medical cannabis research programs. None of them have been cited or censured by the United Nations:

- Argentina
- Australia
- Belgium
- Bermuda
- Brazil
- Canada
- Chile
- Colombia
- Croatia
- Cyprus
- Czech Republic
- Denmark

- Estonia
- Finland
- France
- Georgia
- Germany
- Greece
- Ireland
- Italy
- Jamaica
- Lithuania
- Luxembourg
- Malta
- Netherlands
- New Zealand
- North Macedonia
- Norway
- Peru
- Poland
- Portugal
- San Marino
- Slovenia
- South Africa
- Sri Lanka
- Switzerland
- Thailand
- United Kingdom
- Zimbabwe

In April of 2018, then Attorney General Sessions asserted that the DOJ and DEA were nearly ready to allow cannabis to be produced for research by remarking, "We are moving forward and we will add fairly soon, I believe, the paperwork and reviews will be completed and we will add additional suppliers of marijuana under the controlled circumstances."[213]

BRC's policy positions and comments for the record and for your consideration on cannabis and cannabis-derived products:

---

[213] https://www.marijuanamoment.net/sessions-admits-there-may-well-be-some-benefits-from-medical-marijuana/.

- BRC supports the federally compliant research into cannabis' therapeutic and adverse effects
- BRC supports and advocates for the DEA's Expanded Marijuana program released on 12 August 2016 and 27 August 2019 allowing for the licensing of multiple entities to produce marijuana and its chemical constituents for legitimate research
- BRC supports further research into the analgesic efficacy of cannabis and its potential to displace opioid based therapies for the treatment of chronic pain.
- BRC encourages the FDA, DOJ and DEA to advance the status of scientific research into cannabis by allowing for the registration of legitimate and federally compliant marijuana producers
- We have invested significantly in personnel, physical infrastructure and the development of practices in order to be compliant with Code of Federal Regulations (CFR) Title 21 Chapter 1300 Part C Section 823, the federal government should honor that.

We have refused to violate the CFR and CSA by participating in federally illegal cannabis markets, at great personal and corporate expense, because we have trusted that DOJ and DEA would remain true to their word and federal law. We have undertaken this enterprise as a business, at great risk, because we believe in the importance of compliant and top-quality federal research.

In conclusion, BRC recommends that if the Congress' goal is to ensure cannabis and cannabis-derived products are safe and efficacious, then the DEA and DOJ must register additional producers of federally compliant cannabis for scientific purposes so that legitimate data may be produced.

Sincerely,

G.B. Hodgin

Statement of July 16, 2019, by Kevin A. Sabet, Ph.D., President, Smart Approaches to Marijuana,

Kevin A. Sabet, PhD
President & CEO of Smart Approaches to Marijuana (SAM)

Former White House Senior Drug Policy Advisor (Clinton, Bush, Obama)
http://www.learnaboutsam.org

Thank you Chairman Pallone, Ranking Member Walden, Chairwoman Eshoo, and Ranking Member Burgess for the opportunity to submit testimony on the subject of responsibly researching medicines that may be derived from the marijuana plant. I represent Smart Approaches to Marijuana (SAM), the leading non-partisan national non-profit organization offering a science-based approach to marijuana policy. SAM was founded by former Congressman Patrick Kennedy, senior editor of *The Atlantic* David Frum, and myself, a former White House advisor to the Obama Administration as well as two other U.S. Administrations. SAM is advised by a Science Advisory Board with researchers and physicians from top university research institutions, including Harvard, Yale, and Johns Hopkins.

The Committee is considering legislation that would reduce barriers to researching marijuana (H.R 3797, H.R. 601), and several pieces of legislation that would bypass the research process entirely to legalize recreational marijuana at the federal level without any scientific studies prior to that action (the MORE Act, H.R. 3884, and the Marijuana Freedom and Opportunity Act, H.R. 2843). While the proponents of these legalization bills characterize them as "decriminalization," these bills go far beyond that to completely remove marijuana from the Controlled Substances Act, which would create a pathway for Big Tobacco to take over the marijuana industry as Former Speaker John Boehner has indicated they are poised to do.[214]

Just as there is often confusion over the terms "decriminalization" and "legalization," there is often a lot of confusion concerning the scheduling system within the Controlled Substances Act. Contrary to popular belief, the scheduling system is not a harm index in which marijuana is considered as dangerous as heroin. Rather, the scheduling system is a mechanism for controlling prescription drugs according to their potential for abuse. Because raw plant marijuana has not been proven safe and effective through clinical trials, it cannot be prescribed by doctors and remains in Schedule 1.

In sum, my beliefs after over 25 years of experience can be summed up as such:

---

214 Boehner, John. National Cannabis Summit Marijuana Investing Seminar. (2018) https://www.youtube.com/watch?v=p3FLUuMoFeE.

- Legalization would usher in a new industry similar to Big Tobacco, and would be detrimental to public health and safety.
- There is a false dichotomy between legalization and criminalization. In fact, removing criminal penalties for low-level use can be done without unleashing commercial legalization.
- There has been extensive research on marijuana by the National Academy of Sciences, and other eminent scientific bodies, but the federal government should reduce barriers to research, especially given the escalating potency of marijuana.
- Current medical literature and statistical surveys are clear: marijuana is a drug of abuse, is addictive, and causes clear negative effects in both individuals and society.

It may be helpful to begin with a clarification of terms:

What Is Marijuana?

Marijuana is a complex plant with hundreds of components. Some of those components are called cannabinoids, and affect the brain in different ways. CBD (cannabidiol) and THC (tetrahydrocannabinol) are the two most researched cannabinoids produced by the cannabis (marijuana) plant. Unlike THC, CBD does not produce a state of intoxication and is not addictive. However, CBD has all but been bred out of modern recreational marijuana because it counteracts the intoxication from THC.

Is Marijuana Medicine?

Unfortunately, the issue of marijuana as medicine has become highly politicized rather than adhering to the ordinary scientific process for researching and approving medications. In the mid-1980s, THC was synthesized into a pill form – called Marinol – with a capsule containing THC in sesame oil and approved by the FDA in 1985 for the treatment of nausea and vomiting associated with cancer chemotherapy, supported primarily by the National Cancer Institute (NCI), whose research support goes back to the 1970s. In 1999, the Institute of Medicine (now called the National Academy of Medicine) undertook the most exhaustive review of marijuana's medical potential to date, concluding that smoked marijuana was unlikely the way of the future regarding medical potential, and "should generally not be recommended for long-term medical use…" but that components of marijuana indeed held promise. Since then, there has been interest in how different cannabinoids work together, not only in isolation.

In 2017, the National Academy of Medicine (as a part of the National Academies of Sciences, Engineering, and Medicine) issued an updated report[215] on the current state of knowledge surrounding marijuana by reviewing over 10,000 peer reviewed studies in the international scientific literature that had been conducted since the 1999 report. It is interesting to note that the vast majority of studies showing benefits were conducted with isolated cannabinoids rather than whole-plant marijuana. The report also contained specific guidelines for reducing barriers to researching marijuana.[216]

There are currently four FDA-approved medications based on marijuana (Marinol, Syndros, Cesamet, and Epidiolex). The first three are made from synthesized forms of THC, while the fourth is a purified whole-plant extract CBD. Other potential medications, based on complex plant extracts or isolated cannabinoids, are currently undergoing FDA-approved investigation.

What Is the Definition of a Medicine?

For a drug to be legally considered a medicine, per 57 Fed. Reg. 10499, 10504-10506 (1992), it must pass five common-sense tests:

1) *The Drug's Chemistry Must Be Known and Reproducible.* Doctors must know how much and what they are giving their patients. If the researchers don't know what they are giving test subjects, they cannot record meaningful observations.
2) *There Must Be Adequate Safety Studies.* Measured doses must be tested for safety, usually in animal studies and pre-clinical human trials, to ascertain the pharmacological and toxicological effects of the drug.

---

[215] National Academy of Medicine. The Health Effects of Cannabis and Cannabinoids: The Current State of Evidence and Recommendations for Research. (2017).
[216] *Ibid.* https://www.nap.edu/read/24625/chapter/18.

3) *There Must Be Adequate and Well-Controlled Studies Proving Efficacy.* Measured doses must be tested and provide evidence of efficacy in treating the intended condition. Double-blind, placebo-controlled clinical trials are the gold standard for ascertaining medicinal safety and effectiveness.
4) *Acceptance by Qualified Experts.* The Food, Drug, and Cosmetics Act requires those with scientific training in pharmacology and toxicology to evaluate the safety and effectiveness of drugs before they can be sold to the general public.
5) *The Scientific Evidence Must Be Widely Available.* The supporting scientific evidence must be published in scientific and medical journals so that other experts may evaluate and test the assumptions made in the clinical trials.

Raw marijuana does not pass the five tests to be considered a medicine. Why not?

- *The chemistry of marijuana has not been dosed or standardized.* Approved medicines are the same wherever you buy them. The penicillin tablet bought in a Boston pharmacy is the same as one purchased in San Diego. Not so with the marijuana sold in dispensaries. The marijuana plant grown in Seattle is different from the one grown in Denver. No two are the same—and unlike a pharmacist, the "budtender" selling the product couldn't tell you all the chemicals each plant contained.
- *Raw marijuana contains hundreds of compounds in unknown quantities.* Even if some compounds, if extracted, purified, and standardized, have been proven to treat certain conditions like childhood seizures, raw marijuana contains so many unknown compounds that we do not yet understand their overall effect on humans. That's why even the most basic over-the-counter drugs have a more complex label than pot.
- *Lack of rigorous clinical trials.* As late as 2016, raw marijuana failed the FDA's scientific review to be considered a medicine. Looking at the scientific literature, it's not hard to understand why. Aside from a handful of anecdotal studies, all successful, large-scale clinical trials have been with isolated compounds from the marijuana plant, not raw marijuana itself. The science on raw marijuana just isn't there.

What About the Terminally Ill and Those Who Say Marijuana Helps Them?

No one suggests that the government should arrest or imprison the intractably or terminally ill for trying a substance they think may help them. But decriminalizing small amounts of marijuana for use by cancer patients is very different from legalizing "medical marijuana" for the treatment of everything from headaches to insomnia. These legalization efforts have led to the creation of a new industry that lobbies to expand the use of raw marijuana as a miracle drug that treats all symptoms, with the eventual goal of legalizing recreational marijuana without any restrictions on THC content or form. At that point, the ruse is dropped and many of the businesses who were selling medical marijuana convert to recreational stores.

Moreover, patients with side effects from unapproved, untested marijuana products have no recourse against the fly-by-night companies that produce them. This is the reason why we have an FDA process, and why the results can be so heartbreaking when it is circumvented. The good news is that, as noted above, a number of FDA-approved products derived from the marijuana plant already exist, and more are in the process of clinical trials.

How Can We Chart a Path Forward?

Research and compassion should guide us as we seek to help those who are suffering. Regulations on marijuana research can be streamlined and improved to speed research and development of new, FDA-approved drugs. Additionally, we should increase federal funding for legitimate research into the medicinal constituents of cannabis and fast-track those medicines so that voters will not seek to bypass the FDA.

Unfortunately, bypassing these controls opens the door to a dangerous form of unregulated "medicine" that exposes Americans to unsafe and unscrupulous practices.

How Do State Medical Marijuana Programs Work?

In the absence of medication development, legalization advocates have waged political campaigns to deem marijuana as medicine in various states. Some states have small, highly regulated regimes for a limited number of very sick individuals. But the vast majority of medical marijuana users in the US are not seriously ill. Many studies have found that fewer than 5% of people with medical marijuana recommendation cards have cancer, AIDS, MS, or other serious illnesses.[217]

Why Not Just Reschedule Marijuana or Get It out of the Food, Drug, and Cosmetic Act?

Neither of those proposed solutions would solve the problem of the need for more research, and instead would likely encourage illegal operators to continue to manufacture harmful products. Rescheduling is a red herring in this discussion since many better options exist to expedite research. Rescheduling would not have any effect on specific marijuana penalties and would not permit doctors to prescribe it.[218]

In the case of marijuana, rescheduling the drug to Schedule II or lower would immediately trigger requirements that the FDA regulate the safety and efficacy of the drug. Because the marijuana industry has realized that whole plant marijuana is unlikely to ever pass through FDA trials since they have not dosed or standardized their products, they now vociferously argue against rescheduling the drug. Rescheduling would also not effectively reduce barriers to research, as researchers for Schedule II drugs face nearly all of the same requirements and restrictions as those who research Schedule I drugs.

Current Science Argues against Removing Marijuana from CSA

Current medical literature and statistical surveys are clear: marijuana is a drug of abuse, is physiologically and psychologically addictive, and causes clear negative effects in both individuals and society. Regular use of marijuana can cause permanent changes in the brain, increasing the mass of the *nucleus*

---

217 See for example Nunberg H, et al. "An Analysis of Applicants Presenting to a Medical Marijuana Specialty Practice in California." *Journal of Drug Policy Analysis,* 4(1); (2011). http://www.bepress.com/jdpa/vol4/iss1/art1.

218 See Sabet, K. Should Marijuana Be Rescheduled? *HuffingtonPost.* (2014). http://www.huffingtonpost.com/kevin-a-sabet-phd/should-marijuana-be-resch_b_3745354.html.

accumbens (reward center),[219] similar to the effect of other addictive drugs. Cessation of use may result in physical withdrawal symptoms, including cravings, decreased appetite, sleep difficulty, and irritability.[220] Surveys show that regular marijuana users report more severe consequences than alcohol in most categories, including serious problems at work or school, taking time away from work or school, causing problems with family or friends, or spending a lot of time getting/using drugs.[221] Drugged driving fatalities have markedly increased in states which have legalized marijuana, posing a hazard to the general public.[222] The current body of evidence strongly reinforces current classification of marijuana as a controlled substance under the Controlled Substances Act, particularly with respect to modern, high-potency marijuana and extracts.

In addition, emerging research demonstrates a link between heavy use of high potency marijuana and the development of serious mental illness. A European study from 2019 showed these factors contributing to a five times greater likelihood of having an episode of cannabis induced psychosis.[223] And a recent meta-analysis of peer-reviewed research demonstrated that over one-third of patients experiencing cannabis induced psychosis transitioned to schizophrenia, higher than any other drug.[224]

---

[219] Gilman, et al., Cannabis Use Is Quantitatively Associated with Nucleus Accumbens and Amygdala Abnormalities in Young Adult Recreational Users, *Journal of Neuroscience.* 16 April 2014, 34 (16):5529-5538.

[220] Gorelick DA, Levin KH, Copersino ML, et al. Diagnostic Criteria for Cannabis Withdrawal Syndrome. *Drug Alcohol Depend.* 2012;123(1-3):141-147.

[221] Caulkins, Johnathan P., The Real Dangers of Marijuana. National Affairs. Winter 2016 (30).

[222] AAA Foundation for Traffic Safety. Prevalence of Marijuana Involvement in Fatal Crashes: Washington, 2010-2014. May 2016. Web. 23 Oct. 2016.

[223] Di Forti, et al. The contribution of cannabis use to variation in the incidence of psychotic disorder across Europe (EU-GEI): a multicentre case-control study. *Lancet Psychiatry.* Vol. 6, Iss. 5. May 1, 2019. https://www.thelancet.com/journals/lanpsy/article/PIIS2215-0366(19)30048-3/fulltext.

[224] Murrie B, Lappin J, Large M, Sara G. Transition of substance-induced, brief, and atypical psychoses to schizophrenia: a systematic review and meta-analysis. *Schizophrenia Bulletin.* 2019 October 16. https://academic.oup.com/schizophreniabulletin/advance-article-abstract/doi/10.1093/schbul/sbz102/5588638?redirectedFrom=fulltext.

What Can Be Done to Facilitate Research on Marijuana's Medical Potential?

Recommendation: Allow DEA/NIDA to Issue Multiple Authorizations for Growing Marijuana for Research Purposes

Under international agreements, the US NIDA– the National Institute on Drug Abuse is the sole source for research marijuana, which NIDA procures by contract from the University of Mississippi. According to NIDA, demand for marijuana for research purposes is generally low at this time. Still, multiple states have set up their own marijuana grow operations because of a purported need for marijuana rich in certain components, like CBD. Though the University of Mississippi is now growing marijuana rich in CBD, it is not unreasonable for other NIDA-approved sites to be able to grow different strains of marijuana. Therefore, SAM endorses the idea of NIDA (or other NIH-entities) to be able to grant multiple contracts for research purposes under strict supervision, in coordination with DEA. This is a key part of H.R. 3797, the Medical Marijuana Research Act and H.R. 601.

Recommendation: Waive DEA Registration Requirements for Non-Intoxicating Cannabinoid Research

Under the CSA, the DEA has the authority to issue a regulation *waiving the registration requirement* for certain manufacturers, distributors or dispensers, if the DEA determines that it is "consistent with the public health and safety." 21 USC Sec. 822(d). In theory, DEA could waive the Schedule I research registration requirement for physician researchers working under FDA-approved INDs and using products that have met FDA quality standards. Currently, Epidiolex® (a botanically-derived CBD drug) has been approved by the FDA for treatment of children with epilepsy that is resistant to other medications. Each of the physicians with such a program had to go through a burdensome and time-consuming process to secure a Schedule I research registration. As researchers seek to research other cannabinoids to better understand their potential as new drugs or how they interact with other medications, DOJ/DEA could issue a statement that DEA would issue Schedule I research registrations to all teaching hospitals and clinics with the appropriate field of researchers, allowing them to possess and dispense cannabinoid formulations that have passed some FDA standards. Such registrations could be time-limited, e.g., one year, with a possibility of renewal. If the FDA approves a drug made from those cannabinoids, it then has a medical use and must be moved out of Schedule I. At that point, there would no longer be a need for such special registrations for that product.

Recommendation: Make Permanent the Elimination of the Public Health Service (PHS) Review for Marijuana Research Applications

In 1999, the Department of Health and Human Services (HHS) announced that it intended to establish new procedures "to make available a sufficient amount of research-grade marijuana to support those studies that are the most likely to yield usable, essential data." Marijuana is the only drug that had this new procedure attached to it. HHS explained that "the scientific merits of each protocol will be evaluated through a Public Health Service (PHS) interdisciplinary review process [which] will take into consideration a number of factors, including the scientific quality of the proposed study, the quality of the organization's peer-review process, and the objective of the proposed research."[225] The intention was to streamline and increase research, but the general consensus is that it has had the unintended consequence of stalling research. Since research proposals still have to go through FDA and individual Institutional Review Board (IRB) protocols, many have questioned the wisdom of the PHS process, since it seemingly adds an extra step for no reason. Given that research protocols would still need to go through the FDA and other entities, NIH administratively eliminated the PHS review process for marijuana research applications in 2015. SAM supports making this elimination permanent as Section 5 of H.R. 3797, the Medical Marijuana Research Act, proposes.

Recommendation: DOJ and HHS Should Establish Special Federal Research Programs for Seriously Ill Individuals That Do Not Respond to Other Medications

The CSA authorizes the DOJ/DEA to carry out educational and research programs "directly related to enforcement of the laws...concerning drugs, which may include... (2) studies or special projects to compare the deterrent effects of various enforcement strategies on drug use and abuse; ... and (5) studies or special projects to develop more effective methods to prevent diversion of controlled substances into illegal channels" 21 USC sec. 872 (a).

DOJ/DEA could collaborate with the National Institute for Neurological Diseases and Stroke (NINDS) on a program similar to NCI's Group C program

[225] Health and Human Services Guidance. See: http://grants.nih.gov/grants/guide/notice-files/not99-091.html.

for Marinol. In that program, *over 20,000 patients received the drug over a period of four years under a "Group C" program.* The Group C program was closed when Marinol was approved. Here's how such a program was described in the 1980s:

> "The National Cancer Institute (NCI) is initiating a national THC distribution program by applying to the FDA for its classification as a Group C investigational agent. Since THC is also a Schedule I drug, the distribution system requires strict adherence to Drug Enforcement Agency (DEA) security and safety regulations. Contrary to the usual distribution of Group C drugs, THC will not be available directly to physicians. THC will be made available to hospital pharmacies which are: (1) an NCI recognized Cancer Center (P-30 grant supported), (2) an NCI designated New Drug Study Group, (3) a member of the Council of Teaching Hospitals. Hospital pharmacies that are located in inadequately represented geographic areas when certain criteria are met by them will also be considered. Physicians desiring to prescribe THC need not have Schedule I registration, but should (1) have experience in cancer chemotherapy, (2) have a current DEA registration number, (3) agree to abide by the Guidelines for Use of THC, and (4) be registered with a participating pharmacy. A registered physician may prescribe THC by writing a Research Order for Medication on a usual prescription blank, including, in addition to normal required information, confirmation that patient consent has been obtained and the name of the hospital at which the physician is registered to prescribe THC."

Recommendation DOJ/DEA Could Enter into Agreements with Interested State and Local Agencies to Allow for Research of Cannabinoids

The federal government could (*without the need for changing the CSA*) enter into a cooperative agreement with the states. The CSA, 21 USC sec. 873(a), provides:

> "The Attorney General *shall cooperate* with local, State, and Federal agencies concerning traffic in controlled substances and in suppressing the abuse of controlled substances. To this end, he is *authorized to. notwithstanding any other provision of law,* enter into contractual agreements with State and local law enforcement agencies to provide for cooperative enforcement and regulatory activities under this chapter."

Under this section, the Attorney General is mandated to cooperate and permitted to enter into contractual cooperation agreements "notwithstanding any other provision of law."

DOJ could in theory enter into such agreements with state and local agencies in order to expand current research protocols. The argument would be that, by making CBD or other cannabinoids of research interest (that meet FDA quality standards) more available, patients would not have to resort to federally-unlawful channels, such as dispensaries and other purveyors, where they might purchase cannabis with significant amounts of THC; such agreements would thereby "suppress the abuse of controlled substances."

Recommendation: Crack Down on Illegal Operators

Currently, illegal purveyors of cannabis products are making rich profits from wild health claims, which they falsely promote to patients and other consumers as "legal dietary supplements," resulting in public health hazards. DOJ and FDA should work together to take these products off the online "shelf."

While the FDA has sent warning letters to some companies manufacturing CBD products illegally, FDA has traditionally resisted taking enforcement action in the area of medical marijuana, claiming that since marijuana is a Schedule I drug, jurisdiction is left solely to DEA.

However, medical marijuana companies routinely and blatantly violate the Food, Drug and Cosmetic Act by selling foods and/or "medicines" that are *dangerous, contain illegal components, and have not been reviewed by FDA.* Virtually none of these purveyors is complying with FDA requirements for proper manufacturing (GMP, registration with FDA), labeling and advertising/promotion. Manufacturers and other purveyors of marijuana products make many therapeutic claims that bring those products within the scope of the Food, Drug, and Cosmetic Act (FDCA).

Conclusions

The legalization of marijuana has far outpaced what a sober survey of the scientific literature would indicate. It is time to hit the pause button on further recreational and medical legalization initiatives until we can collect meaningful data from state experiments that are bypassing currently accepted medical practices (see Appendix A for the positions of major medical societies on marijuana legalization). It is also time for the FDA to assert its authority in regulating medications to stop the marketing of marijuana as a cure-all for any and all conditions.

Recently, the Surgeon General issued an advisory that pregnant women should refrain from marijuana use during pregnancy because of the effect of THC on the developing brain.[226] This was tragically necessary because 70% of marijuana stores in Denver were recommending marijuana to pregnant women for morning sickness.[227]

There is still much we do not understand about the hundreds of chemical compounds within the marijuana plant, some of which may hold great promise to treat medical conditions. But there is a right way and a wrong way to go about meaningful and responsible research. We do not need to legalize recreational marijuana in order to study it. We should reduce barriers and make marijuana easier to research within the scheduling system.

Thank you for your consideration.

Appendix A: Medical Association Positions on Marijuana

American Society of Addiction Medicine[228]: "ASAM does not support the legalization of marijuana and recommends that jurisdictions that have not acted to legalize marijuana be most cautious and not adopt a policy of legalization until more can be learned from the 'natural experiments' now underway in jurisdictions that have legalized marijuana."

American Cancer Society[229]: "The ACS is supportive of more research into the benefits of cannabinoids. Better and more effective treatments are

---

[226] https://www.hhs.gov/surgeongeneral/reports-and-publications/addiction-and-substance-misuse/advisory-on-marijuana-use-and-developing-brain/index.html.

[227] Dickson, et al. Recommendations from Cannabis Dispensaries About First-Trimester Cannabis Use. *Obstetrics & Gynecology*. Vol. 131, No. 6, (2018). https://www.denverhealth.org/-/media/denver-health-marijuana-pregnancy-study.pdf?la=en&hash=7CF1182B6937B9E4267378A1E5F04D8ED221DC6C.

[228] American Society of Addiction Medicine. "Public Policy Statement on Marijuana, Cannabinoids, and Legalization."https://www.asam.org/docs/default-source/public-policy-statements/marijuana-cannabinoids-and-legalization-9-21-2015.pdf?sfvrsn=38e06fc2_0#search="public%20policy%20statement%20on%20medical%20marijuana" (2015).

[229] American Cancer Society. "Should Medical Marijuana Be a Medical Option?" http://medicalmarijuana.procon.org/view.source.php?sourceID=001399 (March 27, 2014). American Glaucoma Society. "Position Statement on Marijuana and the Treatment of Glaucoma" https://www.americanglaucomasociety.net/about/statements (August 10, 2009).

needed to overcome the side effects of cancer and its treatment. The ACS does not advocate the use of inhaled marijuana or the legalization of marijuana."

American Glaucoma Society: "Marijuana, or its components administered systemically, cannot be recommended without a long term trial which evaluates the health of the optic nerve… Although marijuana can lower IOP, its side effects and short duration of action, coupled with a lack of evidence that its use alters the course of glaucoma, preclude recommending this drug in any form for the treatment of glaucoma at the present time."

The American Academy of Pediatrics (AAP)[230] opposes "medical marijuana" outside the regulatory process of the US Food and Drug Administration. Notwithstanding this opposition to use, the AAP recognizes that marijuana may currently be an option for cannabinoid administration for children with life-limiting or severely debilitating conditions and for whom current therapies are inadequate. The AAP strongly supports research and development of pharmaceutical cannabinoids and supports a review of policies promoting research on the medical use of these compounds.

The American Medical Association (AMA)[231] "has urged legislatures to delay legalizing cannabis until further research is completed on the public health, medical, economic, and social consequences of its use. In states that have already legalized cannabis, the AMA has urged jurisdictions to take steps to regulate the product effectively to protect the health and safety of high risk populations and the public."

The American Psychiatric Association (APA)[232] *states:*"There is no current scientific evidence that cannabis is in any way beneficial for the treatment of any psychiatric disorder. In contrast, current evidence supports, at minimum, a strong association of cannabis use with the onset of psychiatric disorders. Adolescents are particularly vulnerable to harm, given the effects of cannabis on neurological development. Further research on the use of cannabis-derived substances as medicine should be encouraged and facilitated by the federal government."

---

[230] The American Academy of Pediatrics. "The impact of Marijuana Policies on Youth: Clinical, Research, and Legal Update." http://pediatrics.aappublications.org/content/early/2015/01/20/peds.2014-4146.full.pdf (March 20, 2015).

[231] The American Medical Association. "AMA Applauds Surgeon General's Advisory on Cannabis" https://www.ama-assn.org/press-center/ama-statements/ama-applauds-surgeon-general-s-advisory-cannabis (2019).

[232] The American Psychiatric Association. "Position Statement on Marijuana as Medicine" https://www.psychiatry.org/File%20Library/About-APA/Organization-Documents-Policies/Policies/Position-Cannabis-as-Medicine.pdf (2019).

* * *

Letter of September 19, 2018, from Ted Thompson, JD, Senior Vice President of Public Policy, the Michael J. Fox Foundation

September 19, 2018
The Honorable Matt Gaetz
United States House of Representatives
507 Cannon House Office Building
Washington, DC 20515

Dear Representative Gaetz,

On behalf of The Michael J. Fox Foundation for Parkinson's Research (MJFF), I write to express my support and appreciation for your legislation, H.R. 5634, the *Medical Cannabis Research Act of 2018*. It is estimated that nearly 1 million people in the United States are living with Parkinson's disease (PD), with an estimated annual economic burden of $26.4 billion. MJFF is dedicated to safeguarding access to appropriate health care services and treatments for PD patients.

MJFF advocates on behalf of the PD community, including both patients and families, and is committed to exploring new treatment options for those living with the disease. This includes conducting research on cannabis to determine potential therapeutic use. At this time, there has not been enough research done on cannabis to determine whether it is an effective treatment option. Easing barriers to research invites scientists to determine if cannabis may or may not safely and effectively help patients manage the symptoms associated with Parkinson's.

Current regulations surrounding cannabis block comprehensive medical research on the drug. Because of its federal classification as a Schedule I drug, coupled with the low quantity produced by the sole federally-approved growing site, researchers do not have the proper materials to conduct the necessary research. H.R.5634 calls for additional growing sites to produce cannabis for the purpose of conducting medical research. This allows researchers the opportunity to potentially unlock new therapies and treatments for patients with PD.

MJFF applauds you for authoring this important piece of legislation, and thanks you for your support of advancing medical research. The PD community is looking for a research breakthrough and is hopeful that one is found soon. Should you have any questions, please feel free to contact Aaron Polacek at apolacek@michaeljfox.org or by phone at 202-638-4101 ext.252.

Sincerely,

Ted Thompson, JD;
Senior Vice President of Public Policy

Statement of the Consumer Brands Association, Presented by Dr. Betsy Booren, Senior Vice President, Regulatory and Technical Affairs

Thank you, Chairwoman Eshoo and Ranking Member Burgess, and members of the subcommittee for the opportunity to submit this statement for the record on behalf of the Consumer Brands Association. The Consumer Brands Association represents the $2 trillion consumer packaged goods industry and the 20 million jobs it supports. Consumer Brands advocates for smart regulatory polices that protect public health and open pathways for industry innovation and growth. Our member companies are committed to demonstrating shared values with American consumers on health and supporting standards that bolster consumer confidence in the products we all use every day.

One of the two primary cannabis derivatives, cannabidiol (CBD), has gone mainstream. Almost overnight, CBD products seem to be for sale everywhere — from gas stations and strip malls to grocery stores and online retailers.

Despite the robust market for CBD, few consumers know much about the ingredient. Law enforcement must contend with conflicting guidance about which products are legal and government regulators are resource-challenged as they work to protect consumers from misleading marketing and potentially unsafe products.

Lacking clear federal oversight, a patchwork of inconsistent, often contradictory, state and local regulations has emerged, generating profound consumer confusion. Consumers are unclear or mistaken about what CBD is, what it does and whether all products made with CBD are safe to consume or apply.

Consumer demand for CBD products has skyrocketed since hemp was legalized in the 2018 federal Farm Bill. To understand what is motivating consumers, we conducted a national survey of 2,000 adults across the United States, probing their awareness and overall knowledge of CBD and CBD products. We were surprised by our findings:

- One-in-three Americans report using CBD.
- Four-in-ten Americans who have heard of CBD believe it's another name for marijuana.
- More than half think it has the potential to cause a high sensation.
- Seventy-seven percent assume CBD is regulated at the federal level, including 51 percent who rest easy thinking the Food and Drug Administration (FDA) oversees CBD's safe use and marketing.

As the market continues to grow, the lack of federal regulations around CBD will continue to cause several issues.

First, product safety and quality. Consumers must be assured that the products they're buying are high-quality and safe. But today, without the research needed to show CBD products are safe — or assurances that CBD products have been produced under applicable good manufacturing practices — consumers have no idea if they're purchasing safe products or whether they have been produced to consistently contain a certain amount of CBD, if any.

Second, without rigorous testing requirements, consumers have no idea if they're purchasing pure CBD, CBD with trace amounts of THC or just olive oil with a new name and package.

Finally, there isn't any guarantee of safety despite myriad ailments CBD claims to alleviate. Right now, CBD is approved for one thing only — the treatment of epilepsy as an active ingredient in the drug Epidiolex. Just last month, FDA sent another round of warning letters to companies who were claiming their CBD products could treat a range of health conditions including schizophrenia, cancer, diabetes, arthritis, acne, alcoholism, bipolar disorder, fibromyalgia, irritable bowel syndrome, Parkinson's, PTSD, multiple sclerosis, glaucoma and high cholesterol.

Given the "Wild West" CBD environment, it's important that we look toward developing the critical science and the appropriate regulatory structure so that good actors are provided the opportunity to ensure consumer safety and deliver a product that consumers are clearly demanding. That's why we are calling for a two-pronged approach to clarifying the CBD marketplace.

First, Congress must ensure there is adequate funding for federal research on the health and safety of CBD products. It is important that Congress works to ensure scientific gaps are filled so that our regulators can make informed decisions. As Dr. Peter Grinspoon of the Harvard Medical School explained, "Without sufficient high-quality evidence in human studies we can't pinpoint effective doses, and because CBD is currently mostly available as an unregulated supplement, it's difficult to know exactly what you are getting."

Second, Congress should ensure FDA has the resources necessary to continue its market surveillance and enforcement activities, which include sampling and testing of available CBD products to root out egregious activities and protect consumers. Ultimately, our government regulators must establish a clear, consistent regulatory framework that settles this chaotic market.

Americans support this approach. Our research indicates nearly eight-in-ten (79%) Americans believe CBD should be regulated at the federal level, or federally in concert with the states. The FDA has pledged to act, but the agency estimates it could take five years to establish federal CBD regulations. It is our hope that, by working with Congress, the process can be expedited.

Consumers want FDA to have a regulatory program in place underpinned by sound, risk-based science so they can make smart choices about CBD products. Law enforcement deserves clear guidelines about what's legal and illegal. And America's most trusted brands want to work with Congress to assist FDA in achieving a regulatory framework every consumer can have confidence in.

* * *

Letter of August 26, 2019, from Neil D. Doherty, Acting Assistant Administrator, Drug Enforcement Administration

U.S. Department of Justice
Drug Enforcement Administration
8701 Morrissette Drive
Springfield, Virginia 22152
www.dea.gov

Biophannaceutical Research Company, LLC
BRC 27 Laurel Street
Atherton, California 94027

Dear George B. Hodgin:

On August 12, 2016, the Drug Enforcement Administration (DEA) published a policy statement in the Federal Register (81 FR 53846) ("2016 Policy Statement"). The 2016 Policy Statement concerned applications by persons seeking to become registered under the Controlled Substances Act (CSA) to grow (manufacture) marijuana in order to supply DEA-registered researchers in the United States. You are receiving this letter because you submitted such an application.

DEA supports research into the effects of marijuana and the potential medical utility of its chemical constituents. Under the CSA, DEA is responsible for registering growers to produce an adequate and uninterrupted supply of marijuana under adequately competitive conditions for such research. Since publication of the 2016 Policy Statement, the Department of Justice, of which DEA is a component, has determined that adjustments to DEA's policies and practices may be necessary. This letter serves two main purposes. First, we wish to inform you ofDEA's intent to issue a Notice of Proposed Rulemaking (NPRM) that, if finalized, would supersede the 2016 Policy Statement. This rulemaking process will provide applicants and other interested parties an opportunity to comment on the regulations that should govern the program of growing marijuana for scientific and medical research under DEA registration consistent with applicable law. Second, this letter provides you with instructions on how to withdraw your application if you no longer wish to have your application considered by DEA, or if you no longer seek registration because of recent changes in federal law with respect to "hemp" under the Agricultural Improvement Act of 2018.

Notice of Proposed Rulemaking

Applications for registration to manufacture controlled substances in schedule I or II are governed by 21 U.S.C. § 823(a). Under section 823(a), the DEA Administrator (through a delegation from the Attorney General) may register such an applicant only if the Administrator determines that the registration is consistent with the public interest and with applicable laws and treaties. DEA intends to propose regulations that govern the program of growing marijuana for scientific and medical research under DEA registration, consistent with applicable law.

The 2016 policy statement provided information on how it intended to expand the number of registrations, and described in general terms the way it would oversee those additional growers. Therein, DEA recognized the need to move past the single grower system and register additional growers. DEA has received 33 pending applications; the most recent was filed in May 2019.

Because the size of the applicant pool is unprecedented in DEA's experience, DEA has determined that adjustments to its policies and practices with respect to the marijuana growers program are necessary to fairly evaluate the applicants under the 823(a) factors, including 823(a)(l).

In addition, since publication of the 2016 policy statement, the Department of Justice, in consultation with other federal agencies, has been engaged in a policy review process to ensure that the marijuana growers program is consistent with applicable laws and treaties. That review process remains ongoing; however, it has progressed to the point where DEA is able to issue a notice of applications. Over the course of this policy review process, the Department of Justice has also determined that adjustments to DEA's policies and practices related to the marijuana growers' program may be necessary. Accordingly, before DEA completes this evaluation and registration process, DEA intends to propose regulations in the near future that would supersede the 2016 policy statement and govern persons seeking to become registered with DEA to grow marijuana as bulk manufacturers, consistent with applicable law.

Recent Amendment to the CSA Regarding Hemp

As the result of a recent amendment to federal law, certain fonns of cannabis no longer require DEA registration to grow or manufacture. The Agriculture Improvement Act of 2018, which was signed into law on December 20, 2018, changed the definition of marijuana under the CSA. As amended, the definition of marijuana no longer includes "hemp," which is defined as "the plant Cannabis sativa L. and any part of that plant, including the seeds thereof and all derivatives, extracts, cannabinoids, isomers, acids, salts, and salts of isomers, whether growing or not, with a delta-9 tetrahydrocannabinol [THC] concentration of not more than 0.3 percent on a dry weight basis."[233] Pursuant to the amended definition, cannabis plant material that contains 0.3 percent or

[233] 7 u.s.c. § 1639o(l); 21 u.s.c. § 802(16XBXi).

less delta-9 THC on a dry weight basis is not a controlled substance and does not require a DEA registration to grow. Accordingly, if you have applied for a DEA registration exclusively for the purpose of growing cannabis that contains no more than 0.3 percent delta-9 THC on a dry weight basis, including cannabis that contains cannabidiol and falls below the delta-9 THC threshold, you no longer need to register with DEA for that purpose.

Next Steps

In accordance with DEA regulations[234], a notice of applications will be published in the Federal Register shortly. However, if, as a result of the Agriculture Improvement Act or for any other reason, you no longer wish to have your application considered by DEA, please submit a written statement indicating your desire to withdraw your application.[235] Upon receipt of such a request on or before November 1, 2019, DEA will refund any applicable application fees.[236] If you still wish to seek registration, no further action *is* required as of this time. DEA will provide additional information through the forthcoming NPRM and future letters to applicants, as needed.

Contact Information

Please submit your written correspondence regarding any of the above matters to the following address:

Drug Enforcement Administration
Diversion Regulatory Section (DRG)
Attn: Charlotte D. Barron, Section Chief
8701 Morrissette Drive
Springfield, Virginia 22152

If you have any questions about this letter, please contact Deputy Assistant Administrator Donetta Spears at (202) 307-7165.

---

[234] 21 C.F.R. § 1301.33.
[235] 21 C.F.R. § 1301.16.
[236] DEA is granting a temporary exception to 21 C.F.R. § 1301.13(e) in order *to* issue refunds to those applicants who wish to withdraw their application as a bulk marijuana manufacturer.

Sincerely,

Neil D. Doherty
Acting Assistant Administrator
DEA Diversion Control Division

Fact Sheets, by Nora D. Volkow, M.D., Director, National Institute on Drug Abuse

CBD - epileptic TX
THC - no epileptic TX benefit

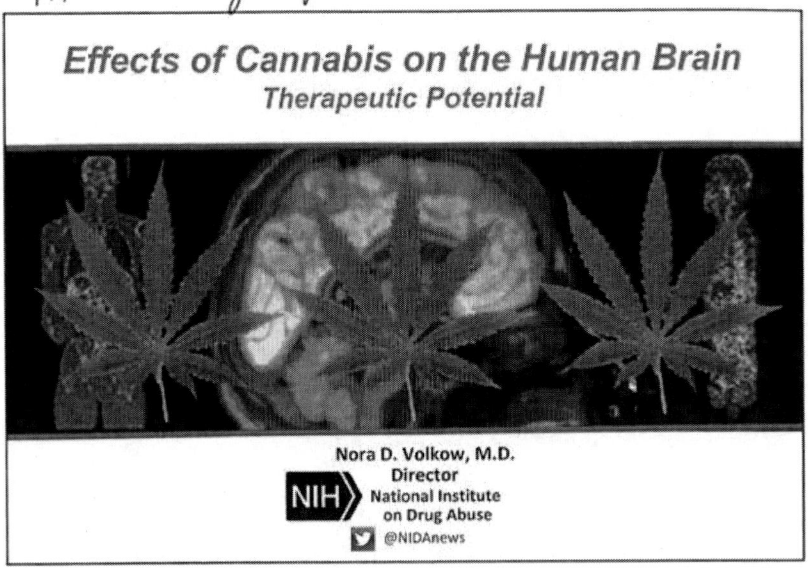

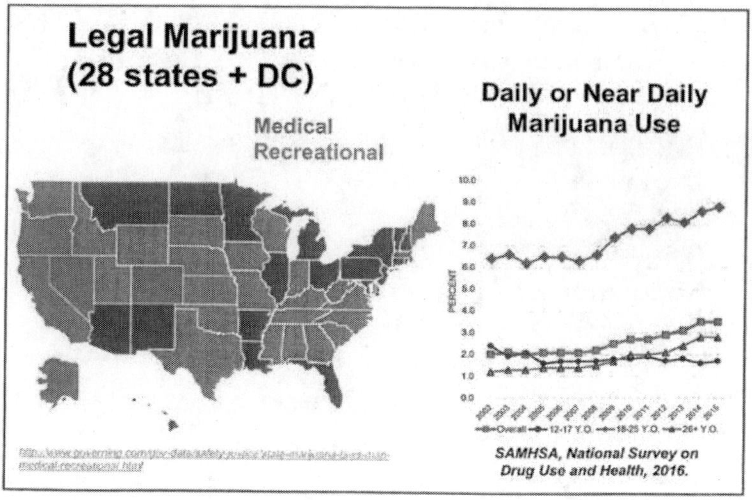
Legal Marijuana
(28 states + DC)
Medical
Recreational
Daily or Near Daily
Marijuana Use
PERCENT
10.0
9.0
8.0
7.0
6.0
5.0
4.0
3.0
2.0
1.0
0.0
Overall
12-17 Y.O.
18-25 Y.O.
26+ Y.O.
SAMHSA, National Survey on
Drug Use and Health, 2016.

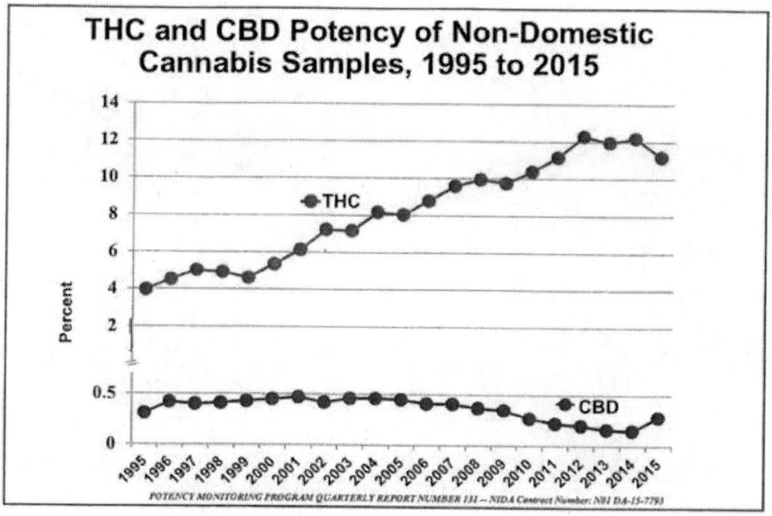
THC and CBD Potency of Non-Domestic
Cannabis Samples, 1995 to 2015
Percent
14
12
10
8
6
4
2
0.5
0
THC
CBD
1995
1996
1997
1998
1999
2000
2001
2002
2003
2004
2005
2006
2007
2008
2009
2010
2011
2012
2013
2014
2015
POTENCY MONITORING PROGRAM QUARTERLY REPORT NUMBER 131 – NIDA Contract Number: N01 DA-15-7793

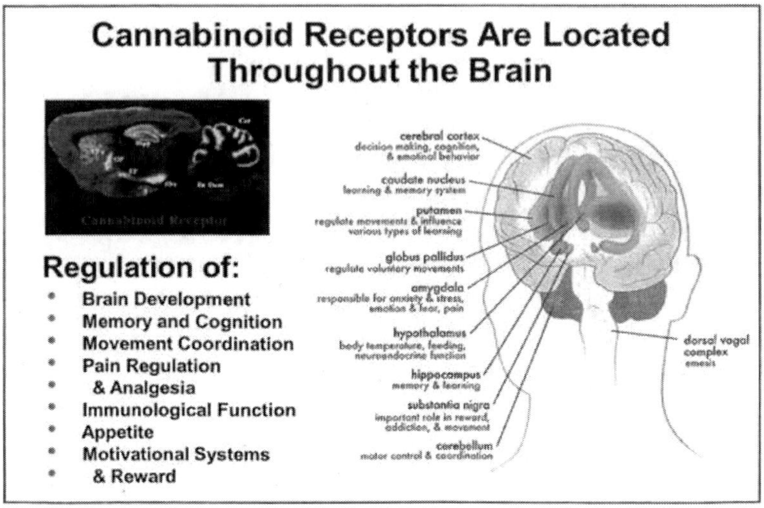
Cannabinoid Receptors Are Located Throughout the Brain
Regulation of:
• Brain Development
• Memory and Cognition
• Movement Coordination
• Pain Regulation & Analgesia
• Immunological Function
• Appetite
• Motivational Systems & Reward
cerebral cortex
decision making, cognition, & emotinal behavior
caudate nucleus
learning & memory system
putamen
regulate movements & influence various types of learning
globus pallidus
regulate voluntary movements
amygdala
responsible for anxiety & stress, emotion & fear, pain
hypothalamus
body temperature, feeding, neuroendocrine function
hippocampus
memory & learning
substantia nigra
important role in reward, addiction, & movement
cerebellum
motor control & coordination
dorsal vagal complex
emesis

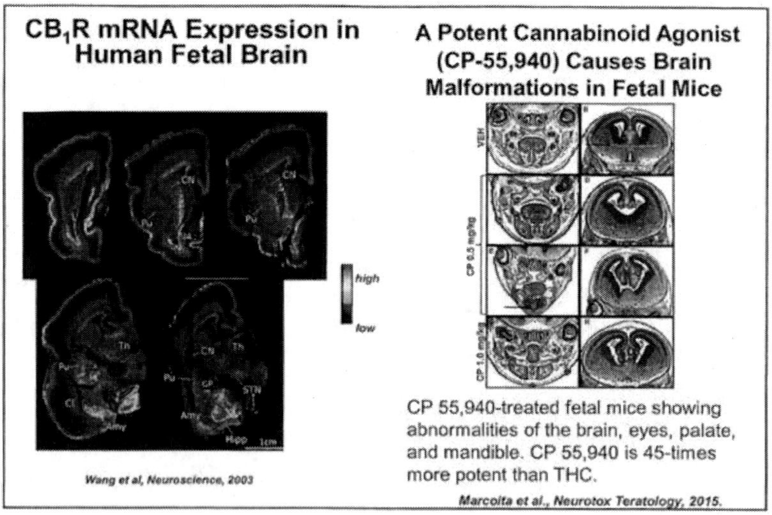
CB1R mRNA Expression in Human Fetal Brain
high
low
Wang et al, Neuroscience, 2003
A Potent Cannabinoid Agonist (CP-55,940) Causes Brain Malformations in Fetal Mice
VEH
CP 0.5 mg/kg
CP 1.0 mg/kg
CP 55,940-treated fetal mice showing abnormalities of the brain, eyes, palate, and mandible. CP 55,940 is 45-times more potent than THC.
Marcolta et al., Neurotox Teratology, 2015.

Marijuana and the adolescent brain

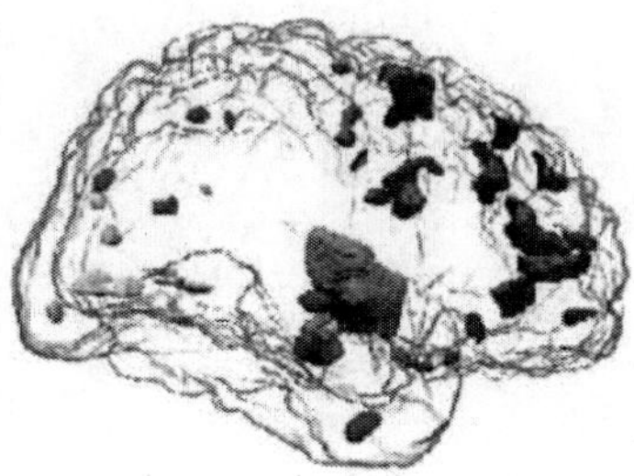

Targeting the Cannabinoid System for Therapeutic Purposes

- Exogenous compounds
  - Phytocannabinoids
    - THC, CBD, combinations
  - Synthetic cannabinoids
    - Dronabinol
- Endogenous manipulation
    - FAAH inhibitors
    - MAGL inhibitors
    - Allosteric modulators
- Receptor targets
  - CB1, CB2, TRPV1, PPAR, 5-HT, peripheral, others…

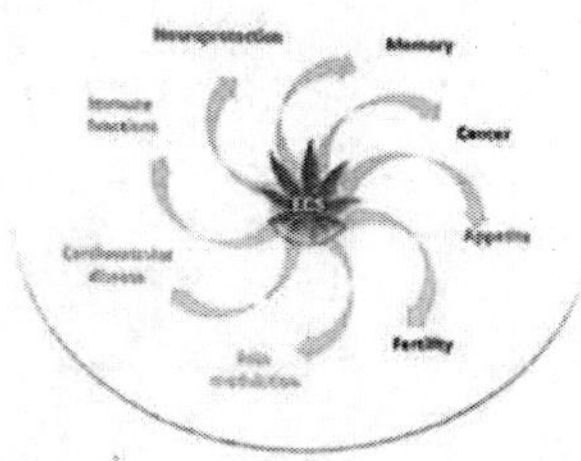

Strength of the Evidence For Marijuana/Cannabinoid Medical Applications

Strongest Evidence

- Nausea (Cancer chemotherapy)
- Spasticity & Pain (MS)
- Appetite Stimulant (AIDS-associated wasting)
- Pain esp. neuropathic
- Glaucoma (decreases intraocular pressure; no evidence it slows disease progression; & short acting)

Modest Evidence

- Anticonvulsant (CBD)
- Anti-inflammatory (CBD)
- Antitumor (THC/CBD) (animal models/cell cultures: glioblastoma; breast cancer cells; others (mechanisms: apoptosis; inhibition of tumor angiogenesis)

Weakest Evidence

- PTSD
- ADHD
- Alzheimer's
- Depression

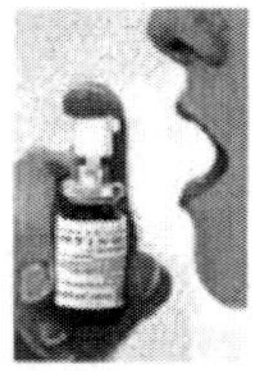

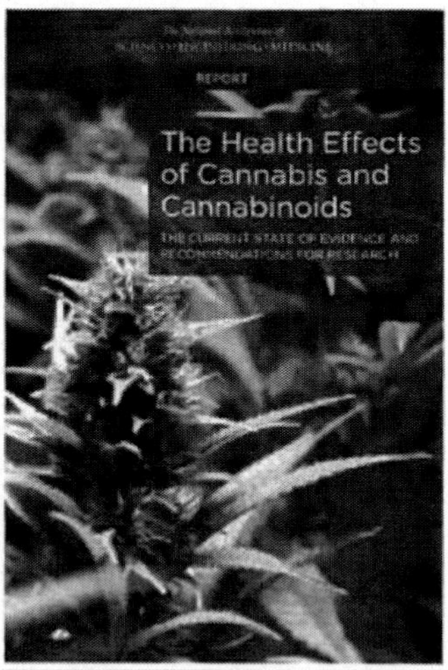

National Academy of Sciences Report

Released: January 12, 2017

PURPOSE:

To provide a comprehensive review of the current evidence regarding the health effects of using cannabis and cannabis-derived products

RECOMMENDATIONS:

1. ***Address Research Gaps***
2. ***Improve Research Quality***
3. ***Improve Surveillance Capacity***
4. ***Address Research Barriers***

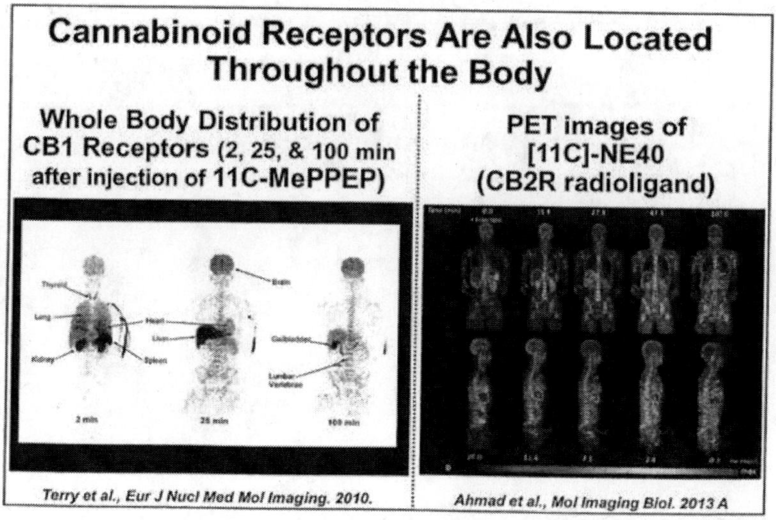
Cannabinoid Receptors Are Also Located Throughout the Body
Whole Body Distribution of CB1 Receptors (2, 25, & 100 min after injection of 11C-MePPEP)
PET images of [11C]-NE40 (CB2R radioligand)
Terry et al., Eur J Nucl Med Mol Imaging. 2010.
Ahmad et al., Mol Imaging Biol. 2013 A

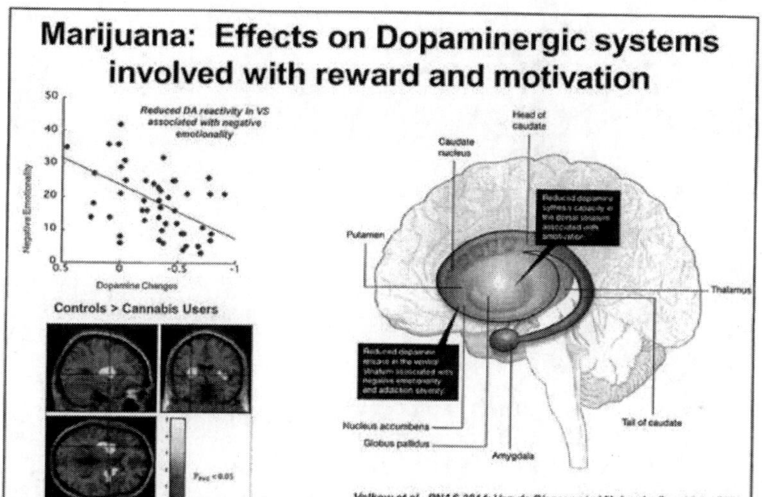
Marijuana: Effects on Dopaminergic systems involved with reward and motivation
Reduced DA reactivity in VS associated with negative emotionality
Negative Emotionality
Dopamine Changes
Controls > Cannabis Users
Head of caudate
Caudate nucleus
Putamen
Thalamus
Nucleus accumbens
Globus pallidus
Amygdala
Tail of caudate
Volkow et al., PNAS 2014; Van de Giessen et al Molecular Psychiatry 2016

Marijuana and mental illness

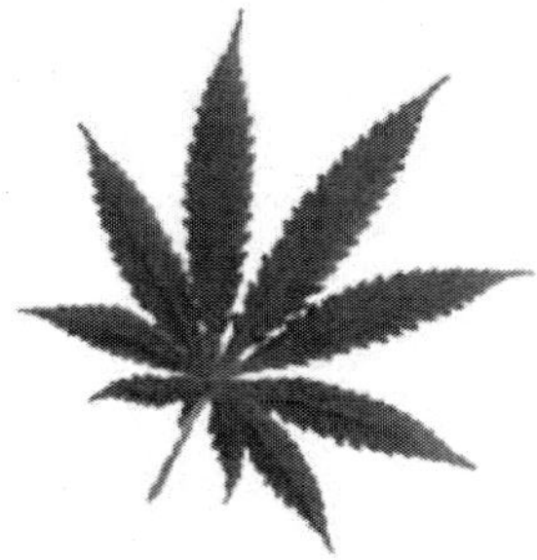

Early (<18y) Long-Term Cannabis Use Decreases Axonal Fiber Connectivity

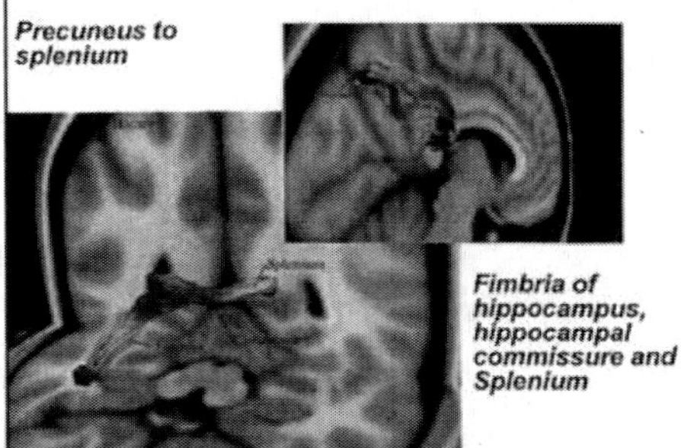

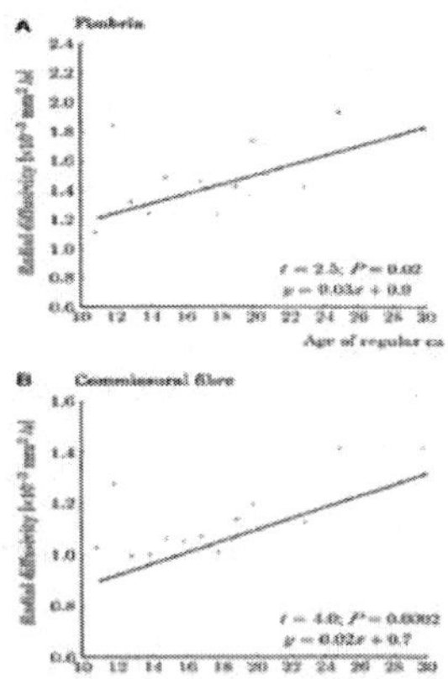

Axonal paths with reduced connectivity (measured with diffusion-weighted MRI) in cannabis users (n=59) compared to controls (N=33). Zalesky et al Brain 2012.

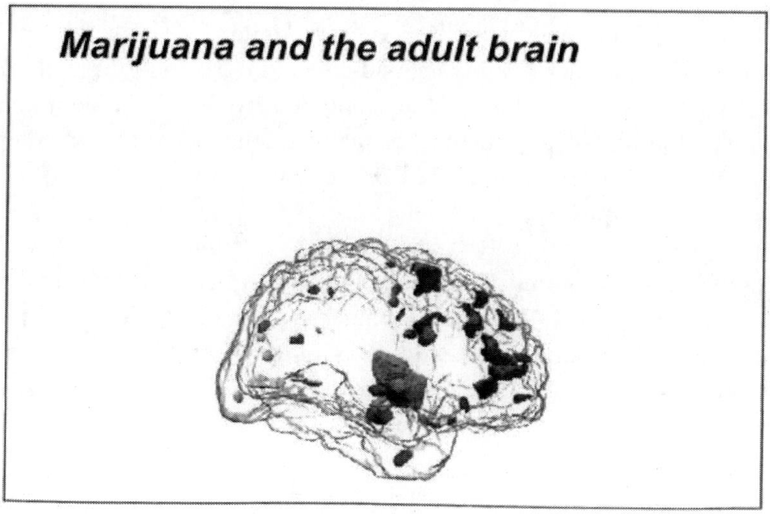

Answers to Submitted Questions for Nora D. Volkow, M.D., Director of the National Institute on Drug Abuse, National Institutes of Health

The Honorable Frank Pallone, Jr, (D-NJ)

1. In your testimony, you discuss the therapeutic potential of cannabis to treat other health conditions. What additional evidence or types of research do we need to ensure the safety and efficacy of medical cannabis products?

Response

Before an intervention (e.g., a drug or other potential medical product) can be tested in people, researchers perform laboratory and animal tests to discover how the drug works and whether it is likely to be safe and work well in humans. Next, a series of clinical trials is performed to assess whether the intervention is safe when used to treat a disease and whether it provides a real health benefit. In Phase I trials, researchers test an intervention in a small group of people (20–80) for the first time to learn about its safety and identify any side effects. In Phase II trials, the intervention is given to a larger group of people (100–300) to determine its effectiveness and to further study its safety. In Phase III trials, the intervention is given to large groups of people

(1,000–3,000) to confirm its effectiveness, monitor side effects, compare it with standard or similar treatments, and collect information that will allow it to be used safely. As with any drug approved by the U.S. Food and Drug Administration (FDA), any medical cannabis product would have to be tested in similar ways. We refer you to the FDA for more information on the medical product approval process.

2. What do we know about the health consequences of cannabis arrests and convictions today and what has your agency done to promote research around the health consequences of cannabis arrests and convictions?

Response

Involvement with the criminal justice system is often associated with poor health outcomes. Studies have shown that having been formerly incarcerated is associated with poor mental health and physical health outcomes, as well as elevated mortality risk.[237] Social isolation, which may occur during or after incarceration, is known to have profound consequences on mental health[238] and increase the chance of future substance use.[239] It also can lead to disparities in access to effective, continuing healthcare.[240] NIDA supports research to understand how cannabis policies affect cannabis use and cannabis use disorder, arrests, and incarceration, including disparities in adolescent marijuana arrests and use.

3. What ways is NIDA advancing research on various CBD products that consumers use?

Response

In Fiscal Year 2019, NIH spent $189 million on cannabinoid research, including $31 million in research on cannabidiol (CBD). NIH has a long history of supporting observational studies of individuals who use CBD and other cannabinoids to understand the health effects of such substances, to characterize patterns of use, and to understand whether individuals are using them to substitute for other drugs. In addition, NIH has been able to support

---

[237] https://www.ncbi.nlm.nih.gov/pubmed/28402828.

[238] https://www.ncbi.nlm.nih.gov/pmc/articles/PMC5975705/.

[239] https://pubmed.ncbi.nlm.nih.gov/31294075/?from_term=social+isolation+substance+use+&from_pos=6.

[240] https://link.springer.com/article/10.1007%2Fs11524-018-0276-0.

research on CBD products produced by DEA-registered manufacturers, including those produced under contract with NIDA, FDA-approved cannabidiol drug products (i.e., Epidiolex), and CBD products imported into the United States with authorization from the DEA. Results from NIH-supported research contributed to the development of Epidiolex, the first FDA-approved CBD therapy, which is used to treat rare pediatric seizure disorders. NIH is also supporting research to examine CBD as a potential therapy for neuropathic pain, arthritis pain, anxiety, other seizure disorders, inflammation, digestive disorders, and opioid addiction.

With the passage of the 2018 Farm Bill, cannabis and cannabis derivatives containing no more than 0.3% delta-9 THC on a dry weight basis are considered "hemp" and are no longer regulated as controlled substances under the Controlled Substances Act. The 2018 Farm Bill explicitly preserved FDA's authority to regulate products containing cannabis or cannabis derived compounds, and at present CBD cannot be legally sold as dietary supplements or added to food. In addition, products containing more than 0.3% delta-9 THC by dry weight, regardless of CBD concentration, remain in Schedule I under the Controlled Substances Act, and unless they are acquired from a DEA-approved source, researchers cannot use NIH grants funds to purchase these products for research.

4. You discuss in your testimony the therapeutic potential of cannabis and cannabis derivatives. Can you discuss how your agency is actively including underrepresented groups in this research?

Response

With limited exceptions, all NIH-funded studies that meet the NIH definition for clinical research must address plans for the inclusion of women, minorities, and individuals of all ages (as appropriate) within the grant application. Using the PHS Human Subjects and Clinical Trial Information Form, applications and proposals should include the minimum and maximum age of potential participants, describe the composition of the proposed study population in terms of sex/gender and racial/ethnic groups, and provide a rationale for selection of such subjects. Any exclusions based on sex/gender or race/ethnicity must include a rationale and justification based on a scientific or ethical basis. Investigators should also plan for appropriate outreach programs and activities to recruit and retain the proposed study population consistent with the purposes of the research project.

The Honorable Doris Matsui (D-CA)

1. Aside from the process the Department of Justice's DEA has set up for researchers to apply for a license to be able to study cannabis, what, if any, other legal means do researchers have to study the public health effects of cannabis?

Response

Researchers may study the health effects of cannabis in a variety of ways that do not require having their own supply of the drug. NIH has a long history of supporting observational studies of individuals who use cannabis to understand the health effects of such substances, to characterize patterns of use, and to understand whether individuals are using them to substitute for other drugs. Such studies may include behavioral and psychological screenings, brain imaging, and other assessments to understand health. For example, NIDA, along with other NIH Institutes, Centers, and Offices, supports the Adolescent Brain Cognitive Development (ABCD) Study, a longitudinal study involving nearly 12,000 adolescents that is examining the impact of substance use, including marijuana use, and other childhood experiences on health and brain development. ABCD and studies like it often rely on an participant's self-reported use and may be limited in their capacity to definitively characterize the products participants are using, which can affect the interpretation of the results. NIH has also supported a robust portfolio of research aimed at understanding how cannabis policies affect health and other outcomes. Indeed, NIH is currently funding studies examining the relationship between cannabis policies and: cannabis and other substance use, misuse, and substance use disorders; opioid prescribing and overdose; racial disparities in cannabis-related arrests; intergenerational transmission of drug use; and other health and economic outcomes. Studies are also examining youth exposure to traditional and social media cannabis promotions and ads.

2. How are federal agencies, and specifically the DEA, currently viewing the applicability of regulations regarding "controlled substances analogues" to synthetically derived non-psychoactive cannabinoids?

Response

We refer you to the DEA for the applicability of controlled substance regulations and the analogue provisions of the Controlled Substances Act to synthetically derived non-psychoactive cannabinoids.

3. What is the position of your agency about the current status of CBD? Does the agency believe there is a distinction between marijuana-derived CBD, which is treated as a Schedule I substance, and hemp-derived and maybe even synthetically-derived CBD which is not a controlled substance? Or, alternatively, do they believe there is federal agency support for an interpretation that any CBD that has less than 0.3% THC is hemp and therefore not regulated as a controlled substance?

Response

It is our understanding that any cannabidiol (CBD) preparation derived from cannabis that contains no more than 0.3% delta-9 THC on a dry weight basis is hemp and is, therefore, not regulated as a controlled substance. On August 26, 2019, the DEA issued a press release stating that "…as the result of a recent amendment to federal law, certain forms of cannabis no longer require DEA registration to grow or manufacture. The Agriculture Improvement Act of 2018, which was signed into law on Dec. 20, 2018, changed the definition of cannabis to exclude 'hemp'—plant material that contains 0.3 percent or less delta-9 THC on a dry weight basis.

Accordingly, hemp, including hemp plants and CBD preparations at or below the 0.3 percent delta-9 THC threshold, is not a controlled substance, and a DEA registration is not required to grow or research it." The press release is available here: https://www.dea.gov/press-releases/2019/08/26/dea-announces-steps-necessary-improve-access-marijuana-research

4. What is the position of your agency on creating some special permissions/exemptions/safe harbor provisions for researchers studying cannabis's properties so they may transport the cannabis they're studying between their various universities without running afoul of federal law?

Response

It is our understanding that current regulations allow for the transfer of Schedule I and Schedule II substances between DEA registrants via the use of the DEA Form 222. We refer you to the DEA for additional information.

The Honorable Robin L. Kelly (D-IL)

The World Health Organization's Expert Committee on Drug Dependence has recognized that cannabis can confer medical benefits and has recommended to the United Nations that international drug control conventions be amended to remove cannabis from the category of strictest control. More than 30 countries have already legalized medical cannabis at the national level. Additionally, 47 U.S. states, the District of Columbia, and four U.S. territories have amended their laws to recognize the therapeutic potential of cannabis. However, there is a gap in research on the impacts of cannabis and possible medical benefits due to many restrictions as a schedule I substance. There are various organizations including Americans for Safe Access (ASA) that promote safe and legal access to cannabis for therapeutic use and research.

1. What changes must be made to the Controlled Substances Act and/or to other aspects of our systems of evaluation and control to enable the U.S. federal government to allow for greater research on the medicinal and therapeutic value of cannabis?

Response

NIDA Director Dr. Nora Volkow recently addressed the United Nations Commission on Narcotic Drugs in support of the U.S.'s recommendation to remove cannabis and cannabis preparations from Schedule IV of the Single Convention. Removal from Schedule IV of the Single Convention would not change the control status of cannabis in the United States where, under the Controlled Substances Act (CSA), "marijuana" and its constituent compounds, excluding hemp, are classified as Schedule I controlled substances – defined as having no currently accepted medical use in the United States, a lack of accepted safety for use under medical supervision, and a high potential for abuse.[241] Researchers have reported that obtaining a new registration can take more than a year, that modifying a registration can also

[241] https://www.deadiversion.usdoj.gov/schedules/.

be time consuming, and that differing interpretations of the Schedule I registration requirements among local Drug Enforcement Agency (DEA) field offices, research institutions, as well as distinct federal and state registration requirements, greatly complicate the process.

It would be useful to clarify aspects of the CSA that have been sources of confusion and administrative burden for the research community, including that it is permissible for one individual to hold a Schedule I registration under which colleagues from the same institution may work even if those colleagues do not work directly for the registrant (e.g., as members of their laboratory); that registered researchers may store, administer, and work with any substances for which they hold a researcher registration at multiple practice sites on a single contiguous campus; and that if a person is registered to conduct research with a controlled substance and applies to conduct research with a second controlled substance that is in the same schedule or in a schedule with a higher numerical designation, an inspection that was performed for purposes of the existing registration shall be sufficient to support the application. Lastly, and specifically relevant to cannabis research, it would be helpful to clarify that individuals registered to conduct research with a controlled substance who need to perform limited manufacturing activities on small quantities of that substance consistent with their research protocol (for example, creating a particular dosage formulation for research purposes) are not required to obtain a separate manufacturing registration. This would be especially helpful in cases in which researchers are required to create dosage formulations in their own laboratories from cannabis products supplied through the NIDA Drug Supply Program.

Research with cannabis and other Schedule I substances can only be carried out with such substances obtained from registered manufacturers as required under the Controlled Substances Act (CSA) or synthesized under a federally approved protocol. The University of Mississippi is the only domestic entity currently registered with the DEA to cultivate cannabis for research purposes, which it does under a contract with NIDA. Researchers supported by NIDA and other federal agencies may not use federal funds to purchase cannabis available through state cannabis dispensaries, as that would violate Federal law. State dispensaries are not registered under the CSA and obtaining material from these dispensaries would be in violation of the CSA. Moreover, some universities have expressed reticence about allowing investigators to purchase dispensary products with non-federal funds or do research with these products on university grounds because doing so would violate federal law. DEA has announced that it intends to review additional grower applications. Having more than one domestic source of research cannabis would likely increase the diversity of products and formulations available to researchers, and may accelerate the development of cannabis-based medications.

It should be noted, these products available to consumers have not been subjected to FDA's drug approval process.

2. Have there been or will there be discussions between federal agency officials and their counterparts at foreign ministries in countries that dispense medical cannabis through their pharmacies to learn how they have been able to provide standardized medical cannabis to patients?

Response

There remains one competent authority in the United States that determines and establishes if a substance has medical use – the FDA. NIDA is a research agency, and the provision of standardized medical cannabis to patients for clinical purposes is outside of our scope.

However, NIDA does support research on the therapeutic potential of cannabis, for which there is a critical need for products standards. Cannabis available through state dispensaries is grown and processed under a variety of conditions and, like other botanical products, may include pesticides, pathogenic microbes, heavy metals, and other contaminants that could be harmful to humans. While most states with legal cannabis require product testing, there is no uniform testing standard. Likewise, product labeling varies, such that it may not be possible to determine the components of a marketed product, including the full range of cannabinoids present. The lack of testing and labeling standards presents challenges to conducting controlled research with these products and poses a potential risk to users.

The Honorable Greg Walden (R-OR)

1. What are the implications of rescheduling marijuana – say to schedule II?

Response

Placement of marijuana would signify a currently accepted medical use. Substances in schedule II-V have an approved medical use. HHS and DEA have reviewed multiple petitions requesting the movement of marijuana from schedule I.

The process for obtaining a Schedule II controlled substance registration is different from and involves fewer steps than the process for conducting research with Schedule I substances. The US Food and Drug Administration (FDA) Controlled Substances Program must review Schedule I research applications submitted to the U.S. Drug Enforcement Administration (DEA) for a determination of the qualifications and competency of the researcher and the merits of the protocol. For clinical research, the FDA's review is in addition to, but separate from, the review it conducts for the purposes of granting an investigational new drug (IND) approval, which is required before the DEA will issue a Schedule I registration. Moreover, each Schedule I substance the researcher is working on must be listed on the registration with authorized amounts the researcher can acquire for approved research. Changes to the protocol, including in the amount of a substance a researcher plans to use, must be reviewed by the FDA. In contrast, Schedule II-V registrations are not specific to a particular study protocol or substance (although some substances may be designated as Code H drugs, requiring additional review), and FDA's Controlled Substances Program does not review Schedule II-V registration applications.

2. How do the current DEA registration processes for modifying a Schedule I registration to conduct research with cannabis impact the ability to do research?
    a. We have heard that it can take up to a year to get a Schedule I registration, and that the process of adding new cannabinoids to an existing registration and getting approval for protocol modifications is time consuming. We have also heard from the research community that differing interpretations of the registration requirements among DEA field offices as well as distinct federal and state requirements can greatly complicate the process. Can you discuss your experience and the experiences of your researchers?

Response

An overarching concern expressed by researchers is a lack of transparency regarding registration requirements for Schedule I and Schedule II-V substances, and differing interpretations of those requirements by DEA field agents and research institutions. In collaboration with ONDCP, HHS, FDA, and DEA, NIDA has also been identifying ways to streamline the Schedule I research registration process.

The challenges associated with conducting cannabis research, which go beyond those related to the registration process, deserve separate mention in light of the increasing availability and potency of cannabis and the proliferation of new cannabis products. Research with cannabis and other Schedule I substances can only be carried out with such substances obtained from DEA registered sources. It would be a violation of Federal law for researchers to purchase or handle products that are being sold in dispensaries or acquired through other sources that are not Federally authorized.

The University of Mississippi is the only entity currently registered with the DEA to cultivate cannabis for research purposes, which it does under a contract with NIDA. This means that researchers supported by NIDA and other federal agencies are unable to use federal funds to purchase cannabis available through state cannabis dispensaries. Moreover, some universities have expressed reticence about allowing investigators to purchase dispensary products with non-federal funds or do research with these products on university grounds for fear of violating federal law. Having only a single source of research cannabis limits the diversity of products and formulations available to researchers and slows the development of cannabis-based medications.

3. Some think that the best way to encourage peer-reviewed research into harms and benefits of marijuana is to completely deschedule it and all of its extracts and derivatives?
   a. Can we improve research without fully descheduling?
   b. What can be done to make it easier to research marijuana without changing its scheduling?

Response

Conducting research with marijuana, as defined under the Controlled Substances Act (CSA), requires a Schedule I registration from the Drug Enforcement Agency. In collaboration with ONDCP, HHS, FDA, and DEA, NIDA has also been identifying ways to streamline the Schedule I research registration process. The process of obtaining a Schedule I registration under the CSA could be improved so as to facilitate and encourage such research. Actions to address the challenges noted in response to question 2 could be helpful.

4. I have heard frustrations from researchers about the inability to research the products sold in marijuana stores and dispensaries. For example, some of the THC vapes associated lung illnesses have been linked to licensed stores in states that have legalized recreational marijuana.
   a. What are some of the challenges to doing ethical research on those products?

Response

A significant challenge to conducting research on these products is that under federal law researchers are unable to access, for research purposes, the products that are being sold in dispensaries or acquired through other Federally unauthorized sources. As a result, permissible research has been restricted to observational studies—or studying health outcomes in people who self-report use of these products. As such, NIH researchers have been unable to definitively characterize the products participants are using or directly test their effects in animal studies or cell cultures. Recently, however, DEA has identified a pathway for a specific program to access dispensary products for activities conducted in conjunction with law enforcement activities. This initial step may lead to additional opportunities for research on such products, including human and animal studies.

All grant applications submitted to the National Institutes of Health, including NIDA, are rigorously reviewed to assess the scientific and technical merit of the application, including the applicants' plans for the protection of human participants or research animals as appropriate. NIH requires that an institutional review board or an institutional animal care and use committee approve the research protocols used in human and animal studies, respectively. And for studies in humans, the FDA would also be required to approve an IND for studies using any THC preparation.

   b. What about in animal models or in vitro?

Response

Animal and in vitro models are often used to assess the effects of substances on a variety of systems. A wide range of physiological effects can be studied in whole animals, and effects on lung cells specifically may be assessed in vivo or in vitro. A recent publication in the New England Journal of Medicine in early 2020 described an animal model of vaping developed to study pulmonary effects of vitamin E acetate exposure.[242] Vitamin E acetate is strongly linked **to** the e-cigarette, or vaping, product use-associated lung injury (EVALI) outbreak, and this model will be a useful tool to investigate its role in this public health crisis.

5. It's my understanding that scientists looking for a diversity of product can get an import permit for schedule I substances, and research those substances from international producers. In fact, three days ago Bloomberg reported on this very issue – that medical researchers are importing marijuana products from companies outside of the US because of the insufficient supply of high quality research-grade marijuana.
   a. Do you think that forcing researchers to import marijuana is better than authorizing licensed and regulated American businesses to produce federally-compliant marijuana for medical research?

Response

The University of Mississippi is currently the only entity in the United States registered with the DEA to cultivate cannabis for research purposes, which it does under a contract with NIDA. Having only a single domestic source of research cannabis limits the diversity of products and formulations available to researchers. We were, therefore, pleased that on August 26, 2019, the DEA signaled that it is moving forward with its review of additional grower applications[243] and that it would promulgate new regulations governing cannabis cultivation.

6. Can you describe what we currently know about the mental health effects of both casual and heavy use of marijuana?
   a. Is there a dose-response effect (the more you take in higher concentrations, the more the effect)?

Response

The association between cannabis use and mental illness is a major concern, particularly in light of the higher content of THC in today's cannabis. High

---

[242] https://www.ncbi.nlm.nih.gov/pubmed/32101656.

[243] https://www.dea.gov/press-releases/2019/08/26/dea-announces-steps-necessary-improve-access-marijuana-research.

doses of THC can trigger acute psychotic episodes, which is one of the main causes for emergency department visits associated with cannabis use.[244] Most of these episodes are short lasting, but some can last from days to weeks after use.[245] While overall risk of developing a lasting psychotic disorder is low, multiple studies have associated adolescent cannabis use (especially use of high potency products) with an increased overall risk for, and early onset of, chronic psychosis such as schizophrenia,[246,247] particularly in those with other risk factors.[248] Both frequent use of cannabis and use of high THC potency cannabis are associated with an increased risk of psychosis, and individuals who use high-potency products at high frequency are at even higher risk. Among patients who sought treatment for their first psychotic episode, daily cannabis users were at three times greater risk for a psychotic disorder than non-users. Daily users of high-potency cannabis were at nearly five times greater risk. Adolescent cannabis use is also associated with increased risk of suicidal behavior.[249]

Cannabis use also can lead to cannabis use disorder (CUD). Data suggest that nearly 10 percent of people who use cannabis will develop CUD.[250] People who begin using cannabis before the age of 18 are four to seven times more likely to develop CUD than adults.[251] The risks of physical dependence, addiction, and other negative consequences increase with frequent use and exposure to high concentrations of THC.[252]

7. How much does the federal government spend on marijuana and cannabinoid research?

Response

In Fiscal Year 2019, NIH spent $189 million on cannabinoid research (which includes marijuana research), including $46 million on therapeutic cannabinoid research.[253]

---

[244] https://www.ncbi.nlm.nih.gov/pubmed/29678279.
[245] https://www.ncbi.nlm.nih.gov/pubmed/31661851.
[246] https://www.ncbi.nlm.nih.gov/pubmed/14754822.
[247] https://www.ncbi.nlm.nih.gov/pubmed/24345517.
[248] https://www.ncbi.nlm.nih.gov/pubmed/15866551.
[249] https://www.ncbi.nlm.nih.gov/pubmed/15866551.
[250] https://www.ncbi.nlm.nih.gov/pubmed/26502112.
[251] https://www.ncbi.nlm.nih.gov/pubmed/17888588.
[252] https://www.ncbi.nlm.nih.gov/pubmed/26213314.
[253] https://report.nih.gov/categorical_spending.aspx.

a. Are there any private sources of funding?

Response

Yes, in addition to industry support for cannabis research (mostly for therapeutic applications), states also fund research on the beneficial and adverse health effects of cannabis and the effects of changes in state policies. One example is the California state-funded Center for Medicinal Cannabis Research at the University of California San Diego[254]. Non-profit organizations also support cannabis research.

b. Can you talk about the process for the Institute of Medicine and National Academies reports on cannabis?

Response

Although the report, "The Health Effects of Cannabis and Cannabinoids: The Current State of the Evidence and Recommendations for Research (2017)," was commissioned and funded by the NIH and other federal agencies, along with state agencies and non-profit groups, the report was conducted independently by the National Academies. The process for developing the report is described in detail in the report's Appendix B. We refer you to National Academies staff for additional details not available therein.

8. Does it matter that marijuana sold today is more potent?

Response

NIDA data suggest that the THC concentration in commonly cultivated cannabis plants increased four-fold between 1995 and 2018 (From 4 to 16 percent in that period), and that cannabis available in dispensaries in some states has average concentrations of THC between 17.7 percent and 23.2 percent. Studies have shown that the potency of cannabis used, the frequency of use, and earlier age of onset of use all are associated with stronger negative effects.[255] Multiple studies have associated adolescent cannabis use with an overall risk for and early onset of chronic psychosis, such as schizophrenia, and both frequent use or use of high THC potency cannabis is associated with a six-fold increased risk of psychosis. Among patients who sought treatment

---

[254] https://www.cmcr.ucsd.edu/, see list of publications at https://www.cmcr.ucsd.edu/index.php/publications/scientific-publications.

[255] https://pubmed.ncbi.nlm.nih.gov/26213314/.

for their first psychotic episode, daily cannabis users were at three times greater risk for a psychotic disorder than non-users. Daily users of high-potency cannabis were at nearly five times greater risk. This raises the concern that more potent cannabis might increase the risk of adverse consequences.

9. Has your agency done any analysis on any sort of addiction concerns to CBD, including work that looks specifically at age or gender?

Response

Yes, NIDA has supported studies to examine the abuse liability of CBD and two recent NIDA-funded publications, published in 2016 and 2017, provide the first rigorous, controlled data on the topic. The 2016 study[256] found that CBD alone produced no significant psychoactive or cardiovascular effects and did not alter the subjective, reinforcing, or cardiovascular effects of smoked cannabis. The 2017 follow-up study[257] re-analyzed the data to examine the abuse liability for CBD alone, and found that CBD alone is no more reinforcing than a placebo control, whereas smoked cannabis reliably produced subjective reinforcing effects (e.g., ratings of being high, mellow, willing to take the drug again). A study published in 2020[258] reporting on the development of an animal model of vaporized cannabis self-administration found that vaporized THC has reinforcing properties and produces drug seeking behavior, but vaporized CBD alone does not. While these studies did not uncover any sex or age specific effects, future research may be able to build on these established results.

The Honorable Gus M. Bilirakis (R-FL)

1. Dr. Volkow – Have use patterns among cannabis users changed over time – and if so, in what ways?

Cannabis is the most widely-used illicit drug in the country.[259] Rates of past-year use remained steady between 2002-2017, but 2018 saw an increase, with 15.9% of the population (43.5M people) reporting past-year use, a figure

---

[256] https://www.ncbi.nlm.nih.gov/pubmed/26708108.

[257] https://www.ncbi.nlm.nih.gov/pubmed/28088032.

[258] https://www.ncbi.nlm.nih.gov/pubmed/31953372.

[259] https://www.samhsa.gov/data/sites/default/files/cbhsq-reports/NSDUHNationalFindingsReport2018/NSDUHNationalFindingsReport2018.pdf.

significantly higher than the prior 15 years. Approximately 1.6% of the population (4.4M) had a cannabis use disorder in 2018, which has remained steady since 2002. Rates of both cannabis use and use disorder are much higher among 18-25-year-olds than other age groups, and the increase in 2018 reflects increased use among 18-25-year-olds and, to a lesser degree, individuals 26 and older.

Cannabis is also the most popular illicit drug used by teens. Data from the 2019 Monitoring the Future (MTF) survey show that overall past year cannabis use rates remain steady among teens (35.7% among 12th graders; 28.8% among 10th graders; and 11.8% among eighth graders).[260] However, 2019 saw two notable increases in cannabis. First, after remaining mostly stable for many years, daily use of cannabis has increased significantly among 8th and 10th graders since 2018. In addition, past year cannabis vaping among adolescents more than doubled in the past two years: in 2019, it was 20.8% among 12th graders, 19.4% for 10th graders, and 7% for 8th graders. Past month cannabis vaping among 12th graders nearly doubled in a single year to 14% from 7.5%–the second largest one-year jump ever tracked for any substance in the history of the MTF survey. This suggests a substantial increase specifically in teens vaping cannabis.

Other modes of consuming cannabis are also increasingly available. One such method is dabbing, which involves heating and vaporizing a concentrated cannabis resin, a process that can deliver large amounts of THC to users quickly. Several studies conducted in Washington state found that sales of cannabis concentrates for vaping or dabbing have been increasing in market share as compared to cannabis flower.[261,262,263].

a. Does a lack of longitudinal research on recreational use and new modes of consumption of cannabis pose a risk to public health – and if so, in what ways?

Longitudinal research on recreational use of cannabis and new modes of consumption is essential to understanding and managing the health risks of cannabis use. There is already some evidence to suggest that some modes of consumption may pose additional risks. For example, one study found that a

---

260 https://www.drugabuse.gov/related-topics/trends-statistics/infographics/monitoring-future-2019-survey-results-overall-findings.

261 https://www.ncbi.nlm.nih.gov/pmc/articles/PMC5673542/.

262 https://www.ncbi.nlm.nih.gov/pmc/articles/PMC6948109.

263 https://pubmed.ncbi.nlm.nih.gov/31522966/.

small but disproportionate fraction of cannabis-related emergency department visits are associated with use of edible cannabis products.[264] Since these products take longer to take effect, individuals may consume more under the assumption that they did not ingest a sufficient dose the first time. This may lead to unpleasant symptoms of intense anxiety, and paranoia. Dabbing, which appears to be increasing, is notable because it exposes users to high concentrations of THC, and the use of higher potency products increases the risk of CUD, addiction, and psychosis. In addition, the outbreak of e-cigarette, or vaping, product use-associated lung injury (EVALI) is strongly linked to vitamin E acetate, an additive in some THC-containing vape products.

NIH is supporting longitudinal research to illuminate the consequences these and other products have for individual and public health. For example, the Adolescent Brain Cognitive Development (ABCD) Study will follow nearly 12,000 9- and 10-year-olds from adolescence into early adulthood, to study the effects of environmental factors, including marijuana and other drug use, on adolescent brain and cognitive development. The Population Assessment of Tobacco and Health (PATH) study, a national longitudinal study of tobacco use behavior, attitudes, and health outcomes in 49,000 people ages 12 and older, also collects data on the use of traditional nicotine delivery products, such as cigars (as blunts), hookah, and electronic devices, to consume cannabis.

b. What role do states play in cannabis-research? Do states have additional requirements for research approvals?

Some states fund cannabis research, states conduct surveillance activities to monitor cannabis related outcomes (e.g., emergency department visits), and states have their own controlled substances laws that researchers are required to follow.

c. On average, how many research solicitations for cannabis and cannabinoids are issued each year?

The NIH Guide for Grants and Contracts is NIH's official publication of notices of grant policies, guidelines and funding opportunity announcements (FOAs). Searching the guide for “cannabis,” “marijuana,” or “cannabinoid” results in 13 announcements in 2017, 22 in 2018, and 13 in 2019, for an

---

[264] https://www.ncbi.nlm.nih.gov/pubmed/30721641.

average of 16 per fiscal year. Importantly, however, the majority of NIH-funded research is investigator-initiated, meaning that many investigators submit meritorious grant applications independent of these specific FOAs.

d. On average, what percentage of NIDA-supported research is investigating the potential medical/therapeutic uses of cannabinoids?

In fiscal year 2019, NIH supported $189 million in cannabinoid research, including $46 million in therapeutic cannabinoid research. NIDA in particular supported $118 million in cannabinoid research, including $25 million in therapeutic cannabinoid research, meaning that therapeutic cannabinoid research accounted for 1.7 percent of NIDA's $1.419 billion FY 2019 budget.[265]

2. Dr. Volkow – 33 states and the District of Columbia have approved cannabis for medical use and 11 others along with the District of Columbia for recreational use. Several states have standards for purity and contamination, while others don't. Many organizations establish voluntary standards for a variety of products, and the use by federal agencies of voluntary consensus standards is widespread.
    a) Do you think that proactive industry efforts to develop appropriate safety standards for cannabis is a good idea – why or why not?
    b) Would your agencies be willing to consider monitoring or participating in the development of these voluntary national consensus standards?

Response

Cannabis available through state dispensaries is grown and processed under a variety of conditions and, like other botanical products, may include pesticides, pathogenic microbes, heavy metals, and other contaminants that could be harmful to humans. While most states with legal cannabis require product testing, there is no uniform testing standard. Likewise, product labeling varies, such that it may not be possible to determine the components of a marketed product, including the full range of cannabinoids present. The

[265] https://report.nih.gov/categorical_spending.aspx.

lack of testing and labeling standards presents health and safety concerns for users and challenges conducting controlled research with these products.

Relatedly, NIDA is soliciting input on the establishment and implementation of a standard unit of THC for cannabis research. Although not intended to serve as a safety standard for consumer products, a standard unit similar to that used for alcohol (the standard drink), tobacco (the cigarette), or opioids (morphine milligram equivalents), would improve measures of THC exposure outcomes and inform policy and public health strategies around cannabis use.

Answers to Submitted Questions for Douglas Throckmorton, M.D., Deputy Director for Regulatory Programs, Center for Drug Evaluation and Research, U.S. Food and Drug Administration

<u>**The Honorable Frank Pallone, Jr. (D-NJ)**</u>

1. **The Food and Drug Administration (FDA) recently received $2 million in federal appropriations to help develop CBD-related policy, including research. How does the FDA plan to use these funds? Given the size of the market, is more funding or authority needed?**

   The Food and Drug Administration (FDA or the Agency) is using these funds to support sampling studies of CBD products, research to better understand the effects of CBD-containing products, and to support policy development, including evaluation of a risk-based enforcement policy that would provide greater transparency and clarity regarding FDA's enforcement priorities within the marketplace for producers, retailers, consumers, and our state, local, territorial, and tribal partners.

   Regarding potential needs for additional funding or authorities, the FY 2021 President's Budget provides $5 million to enable FDA to continue regulating the usage of cannabis-derived substances, such as CBD, in FDA-regulated products. The funding will support regulatory activities, including policy development, review of product applications, inspections, enforcement, and targeted research.

We are also evaluating the impact that potential rulemaking allowing CBD-containing products to be sold legally as dietary supplements might have on FDA's ability to provide adequate and effective oversight, as well as oversight of other dietary supplement products for which we have responsibility. Although the existing regulatory framework for dietary supplements includes certain controls over product safety and quality and labeling standards, there would be certain challenges in overseeing CBD as a dietary supplement. We are mindful of such challenges as we consider potential next steps, with consideration toward issues such as the following:

- Unlike with many other products we regulate, we lack clear authority to require individual participants in the dietary supplement industry to tell FDA what products they are making and selling to consumers. This would limit our ability to provide timely, systematic, and comprehensive oversight over all CBD products marketed as dietary supplements, were we to undertake rulemaking to allow such marketing.

- Rulemaking to allow products containing CBD to be sold legally as dietary supplements would greatly increase the number of dietary supplements products on the marketplace and would have implications for FDA foods program's overall workload and prioritization. In considering potential rulemaking, FDA needs to evaluate potential impacts on existing demands on our resources and work priorities.

- Under the existing framework for dietary supplements, FDA has limited authorities to identify and address violative products that put the public at risk. In any action FDA might take, we would need to ensure that consumers have an accurate awareness of the degree to which FDA is (and is not) able to provide regulatory oversight, so that they are able to make well-informed decisions.

- FDA requested additional authorities in the FY 2021 budget that would help to address the challenges our dietary supplement program faces.

2. **Dr. Throckmorton stated in testimony that "FDA knows from CBD products we have tested that they may not contain the amount of CBD indicated on a label, or they may contain other potentially dangerous compounds that are not listed on the label. Therefore, FDA must consider questions related to good manufacturing practices for CBD products and potential labeling that might be appropriate for these products to address any potential risks to consumers." Did the FDA take any enforcement action against the companies for the products tested and found to contain a presence of "dangerous compounds", or were mislabeled because they did not contain the levels of CBD indicated on the label? Would the agency please provide us a full accounting of the results of any CBD product testing they have performed, and all enforcement action taken against violative products?**

   Please see our webpage "Warning Letters and Test Results for Cannabidiol-Related Products" for the requested information: *https://www.fda.gov/news-events/public-health-focus/warning-letters-and-test-results-cannabidiol-related-products*.

   In accordance with the FY2020 appropriations act and the requirement to submit a report to the Committees on Appropriations regarding a sampling study of CBD products on the market, FDA conducted additional testing of CBD products and provided a report of the sampling study to Congress .

3. **In your testimony, you acknowledge that FDA is "considering the possibility of new legal pathways for CBD products." Given the rapidly growing marketplace and consumer consumption of CBD products, it is crucial that prompt action be taken to assure CBD products are appropriately regulated. What pathways specifically and under what timelines is the agency exploring?**

As stated in our March press release, FDA is currently evaluating issuance of a risk-based enforcement policy that would provide greater transparency and clarity regarding factors the Agency intends to take into account in prioritizing enforcement decisions. Any enforcement policy would need to further the goals of protecting the public and providing more clarity to industry and the public regarding FDA's enforcement priorities while we take potential steps to establish a clear regulatory pathway. A copy of the March press release can be accessed on our website here: *https://www.fda.gov/news-events/press-announcements/fda-advances-work-related-cannabidiol-products-focus-protecting-public-health-providing-market*.

FDA is also evaluating potential rulemaking to allow additional pathways for the marketing of CBD consumer products. Under current law, it is not permitted to add CBD to a food, or market it as a dietary supplement, because CBD was first studied as a drug, and studied clinically before that in investigations the existence of which was made public. FDA has the authority to issue a rule that would create an exception for CBD, and we are currently considering whether it would be appropriate to create such an exception for some category of CBD products.

In considering this question, FDA is looking at safety concerns, as well as other relevant issues, including whether the broader availability of CBD to consumers would disincentivize ongoing and future medical research for new drug development of future CBD-based drugs, which is currently an area of great potential.

4. **FDA officials have indicated that FDA is hampered in its ability to regulate CBD products labeled as dietary supplements because they "may not actually be a dietary supplement at all." This interpretation seems to preclude the agency from enforcing the full range of regulatory requirements, including safety and quality controls set forth in law, for dietary supplements. Does FDA believe that the agency has clear authority to issue warning letters or take other enforcement action related to CBD products that carry dietary supplement labels but do not otherwise meet the definition of a dietary supplement? If so, what actions has the agency taken. If not, please explain why.**

Congress has not updated FDA's dietary supplement authorities since 1994. Since this time, the market has evolved and expanded rapidly, and FDA now faces certain challenges in providing appropriate regulatory oversight of products marketed as dietary supplements. In the FY2021 budget, FDA requested updates to the Agency's dietary supplement authorities. We would be happy to brief your staff on this proposal and how it may assist the Agency in addressing the challenges the Agency faces in regulating dietary supplements.

You can find the warning letters FDA has issued regarding violative CBD products on our webpage "Warning Letters and Test Results for Cannabidiol-Related Products" here: *https://www.fda.gov/news-events/public-health-focus/warning-letters-and-test-results-cannabidiol-related-products*.

5. **Does FDA support establishing a temporary limit on the daily maximum serving size of CBD in dietary supplements based on existing science that could be modified over time based on the results of additional research and analysis? If so, please explain why. If not, please explain why.**

FDA lacks safety data to support establishing a particular daily maximum use level at this time. There are remaining unanswered questions about chronic exposure, meaning the effect on the body if CBD is used every day over time. There are also remaining unanswered questions about cumulative exposure, i.e. the effect of combined use of various different CBD products over time. These safety questions would need to be addressed before a particular daily use level could be appropriately determined.

6. **What are FDA's views on the status of so-called "full-spectrum" CBD that is derived from hemp in which the level of CBD has not been concentrated? Could this form of CBD be a legal dietary ingredient under current FDA policy interpretations?**

The terms "full spectrum" and "broad spectrum" are marketing terms that have been used by industry but are not clearly defined and have not been the subject of a voluntary consensus standard. FDA has no formal definition for these terms. However, FDA is actively working to better understand the range of hemp-derived products on the market, including products that are marketed in this way, and what regulatory and public health implications such products may pose, and we will keep you updated.

7. **Is it FDA's position that it would review and provide feedback to a New Dietary Ingredient (NDI) notification submitted now for hemp-derived cannabidiol for use in dietary supplements? If not, why not? Would the agency provide confidentiality for proprietary evidence of safety provided by companies informally seeking advice about developing and submitting an NDI?**

First, we re-opened our docket in an effort to obtain more safety data on CBD. This docket includes a mechanism for a stakeholder to submit data or information that the stakeholder believes to be confidential. We hope that this will enable responsible industry participants, academic researchers, and other stakeholders to share relevant information with FDA – including information about specific products, which could help inform appropriate regulatory steps.

You may find the docket and information for confidential submissions here: *https://www.federalregister.gov/documents/2020/03/11/2020-04919/scientific-data-and-information-about-products-containing-cannabis-or-cannabis-derived-compounds.*

We note that at present, it is not lawful for a CBD product to be marketed as a dietary supplement. Under 201(ff)(3)(B) of the Federal Food, Drug, and Cosmetic Act, if a product contains a drug ingredient (such as CBD) within the scope of the statute, the product is excluded from the definition of a dietary supplement. FDA's Office of Dietary Supplement Program does not review New Dietary Ingredient Notifications (NDINs) for products that do not meet the definition of a new dietary ingredient. This applies to CBD currently.

FDA has authority to remove this prohibition via notice and comment rulemaking. This would allow CBD products to meet the definition of a dietary supplement, in which case the submission of new dietary ingredient notifications for CBD dietary supplement products would be permitted. FDA is currently evaluating issuance of a risk-based enforcement policy for CBD products while we are also considering the creation of alternative regulatory pathways, such as via rulemaking, for CBD products, and commits to keeping the Committee updated on this work. We are also happy to provide your office a briefing on the new dietary ingredient notification process.

8. **Is FDA anticipating the need for additional authorizations or appropriations in order to effectively regulate dietary supplements containing CBD in a manner that that does not detract from other agency enforcement activities?**

   See response to Question #1. We would be happy to provide the Committee technical assistance on any legislative proposals pertaining to CBD.

The Honorable Doris Matsui (D-CA)

1. **Aside from the process the Department of Justice's DEA has set up for researchers to apply for a license to be able to study cannabis, what, if any, other legal means do researchers have to study the public health effects of cannabis?**

   For the purposes of drug development, for substances that are controlled under the Controlled Substances Act (CSA), researchers must obtain a DEA license and their clinical research protocol must be approved by both FDA and DEA. In addition, in order to conduct clinical studies, researchers must submit an investigational new drug application (IND) to FDA.

2. **How are federal agencies, and specifically the DEA, currently viewing the applicability of regulations regarding "controlled substances analogues" to synthetically derived non-psychoactive cannabinoids?**

   We defer to DEA on this question.

3. **What is the position of your agency about the current status of CBD? Does the agency believe there is a distinction between marijuana-derived CBD, which is treated as a Schedule I substance, and hemp-derived and maybe even synthetically-derived CBD which is not a controlled substance? Or, alternatively, do they believe there is federal agency support for an interpretation that any CBD that has less than 0.3% THC is hemp and therefore not regulated as a controlled substance?**

The Agriculture Improvement Act of 2018 (Farm Bill) removed hemp (defined as cannabis (Cannabis sativa L), and derivatives of cannabis, with extremely low (not more than 0.3% on a dry weight basis) concentrations of delta-9 THC) from the definition of marijuana under the CSA. However, the Farm Bill preserved FDA's authorities, including those under the Federal Food, Drug, and Cosmetic Act (FD&C Act) and section 351 of the Public Health Service Act, such that cannabis products, including hemp products that are not controlled under the CSA, are subject to the same authorities and requirements as FDA-regulated products containing any other substance. This allows FDA to continue enforcing the law to protect patients and the public while also providing potential regulatory pathways, to the extent permitted by law, for products containing cannabis and cannabis-derived compounds.

Under current statute (FD&C Act section 301(ll)), it is prohibited to introduce into interstate commerce a food to which CBD has been added, because CBD was previously authorized for investigation as a drug before being marketed in a food (and was subsequently approved as a drug ingredient in Epidiolex). For the same reasons, CBD also does not meet the definition of a dietary supplement under 201(ff)(3)(B) of the FD&C Act. These provisions allow the agency to make an exception through notice-and-comment rulemaking, but that process would typically take three to five years.

At this time, FDA does not have sufficient data to clarify a distinction in safety between hemp-derived, marijuana-derived, or synthetically-derived CBD. However, FDA has authority over any FDA-regulated products that contain CBD, regardless of whether the CBD is derived from hemp, marijuana, or is synthetically derived. FDA defers to the Drug Enforcement Administration (DEA) on the question of which substances are controlled substances.

4. **What is the position of your agency on creating some special permissions/exemptions/safe harbor provisions for researchers studying cannabis's properties so they may transport the cannabis they're studying between their various universities without running afoul of federal law?**

   We defer to DEA on this question.

The Honorable Robin L. Kelly (D-IL)

The World Health Organization's Expert Committee on Drug Dependence has recognized that cannabis can confer medical benefits and has recommended to the United Nations that international drug control conventions be amended to remove cannabis from the category of strictest control. More than 30 countries have already legalized medical cannabis at the national level. Additionally, 47 U.S. states, the District of Columbia, and four U.S. territories have amended their laws to recognize the therapeutic potential of cannabis. However, there is a gap in research on the impacts of cannabis and possible medical benefits due to many restrictions as a schedule I substance. There are various

organizations including Americans for Safe Access (ASA) that promote safe and legal access to cannabis for therapeutic use and research.

1. **What changes must be made to the Controlled Substances Act and/or to other aspects of our systems of evaluation and control to enable the U.S. federal government to allow for greater research on the medicinal and therapeutic value of cannabis?**

   FDA continues to believe the existing drug approval process represents the best way to ensure that safe and effective new medicines, including any drugs derived from cannabis, are available to patients in need of appropriate medical therapy. The study of cannabis and cannabis-derived compounds in clinical trial settings is needed to assess the safety and effectiveness of these substances for the treatment of any disease or condition. The Agency's role, as laid out in the Federal Food, Drug, and Cosmetic Act, is to review data submitted to FDA in an application for approval to ensure that the drug product meets the statutory standards for approval.

   FDA is committed to supporting the efficient development of new drugs, including cannabis and cannabis-derived drugs, through the investigational new drug and drug approval process.

   We defer to DEA on the questions related to the CSA.

2. **Have there been or will there be discussions between federal agency officials and their counterparts at foreign ministries in countries that dispense medical cannabis through their pharmacies to learn how they have been able to provide standardized medical cannabis to patients?**

   We have hosted foreign regulators here in the U.S. and have held teleconferences with foreign regulators to discuss the regulation of cannabis. Furthermore, we plan to continue to meet with foreign regulatory counterparts to discuss shared interests concerning cannabis and cannabis-derived compounds with a focus on obtaining and evaluating scientific and safety/risk data and understanding our respective countries' regulatory landscapes. For example, in the past two years, we have met with regulatory counterparts from Canada, Israel, and Scotland. We will continue to collaborate and encourage the exchange of safety information with our foreign counterparts in an effort to better understand the broader impact of cannabis and cannabis-derived compounds on the public health and to inform our future surveillance strategies.

<u>The Honorable Greg Walden (R-OR)</u>

1. **There is some confusion over how drugs are scheduled. For example, there are some who do not understand why marijuana is in the same schedule as heroin and LSD.**

   a. **Is the scheduling system a harm index that groups drugs together based on how lethal or dangerous they are?**

Schedule I contains all controlled substances that have a high potential for abuse and no currently accepted medical use in the United States, which is true of marijuana, LSD, and heroin. Schedules II through V are for drugs with a currently accepted medical use in the United States but also some degree of abuse potential. For example, Schedule II drugs have a high potential for abuse but also a currently accepted medical use, which includes many opioid analgesic substances such as oxycodone, hydrocodone, and fentanyl, or stimulants that treat ADHD, such as amphetamine and methylphenidate. Schedules III, IV, and V are for drugs with accepted medical uses but with incrementally less abuse potential. Schedule V drugs have less abuse potential than Schedule IV drugs, which have less abuse potential than Schedule III drugs, which have less abuse potential than Schedule II drugs. Harm to the public health, which encompasses the dangers to individuals who may abuse a substance, is one of the factors considered in a scientific and medical evaluation of a substance as part of the drug scheduling process. In accordance with the process set forth in the Controlled Substances Act (CSA), HHS conducts the scientific and medical evaluation of a drug (referred to as the "Eight Factor Analysis") and submits the Eight Factor Analysis to DEA for a final scheduling determination. Consideration of all eight factors specified in the CSA ultimately leads DEA to make findings related to a drug or substance's relative abuse potential, safety, medical uses, and dependence liability, and to make a scheduling decision in accordance with those findings. Furthermore, 21 USC 811 covers the authority and criteria for classification of substances and outlines that the recommendations of HHS shall include recommendations with respect to the appropriate schedule, if any, under which such drug or other substance should be listed. The recommendations of HHS shall be binding to DEA as to such scientific and medical matters, and if HHS recommends that a drug or other substance not be controlled, DEA shall not control the drug or other substance.

b. Why is marijuana in schedule I?

Marijuana continues to be controlled in Schedule I because it has a high potential for abuse, no currently accepted medical use in treatment in the United States, and lacks accepted safety for use under medical supervision. Significantly, however, the CSA was amended recently to exclude from its definition of "marihuana" any cannabis plants or derivatives of cannabis that have extremely low concentrations of the psychoactive compound delta-9-tetrahydrocannabinol (THC). Such cannabis materials are now defined as "hemp" and, by statutory definition, must have a THC content not more than 0.3 percent on a dry weight basis. Hemp is not a controlled substance under the CSA.

2. What are the implications of rescheduling marijuana – say to schedule II?

If marijuana were to be rescheduled to Schedule II of the CSA, there would not be significant changes in FDA's regulatory approach towards marijuana. We defer to DEA on the implications under the CSA.

3. There have been several attempts to reschedule marijuana through lawsuits or administrative action. Can you discuss the most recent attempts?

There is extensive discussion of this by DEA in a 2016 Federal Register notice (81 FR 53687) that responds to two citizen petitions requesting rescheduling of marijuana. HHS conducted a scientific and medical evaluation to inform DEA's response on those petitions. We refer you to DEA for any additional information.

a. What are the criteria for a substance to be considered a medicine?

The term "medicine" does not have a specific legal or regulatory meaning, but we understand your question to be referring to a drug for medical use. The Federal Food, Drug, and Cosmetic Act (FD&C Act) and FDA regulations define the term *drug*, in part, by reference to its intended use, as "articles intended for use in the diagnosis, cure, mitigation, treatment, or prevention of disease" and "articles (other than food) intended to affect the structure or any function of the body of man or other animals."

b. Does smoked marijuana have a medicinal value?

As mentioned above, marijuana – regardless how it is introduced into the body – has no currently accepted medical use in treatment in the United States.

c. How would that be properly researched according to modern medical practice?

The study of cannabis and cannabis-derived compounds in clinical trial settings is needed to assess the safety and effectiveness of these substances for the diagnosis, prevention, or treatment of any disease or condition. FDA provides extensive guidance as to how adequate well-controlled clinical trials can be designed in order to demonstrate that a substance is safe and efficacious for the particular therapeutic indication to be studied.

4. If marijuana were descheduled do you think that there would be a rush to market the products in consumer-friendly forms like flavored vapes and gummies?

We cannot predict what the market for products would be if marijuana were decontrolled.

a. Following CBD's descheduling when made from hemp, doesn't the recent rush to put CBD into everything with no supporting research give us some indication of how this would go?

We cannot predict what the market for products would be if marijuana were decontrolled.

5. **Do you believe that the barriers to conducting research on marijuana and marijuana-derived compounds because of their Schedule I status have hindered or delayed drug development?**

   Schedule I substances, including drugs that are derived from botanical sources such as cannabis, can be and are the subject of clinical trials under the Federal Food, Drug, and Cosmetic Act. Nevertheless, we recognize that research on such substances is more complicated because of the need to comply with the CSA and DEA regulations. FDA is focused on making certain the processes for drug development using marijuana and marijuana-derived products are efficient and transparent to investigators.

6. **Some think that the best way to encourage peer-reviewed research into harms and benefits of marijuana is to completely deschedule it and all of its extracts and derivatives?**

   a. **Can we improve research without fully descheduling?**

      Yes. FDA believes that scientifically valid research conducted under an IND application is the best way to determine what patients could benefit from the use of drugs derived from cannabis, regardless of CSA schedule. As mentioned above, FDA supports the conduct of that research by:

      - Providing information on the process needed to conduct clinical research using cannabis.

      - Providing information on the specific requirements needed to develop a drug that is derived from a plant such as cannabis. In December 2016, FDA updated its Guidance for Industry: Botanical Drug Development, which provides sponsors with guidance on submitting IND applications for botanical drug products.

      - Providing specific support for investigators interested in conducting clinical research using cannabis and its constituents as a part of the IND process through meetings and regular interactions throughout the drug development process. In July, FDA issued a draft guidance outlining FDA's current thinking on several topics relevant to clinical research related to the development of drugs containing cannabis or cannabis-derived compounds.

      - Providing general support to investigators to help them understand and follow the procedures to conduct clinical research through FDA Center for Drug Evaluation and Research's Small Business and Industry Assistance group.

   b. **What things that can be done to make it easier to research marijuana without changing its scheduling?**

FDA supports licensing additional entities to supply cannabis, including extracts and derivatives, to legitimate researchers and drug product developers in the United States, and enabling researchers holding Schedule I licenses to obtain products from state authorized dispensaries. In July, FDA issued a draft guidance outlining FDA's current thinking on several topics relevant to clinical research related to the development of drugs containing cannabis or cannabis-derived compounds.

7. **There is currently one FDA approved drug that contains CBD as the active ingredient (Epidiolex) and two FDA approved drugs that contain THC as the active ingredient (Marinol and Syndros).**

   a. **Does the accepted medical use of these compounds support the administrative rescheduling cannabis, possibly to schedule II?**

   No. Findings of safety and efficacy from the clinical trials of those FDA-approved drug products cannot extend to cannabis generally. Cannabis contains a large number of cannabinoids and other chemical substances and varies greatly in its composition among different chemovars of the cannabis plant. Safety and efficacy of well-characterized cannabis plant material has not been demonstrated in adequate and well-controlled trials for any therapeutic indication. Therefore, there are no conditions of medical use that have received an FDA approval or can be presumed based on our approvals of those specified products containing pure forms of CBD or THC.

   b. **Does it make a difference if the compounds are synthetic or naturally derived from cannabis?**

   A pure drug substance is generally the same substance whether it is synthetically derived or extracted and purified from the cannabis plant. However, natural and synthetic substances may differ somewhat in their impurity profiles based on the manufacturing steps taken to extract or synthesize the substance. Such minor differences would be considered in FDA's drug review process as we consider any drug substance's purity and the significance of any process impurities it contains.

8. **The DEA occasionally refers scheduling questions to FDA for medical and scientific reviews. The law requires DEA and FDA to consult on these issues together. One example is when DEA refers a rescheduling petition to FDA to for an "Eight Factor Analysis" to determine a compound's potential for abuse.**

   a. **What is your current procedure to ensure timely review of the scheduling status of such compounds, including the completion of medical and scientific reviews as requested by the DEA?**

   Scientific and medical evaluations of a substance referred to FDA often involve a large body of in vitro, animal, and human laboratory studies as well as epidemiology and other types of data and information. The period of time it takes to complete such an evaluation varies, and often depends on the circumstances for the substance in question. Often DEA requests such an evaluation, also referred to as an Eight Factor Analysis, for substances that DEA has already controlled in Schedule I by issuance of a temporary order [under 21 U.S.C. 811(h)]. In such cases the temporary control status is for a two-year period, and the Eight Factor Analysis is conducted in a timely way to respond to DEA before the expiration of the temporary order.

b. **Could communication be improved between DEA and FDA regarding the scheduling status of promising scheduled compounds and, if so, what steps are being taken to do so?**

If a substance is controlled in schedule I and is of interest for scientific research, DEA and FDA coordinate efficiently so that DEA can carry out its registration process for research involving schedule I drugs. FDA and DEA also make frequent use of our memorandum of understanding so that we may discuss any issues and concerns that arise for controlled substances used in research and resolve any specific circumstances impacting the registration of investigators for their research activities.

9. **It is important for FDA to make timely and thoughtful decisions regarding the scheduling status of promising compounds in clinical development. Research on cannabis-derived compounds has increased in the last decade, and so has the promise these compounds hold for patients. Several naturally-derived and synthetic compounds have been added to Schedule I because of their chemical similarity to marijuana and THC. Some of these compounds are already in Phase II and III trials to treat rare diseases with significant unmet medical need, such as cystic fibrosis and scleroderma. Unfortunately, the Schedule I status of cannabis has inhibited the ability of researchers to conduct clinical trials on these promising compounds. Current law only requires FDA to conduct scheduling reviews after a drug has been approved, but no such process exists for drugs that are in advanced clinical development.**

a. **Would it be appropriate for FDA to take a more pro-active approach reviewing these compounds during the clinical trial process?**

Under the current process, FDA reviews drugs for potential scheduling actions in parallel with the review of a new drug application (NDA). Our reviews for drug scheduling purposes are almost always completed within the same review period as the NDA. The process as provided for in the Improving Regulatory Transparency for New Medical Therapies Act of 2015 ensures that drug scheduling occurs in a timely fashion soon after a new drug is approved by FDA. However, it is only because of FDA approval that the drug is considered to have a currently accepted medical use, which is one of the criteria for rescheduling the substance from schedule I to another less restrictive schedule.

b. Should Congress authorize a new process for FDA to evaluate scheduling status of promising drugs with an FDA-approved Investigational New Drug (IND) application?

We do not see a need for a new process. The current drug development process, working through IND applications, provides investigators a mechanism to obtain help in drug development and a recognized pathway to approval with appropriate data. Importantly, the pathway also provides protections for individuals who enroll in clinical trials, a critical element in clinical research. As discussed above, FDA has worked to make this process efficient and to support investigators who use it to study compounds derived from marijuana.

c. Under current law, how will you ensure the scheduling status of promising compounds, particularly those in advanced clinical development for areas of unmet medical need, does not inhibit the clinical trial process?

We will continue to work cooperatively and expeditiously with our DEA partners so that DEA's registration processes do not unduly impede important research.

10. What does FDA know about the possible risks associated with CBD use?

Since passage of the 2018 Farm Bill, FDA has been working proactively to better understand the potential risks associated with use of CBD. There are known risks associated with CBD that include liver injury, metabolic interactions with other drugs, potential testicular injury and infertility (as seen in animal studies), and drowsiness. FDA is working to address questions about these risks, such as whether and how dosage affects their risk of occurrence in different populations.

At the same time, there are important gaps in the scientific understanding regarding CBD, which are relevant to evaluating the safety of CBD in consumer products such as foods or dietary supplements. For example:

- FDA lacks safety data about the impact of CBD use in vulnerable populations, such as the elderly, pregnant and lactating women, and those with chronic illnesses.

- FDA does not have data regarding cumulative or sustained long-term exposure to CBD. For example, we lack information on the risks associated with consuming multiple CBD products in different forms (e.g., topicals, edibles, beverages, gummies), as well as the risks associated with sustained use over an extended period of time (e.g., daily use for months or years). FDA is also concerned about the potential risks associated with high dosages for a short period of time.

11. There are over 1500 CBD products on the market. A report in USA Today stated that 1 of every 7 Americans used a CBD product in 2019.

a. **Are there any concerns that CBD preparations on the shelves could have over 0.3 percent THC?**

FDA is concerned that products containing hemp-derived cannabidiol that are available on shelves could contain more than 0.3 percent THC. Additionally, FDA is concerned that products readily available to consumers contain amounts of CBD other than what is listed on the label, may contain heavy metals, or may contain other contaminants that could be of risk to consumers.

b. **Has anyone conducted any sampling for the presence of THC in CBD products on the shelves?**

FDA has tested some CBD products for the presence of THC. Those test results are available on our website here: *https://www.fda.gov/news-events/public-health-focus/warning-letters-and-test-results-cannabidiol-related-products.*

In accordance with the FY2020 appropriations act, FDA conducted further sampling of CBD products and provided a report of the sampling study to Congress .

12. **There has been significant interest in FDA establishing a legal pathway to market hemp-derived CBD products. One suggested approach is to exempt hemp-derived CBD from the drug exclusion clause in the law governing dietary supplements. This would effectively allow for CBD, an active pharmaceutical ingredient, to be marketed as a dietary supplement and bypass FDA's role in first determining whether this can be done safely.**

a. **Would FDA be concerned about the precedent this would set- that Congress could determine that an active drug ingredient would be appropriate for marketing as a dietary supplement without review and consideration by the FDA?**

FDA is currently evaluating issuance of a risk-based enforcement policy for CBD products while we also evaluate potential new regulatory pathways for these products. A significant challenge is that FDA does not have data regarding longer-term or cumulative exposure to CBD (e.g., the effects of regular and sustained use over a period of years). FDA also lacks data on the safety of CBD use in certain special populations, such as pregnant and nursing mothers. FDA is also concerned that high dosages for a short period of time could present a different risk. FDA also needs further data on the safety of the use of CBD in different routes of administration (such as transdermal and oral uses). FDA is happy to provide Congress technical assistance on any potential legislation regarding CBD.

13. **Would FDA using the World Health Organization's data on CBD help establish whether there may be a safe level for CBD use in dietary supplements and foods?**

When dealing with complex questions like those posed by CBD, FDA's top priority is always our mission of protecting and promoting public health. The Agency is committed to science-based decision making when it comes to CBD. We are considering all safety data available to us as we work to answer remaining unanswered safety questions. This includes meeting with international regulators to understand what steps they are taking, and how their experience can inform FDA action.

14. Some have suggested that Congress should exempt CBD from the drug exclusion clause in the law governing dietary supplements. This would allow for CBD, an active pharmaceutical ingredient, to be legally marketed in dietary supplements and foods by bypassing FDA's role in first determining whether this can be done safely.

a. Is FDA concerned about the precedent this type of proposal would set- that Congress can circumvent FDA and say that a specific drug ingredient can also be included in foods or dietary supplements without review and consideration by your Agency?

FDA is currently evaluating issuance of a risk-based enforcement policy for CBD products while we also evaluate potential new regulatory pathways for these products. A significant challenge is that FDA does not have data regarding longer-term or cumulative exposure to CBD (e.g., the effects of regular and sustained use over a period of years). FDA also lacks data on the safety of CBD use in certain special populations, such as pregnant and nursing mothers. FDA is also concerned that high dosages for a short period of time could present a different risk. FDA also needs further data on the safety of the use of CBD in different routes of administration (such as transdermal and oral uses). FDA is happy to provide Congress technical assistance on any potential legislation regarding CBD.

The Honorable Gus M. Bilirakis (R-FL)

1. **Dr. Throckmorton – Recently, we've seen a proliferation of CBD products on the market. What is the effect of CBD on individuals with daily or sustained use, on the developing brain, and on pregnant or breastfeeding women?**

FDA lacks safety data about cumulative exposure or long-term use of CBD. We also lack safety data about CBD use in vulnerable populations, such as pregnant and lactating women, those with chronic illnesses, children, and the elderly.

a. Does FDA have concerns with CBD from the data its reviewed – and if so, what are those concerns?

There are known adverse events associated with CBD that include liver injury, metabolic interactions with other drugs, potential testicular injury and infertility (as seen in animal studies), and somnolence (drowsiness). FDA is working to address questions about these risks, such as whether and how dosage affects their risk of occurrence in different populations.

FDA also lacks data regarding cumulative exposure to CBD. FDA is concerned that high dosages for a short period of time could present a different risk. FDA also needs further data on the safety of the use of CBD in different routes of administration (such as transdermal and oral uses). The Agency is concerned that broad use of CBD at varying dosages without medical supervision may result in serious illness or injuries.

b. Has FDA approved a marketing application for cannabis for the treatment of any disease or condition?

To date, FDA has not approved a marketing application for cannabis for the treatment of any disease or condition. The Agency has, however, approved one cannabis-derived drug product: Epidiolex (cannabidiol), and three synthetic cannabis-related drug products: Marinol (dronabinol), Syndros (dronabinol), and Cesamet (nabilone).

c. How are cannabis-derived drug products or synthetic cannabis-related drug products applications reviewed and what is the average length of review?

Cannabis-derived products are reviewed using the same processes used for drugs derived from any other source. This includes providing developers the opportunity to meet with FDA on multiple occasions to obtain technical assistance. Once a product is submitted for marketing approval (as a New Drug Application) the timeframes established under the Prescription Drug User Fee Act (PDUFA) for the review of marketing applications for new drugs, including new drugs containing cannabis, are 6 months for applications that are designated a *priority* review and 10 months for applications that are designed a *standard* review. A product is designated a *priority* review by FDA if the product that is the subject of the marketing application demonstrates the potential to provide a significant improvement in the safety or effectiveness of the treatment, diagnosis, or prevention of a serious condition over available therapy. Information on CDER approval times, in general, can be found at: *https://www.fda.gov/drugs/nda-and-bla-approvals/nda-and-bla-approval-times*.

d. Of the applications filed, what percentage are approved and what are the common reasons for denial?

We cannot address this question specific to applications for drug products that contain cannabis, as we may not, under our regulations, disclose the existence of an application before an approval letter is sent to the applicant, unless the existence of the application has been previously publicly disclosed or acknowledged.

Please note that, to date, the Agency has not approved a marketing application for cannabis for the treatment of any disease or condition. FDA has, however, approved one cannabis-derived and three cannabis-related drug products. These approved products are only available with a prescription from a licensed healthcare provider.

FDA has approved Epidiolex, which contains a purified form of the drug substance CBD for the treatment of seizures associated with Lennox-Gastaut syndrome,Dravet syndrome, and tuberous sclerosis complex in patients one year of age and older. That means FDA has concluded that this particular drug product is safe and effective for its intended use.

The Agency also has approved Marinol and Syndros for therapeutic uses in the United States, including for the treatment of anorexia associated with weight loss in AIDS patients. Marinol and Syndros include the active ingredient dronabinol, a synthetic delta-9- tetrahydrocannabinol (THC) which is considered the psychoactive component of cannabis. Another FDA-approved drug, Cesamet, contains the active ingredient nabilone, which has a chemical structure similar to THC and is synthetically derived.

FDA may refuse to approve an NDA for any of the reasons described in section 505(d) of the Federal Food, Drug, and Cosmetic Act and in our regulations at 21 CFR 314.125(b), including, among other reasons, that the results of the studies that support the application do not show that the drug product is safe for use under the conditions prescribed, recommended or suggested in the drug's proposed labeling and there is a lack of substantial evidence consisting of adequate and well-controlled investigations that the drug product will have the effect it purports or is represented to have under the conditions of use prescribed, recommended or suggested in its proposed labeling.

2. **Dr. Throckmorton – 33 states and the District of Columbia have approved cannabis for medical use and 11 others along with the District of Columbia for recreational use. Several states have standards for purity and contamination, while others don't. Many organizations establish voluntary standards for a variety of products, and the use by federal agencies of voluntary consensus standards is widespread.**

   a. **Do you think that proactive industry efforts to develop appropriate safety standards for cannabis is a good idea – why or why not?**

   In general, FDA recognizes the value of uniform standards for manufacturing and marketing of drug products, including standards related to product quality. An industry-lead effort is one of several approaches to the development of such standards. It would be premature to speculate on any federal adoption of such standards.

   b. **Would your agencies be willing to consider monitoring or participating in the development of these voluntary national consensus standards?**

   FDA is focused on the identification of an appropriate framework for federal regulation of cannabis-derived products. FDA believes that such a framework is critical to the ordered development of a robust industry. Such a framework is important as initial work, since the development and adoption of standards, including manufacturing standards, will reflect the approaches chosen for federal product marketing.

Chapter 2

The Schedule I Status of Marijuana*

Lisa N. Sacco

The Controlled Substances Act (CSA) places various substances in one of five schedules based on their medical use, potential for abuse, and safety or risk for dependence. The five schedules are progressively ordered with Schedule V substances regarded as the least dangerous and addictive and Schedule I substances considered the most dangerous and addictive. Schedule I substances are considered to have a "high potential for abuse" with "no currently accepted medical use in treatment in the United States." The CSA prohibits the manufacture, distribution, dispensation, and possession of Schedule I substances except for federal government-approved research studies.

Marijuana is listed as a Schedule I controlled substance under the CSA, and has been on Schedule I since the CSA was enacted in 1970 (P.L. 91-513).

The Schedule I status of marijuana means that the substance is strictly regulated by federal authorities.

Yet, over the last several decades, most states and territories have deviated from across-the-board prohibition of marijuana, and now have laws and policies allowing for some cultivation, sale, distribution, and possession of marijuana.

---

* This is an edited, reformatted and augmented version of Congressional Research Service Publication No. IN11204, updated March 25, 2022.

In: New Policies on Marijuana's Status
Editor: Jack M. Lee
ISBN: 979-8-88697-870-4

Select Issues Surrounding the Schedule I Status of Marijuana and the Policy Gap with States

Select key issues related to the Schedule I status of marijuana and the gap between federal and state marijuana policies are highlighted below.

- *Institutions of Higher Education (IHEs).* It has been reported that IHEs may decline to permit research on marijuana on their campuses, because doing so may put them at risk of losing federal funds. An IHE's policy prohibiting marijuana on campus may also affect students for whom their states have authorized the use of medical marijuana. Under the Higher Education Act of 1965, each IHE must adopt a program to prevent the use of illicit drugs and alcohol and annually distribute standards of conduct that prohibit the unlawful possession, use, or distribution of illicit drugs and alcohol on the institution's property or as part of any of its activities and that describe applicable legal sanctions.
- *Financial Services for Marijuana-Related Businesses.* Despite the guidance issued by the Treasury Department's Financial Crimes Enforcement Network (FinCEN) on how financial institutions may provide banking services to marijuana-related businesses, many financial institutions remain reluctant to openly enter into relationships with state-authorized marijuana businesses due to the Schedule I status of marijuana.
- *Research on Marijuana.* The Schedule I status has reportedly created difficulty for researchers who seek to study marijuana, but are potentially unable to meet the strict requirements of the CSA, or seek a different strain, potency, or quality of marijuana for their research than what is lawfully available.
- *Legal Consequences for Individuals.* Violations of federal marijuana laws, even in instances where individuals are using marijuana consistent with state laws, give rise to a range of other issues including eligibility for housing and food assistance, gun ownership, visas, and employment.

Drug Enforcement Administration (DEA) Rejection of Petitions to Reschedule

Over the years, several entities have submitted petitions to the DEA to reschedule marijuana. In August 2016, after a five-year evaluation process done in conjunction with the Food and Drug Administration (FDA), the DEA rejected two petitions—one submitted by two state governors and the other submitted by a New Mexico health provider—to move marijuana to a less-restrictive schedule under the CSA. Consistent with past practice, the rejections were based on a conclusion by both the FDA and DEA that marijuana continues to meet the criteria for inclusion on Schedule I—namely that it has a high potential for abuse, has no currently accepted medical use, and lacks an accepted level of safety for use under medical supervision.

Authority to Alter the Schedule I Status of Marijuana

Both Congress and the Administration have the ability to alter marijuana's status as a Schedule I substance. The Administration could make such changes on its own, though it is bound by the CSA to consider factors including a substance's medical utility and risk of abuse and dependence prior to altering its scheduling status. Congress could also alter marijuana's status by amending the CSA but without such confines. Of note, in congressional hearings and other forums, some Members of Congress in both major parties have questioned the Schedule I status of marijuana while other Members have maintained that marijuana should remain illegal. Those questioning its status have expressed support for, at minimum, moving it to a lower schedule. Some have gone further and supported its removal from the CSA altogether. Those continuing to support its Schedule I status express concern over the negative implications of its widespread use.

Options for Congress

Congress could choose to maintain the federal prohibition on marijuana, but if it wanted to address the Schedule I status, it could do a number of things: (1) amend the CSA to move marijuana to a less restrictive schedule; (2) create an entirely new schedule or other category for marijuana; or (3) remove it entirely from the CSA. If marijuana *remains* a controlled substance under the CSA *under any schedule*, that would maintain the existing conflict between the federal government and states that have legalized *recreational* marijuana, though moving marijuana to a less restrictive schedule could help mitigate conflicts between federal law and state *medical* marijuana laws. The creation of a new schedule solely for marijuana would give Congress an opportunity to modify the criminality of marijuana under the CSA. If Congress chose to remove marijuana from the CSA entirely, it could seek to regulate and tax commercial marijuana activities.

In 2021, the House Judiciary Committee marked up and ordered to be reported H.R. 3617, the Marijuana Opportunity Reinvestment and Expungement Act of 2021 (the MORE Act). Among other things, the bill would remove marijuana from the CSA. Other bills introduced in the House in the 117th Congress, including H.R. 365 and H.R. 2649, would remove marijuana from, or move it to a lower schedule of, the CSA.

Index

A

B

C

D

E

F

H

I

R

S

T

V

W